COVID-19: Diagnosis and Management-Part II

Edited by

Neeraj Mittal

Department of Endocrinology
Postgraduate Institute of Medical Education and Research
Chandigarh-160012
India

Sanjay Kumar Bhadada

Department of Endocrinology
Postgraduate Institute of Medical Education and Research
Chandigarh-160012
India

O.P. Katare

University Institute of Pharmaceutical Sciences
UGC Centre of Advanced Studies
Punjab University
Chandigarh-160014
India

&

Varun Garg

Department of Medical Affairs
Cadila Healthcare Limited
Ahmedabad 382421
Gujarat
India

COVID-19: Diagnosis and Management-Part II

Editors: Neeraj Mittal, Sanjay Kumar Bhadada, O. P. Katare and Varun Garg

ISBN (Online): 978-1-68108-805-1

ISBN (Print): 978-1-68108-806-8

ISBN (Paperback): 978-1-68108-807-5

need for a court order if at any point you breach any terms of this License Agreement. In no event will any delay or failure by Bentham Science Publishers in enforcing your compliance with this License Agreement constitute a waiver of any of its rights.

3. You acknowledge that you have read this License Agreement, and agree to be bound by its terms and conditions. To the extent that any other terms and conditions presented on any website of Bentham Science Publishers conflict with, or are inconsistent with, the terms and conditions set out in this License Agreement, you acknowledge that the terms and conditions set out in this License Agreement shall prevail.

Bentham Science Publishers Ltd.
Executive Suite Y - 2
PO Box 7917, Saif Zone
Sharjah, U.A.E.
Email: subscriptions@benthamscience.net

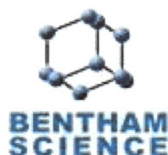

BENTHAM SCIENCE

CONTENTS

CHAPTER 2 CURRENT TREATMENT METHODS FOR CORONAVIRUS DISEASE-19 27

Kuldeep Kumar, Sonal, Pankaj Bhatia, Dhandeep Singh, Amteshwar S. Jaggi and Nirmal Singh

FOREWORD

It is my proud privilege to introduce the book "Covid-19: Diagnosis and Management," which is authored by a group from PGIMER, Chandigarh. The timing of this monograph is very apt as it has been about 9 months since the start of the COVID-19 pandemic, and it is now that we are starting to unravel the various mechanisms of disease pathogenesis and treatment modalities for this viral infection which has infected 29 million people, out of which about 1 million have died globally.

It has been the need of the hour to come up with a treatment for this pandemic disease. Moreover, it is of utmost importance that all the information related to COVID -19 should be compiled in one place, a goal which this book will fulfill.

Though the tests for diagnosis of the infection have been developed in the start of the pandemic, there are still some issues in diagnosis, including the sensitivity of the best test available, *i.e.*, Real-Time Polymerase Chain Reaction.

The book is very well organized and has been divided into two parts; each part is comprised of 6 chapters and covers all the aspects of COVID-19 from the history to the treatment of the disease. Based on the best scientific studies available, the editors and authors have used their vast professional experience to discuss the all clinical aspects of COVID-19, including clinical presentation to diagnosis in the first part and treatment of COVID-19 in the second part, and I am very sure that this compendium will become the benchmark to refer to for any information required on COVID-19.

Whenever we write books, we must have in our minds, as clearly as possible, the affirmation of Carlyle Guerra de Macedo, who was the Director of Pan American Health Organization, relative to the responsibility of what is being published: "It must be remembered that behind each table, every report or material examined, there are lives, there are people, there is suffering, waiting for our efforts and human solidarity." Both the parts of the book are very well organized, and the readers will get a mine of information available to date on COVID-19 in one place, and it would be helpful to both the clinicians and the lab professionals for day-to-day guidance in various matters. The monograph is comprehensive but is written in a lucid manner that is easy to grasp, and even complex topics are made simple for understanding.

I am also sure that as the knowledge of the virus evolves further, the authors will certainly keep updating the work from time to time, further adding to the importance of the book. I would like to congratulate the editors/authors for this tremendous effort, and I am very sure that this book will surely be of use to readers around the world and help them in the diagnosis and management of patients with COVID-19 and will also go a long way in the efforts to help fight the pandemic, which is being faced by the humanity now.

Prof. R. Sehgal
Department of Medical Parasitology
Chairperson Group D Departments
Postgraduate Institute of Medical Education & Research
Chandigarh-160012
India

PREFACE

The coronavirus disease 2019 (COVID-19) outbreak has spread throughout the globe and declared as a pandemic by the World Health Organization (WHO) on 11th March, 2020. Till date on 1st September 2020, there are more than 25,327,098 confirmed cases of COVID-19 worldwide and around 848,255 deaths have been reported. The clinicians and scientists across the globe need all the information on this pandemic disease on one platform. We have already discussed history, epidemiology, and diagnosis in part I of this book. Part II of the book "COVID-19: Diagnosis and Management" is a concise and visual reference for this viral disease. It will provide comprehensive knowledge that will cover all the aspects related to the prevention and treatment methodology of this communicable disease COVID-19.

Key Features:

1. Chapter vise description and segregation of all the areas of management of COVID-19.
2. Six chapters cover prevention and treatment aspects of COVID-19.
3. Multiple tables and figures summarize and highlight important points.
4. Covering all the aspects of COVID-19 making this a perfect textbook for Virologist and medical students.
5. A summary of the current standards for the evaluation and clinical management of COVID-19.
6. A detailed list of references, abbreviations and symbols.

This book is an essential reference for practicing and training virologists, pulmologists, medical students, scientists working in various research labs, pharmaceutical and biotechnology industries on COVID-19.

Neeraj Mittal

Department of Endocrinology
Postgraduate Institute of Medical
Education and Research,
Chandigarh-160012
India

Sanjay Kumar Bhadada

Department of Endocrinology
Postgraduate Institute of Medical
Education and Research,
Chandigarh-160012
India

O. P. Katare

University Institute of Pharmaceutical Sciences
UGC Centre of Advanced Studies
Punjab University
Chandigarh-160014
India

Varun Garg

Department of Medical Affairs
Cadila Healthcare Limited
Ahmedabad 382421
Gujarat
India

List of Contributors

Aishwarya Joshi	Institute of Science, Nirma University, Ahmedabad, Gujarat, India
Amteshwar S. Jaggi	Department of Pharmaceutical Sciences and Drug Research, Punjabi University, Patiala, India
Anamika Gautam	School of Pharmaceutical Sciences, Lovely Professional University, Phagwara, Punjab, India
Ankita Sood	School of Pharmaceutical Sciences, Lovely Professional University, Phagwara, Punjab, India
Archit Sood	Panjab University, Chandigarh, Punjab, India
Bimlesh Kumar	School of Pharmaceutical Sciences, Lovely Professional University, Phagwara, Punjab, India
Dhandeep Singh	Department of Pharmaceutical Sciences and Drug Research, Punjabi University, Patiala, India
Dhara Patel	Topicals Research and Development, Amneal Pharmaceuticals, Piscataway, New Jersey, USA
Indu Melkani	School of Pharmaceutical Sciences, Lovely Professional University, Phagwara, Punjab, India
Kardam Joshi	Topicals Research and Development, Amneal Pharmaceuticals, Piscataway, New Jersey, USA
Kuldeep Kumar	Department of Pharmaceutical Sciences and Drug Research, Punjabi University, Patiala, India
Mangesh Pradeep Kulkarni	School of Pharmaceutical Sciences, Lovely Professional University, Phagwara, Punjab, India
Manvendra Kumar	Department of Pharmaceutical Sciences and Natural Products, Central University of Punjab, Bathinda, India
Nikunj Tandel	Institute of Science, Nirma University, Ahmedabad, Gujarat, India
Nirmal Singh	Department of Pharmaceutical Sciences and Drug Research, Punjabi University, Patiala, India
Pankaj Bhatia	Department of Pharmaceutical Sciences and Drug Research, Punjabi University, Patiala, India
Pankaj Prashar	School of Pharmaceutical Sciences, Lovely Professional University, Phagwara, Punjab, India
Priya Sharma	Institute of Science, Nirma University, Ahmedabad, Gujarat, India
Raj Kumar	Department of Pharmaceutical Sciences and Natural Products, Central University of Punjab, Bathinda, India
Rajeev K. Tyagi	Division of Gastroenterology, Hepatology and Nutrition, Department of Medicine, Vanderbilt University Medical Center, Nashville, TN, USA Biomedical Parasitiology and Nano-immunology Lab, CSIR Institute of Microbial Technology (IMTECH), Chandigarh, India

Rajesh Kumar   School of Pharmaceutical Sciences, Lovely Professional University, Phagwara, Punjab, India

Rimesh Pal   Department of Endocrinology, Post Graduate Institute of Medical Education and Research, Chandigarh, India

Sahil Arora   Department of Pharmaceutical Sciences and Natural Products, Central University of Punjab, Bathinda, India

Sanjay Kumar Bhadada   Department of Endocrinology, Post Graduate Institute of Medical Education and Research, Chandigarh, India

Sheetu Wadhwa   School of Pharmaceutical Sciences, Lovely Professional University, Phagwara, Punjab, India

Shivani Joshi   Institute of Science, Nirma University, Ahmedabad, Gujarat, India

Sonal   Department of Pharmaceutical Sciences and Drug Research, Punjabi University, Patiala, India

Soundappan Kathirvel   Department of Community Medicine and School of Public Health, Postgraduate Institute of Medical Education and Research, Chandigarh, India

CHAPTER 1

Prevention of COVID-19: Facts to Overcome the Myths

Rajesh Kumar[1], Mangesh Pradeep Kulkarni[1], Sheetu Wadhwa[1] and **Soundappan Kathirvel[2,*]**

[1] *School of Pharmaceutical Sciences, Lovely Professional University, Phagwara, Punjab, India*

[2] *Department of Community Medicine and School of Public Health, Postgraduate Institute of Medical Education and Research, Chandigarh-160012, India*

Abstract: The entire world has slowed down since the outbreak of a highly contagious virus, *i.e.*, Severe Acute Respiratory Syndrome Coronavirus 2 (SARS-CoV-2). Extensive efforts are being made to reduce disease transmission, optimize the management strategy to reduce deaths and to come up with a vaccine as a preventive measure. Though several scientists across the globe are working tirelessly for developing an effective vaccine, it may still take several months to launch it successfully in the market. The behavioural interventions like maintenance of physical distancing (at least one meter), hand hygiene and cough etiquette, and use of personal protective equipment (PPE) are the currently available effective strategies to break the chain of disease transmission. All these interventions have been implemented at the population and individual level with or without linking with regulations. Based on the risk of exposure, provision and use of appropriate PPE is the need of the hour. The healthcare professionals working in COVID-19 areas have been recommended to use full PPE, which includes gloves, N-95 face masks, face shields, goggles, full-body gowns, and shoe covers. The general population has been asked to use homemade or triple-layered surgical masks in addition to the maintenance of physical distancing and hand hygiene. There are other additional strategies or measures which may or may not prevent the COVID-19 transmission. This chapter attempts to clarify the important and effective measures for the prevention of COVID-19 at the individual and community levels. It also tried to demystify the myths related to COVID-19.

Keywords: COVID-19, Diet, Disinfection, Face mask, Face shield, Filtering facepiece, Gloves, Hand hygiene, Home quarantine, Hydroxychloroquine, Institutional quarantine, N95 mask, Pandemic, Personal protective equipment, Physical distancing, Prevention, Sanitization, Screening, Transmission, Travel.

* **Corresponding author Soundappan Kathirvel:** Department of Community Medicine and School of Public Health, Postgraduate Institute of Medical Education and Research, Chandigarh-160012, India; Tel: +91-7087003412; E-mail: selvkathir@gmail.com

Neeraj Mittal, Sanjay Kumar Bhadada, O. P. Katare and Varun Garg (Eds.)

INTRODUCTION

As it has been well-said, "Prevention is better than cure", the same applies to the pandemic situation of COVID-19 as the causative virus is novel, and there is no specific treatment available. In this situation, only the preventive measures applicable to the community and individual level will help control the spread of infection and its impact. There are several preventive measures, specifically behavioural interventions like use of face masks or personal protective equipment, maintaining hand hygiene and physical distancing, practicing cough etiquette and others to contain the spread of Severe Acute Respiratory Syndrome Coronavirus 2 (SARS-CoV-2), which have been discussed throughout this chapter (World Health Organization, 2020c). A thorough understanding of existing evidence on the mode of transmission of the infection is important to practice the preventive measures further.

The modes of transmission of coronavirus can be broadly categorized into two types. Direct transmission is characterized by close and direct contact of a healthy person with asymptomatic (less likely) or symptomatic COVID-19 patient, especially when a healthy individual comes into close contact (up to 2 meters) and has been exposed to the respiratory droplets (>5-10µm diameter) produced by sneezing, coughing, talking and other activities (Bai *et al.*, 2020). Indirect transmission of infection happens through contact with fomites. It is generated during sneezing and coughing, which may deposit on clothes and even surfaces or objects, making it viable for transmission (Guo *et al.*, 2020). However, the evidence on airborne transmission (through droplet nuclei-diameter <5µm) and transmission through the faeco-oral route is extremely limited. Though mother-to-child transmission is highly unlikely, the newborn baby is equally at risk of acquiring the disease like others for the person-to-person transmission through respiratory droplets or through contact with fomites (Sohrabi *et al.*, 2020; World Health Organization, 2020b). Table **1** summarizes the myths and facts related to the transmission of COVID-19 (Fong, 2020).

Table 1. COVID-19 transmission associated myths and facts.

Sr. No.	Myth	Fact
1	Coronavirus cannot be transmitted in extreme weathers like hot and humid or cold/freezing temperatures	There is no evidence till date that supports these theories and has been denied by WHO as well. The virus can stay viable even at significantly high temperatures, and this fact is supported by the increasing number of cases in India.
2	The novel coronavirus can spread through mosquitoes and houseflies	No. It is not. It is spread by respiratory droplets and through contacts.

(Table 1) cont.....

Sr. No.	Myth	Fact
3	Only people with symptoms of this disease can spread it	Though transmission by an asymptomatic person is unlikely and no robust evidence available, it is possible.
4	Tobacco smoking prevents from corona infection	No. Actually, it may increase the risk of severe disease due to lowering lung function and hence increased mortality.
5	Being able to hold the breath for more than 10 seconds is a sign of the absence of virus	As more than 80% of patients present without any symptoms or with mild disease, they can hold the breath even during the acute stage.
6	Use of hand dryers can kill the virus	Hand dryers are not an effective disinfectant method against coronavirus. Alcohol-based sanitizers or hand wash using soap and water is an effective method.

MEASURES TO PREVENT THE SPREAD, ASSOCIATED MYTHS AND FACTS

The preventive measures ranged from using a simple face mask to using a full set (from head to toe) of personal protective equipment. Similarly, the preventive measures work together and effectively prevent the transmission of the disease like the use of face mask, physical distancing, maintenance of hand hygiene and others. Further, most of the measures are related to changing the behaviour and practice, some of which are linked with regulations.

Personal Protective Equipment (PPE)

The PPE can act as a physical barrier, or it is something that protects a person from any lethal biological agent when used properly (World Health Organization, 2020d).

PPE can be divided into various components, such as:

1. Head Cap/cover
2. Face Shield
3. Mask
4. Goggles
5. Gloves
6. Shoe Cover
7. Gowns or Coveralls

All the above-mentioned components together make a complete PPE, and a brief explanation on them, rationale of their use and the standards thereof are discussed below:

Head Covers

This works as a primary covering for the head and also the hair to prevent cross-contamination between the patients and healthcare providers.

Face Shield

Face shields are like the primary walls for the protection of the face, *i.e.,* nose, eyes and mouth, which are vulnerable to getting infected by the droplet transmission that is generated as a result of sneezing or coughing or talking and protects the face from direct exposure to infectious droplets as well as refrains a person from touching the face (Gupta, 2020).

The standards and specification for face shields are following:

- Must be made of a transparent plastic/polymer and provide clear visibility from either side and should be preferably fog-resistant.
- Should cover the sides and length of the face.
- An adjustable/elastic in nature band for its snug fitting to the forehead.
- May be disposable or preferably reusable after appropriate disinfection.

Mask

A face mask is the most common PPE used by all groups of population based on the risk of exposure or type of setting, *i.e.,* at the community or healthcare setting. It varies from simple homemade cloth mask or advanced masks like filtering facepiece (FFP) 3. As the cloth masks or non-medical masks are not fluid resistant and have low filtration efficiency, they are not considered to be a PPE. Further, masks can be disposable or reusable after adequate and appropriate disinfection.

Classification of Masks

Single-Use Masks

Usually with a single layer, and prevents larger dust particles. The filtration efficiency of this mask is 95% for particles above 3.0 microns.

Surgical Masks

It is usually triple-layered and the filtration efficiency up to 98% for particles above 0.1 microns. However, effectiveness in the prevention of infection is low in case of exposure with confirmed COVID-19 patient.

Respirator or FFP Masks

These are effective masks, especially in preventing the airborne transmission of infections and smaller particles. Further, it is available with or without an exhaling valve.

Non-respirator or Dust Masks

These are worn to prevent non-toxic nuisance dust generated from various activities. However, it will not provide adequate protection from hazardous dust or infectious agents (Robertson, 2020).

FFP (Filtering Face Piece) Classification

FFP is classified into three types based on the filtering capacity and total inward leakage of a mask. The lesser the inward leakage better is the protection offered (Bode Science Center, 2020).

- FFP-1: Maximum of 22%
- FFP-2: Maximum of 8%. The N95 mask is a type of FFP2 mask.
- FFP-3: Maximum of 2%

Masks used for Prevention of COVID-19 Transmission

Masks are of several types, but specifically, two types of masks are used in the present conditions of COVID-19, which are:

N-95 Mask

It is the best suiting mask for the present situation as it has good aerosol filtration percentage, *i.e.,* 95% and it closely fits the face of one wearing it with a tighter and better seal than any other mask. These are available with and without an exhalation valve. The valve allows free movement of exhaled air and reduces the discomfort when worn. It is recommended in place of moderate to high risk of exposure to COVID-19.

The standards that a N-95 mask should meet are:

- High filtration capacity with good breathability with or without expiratory valve.
- Ensuring shape that does not collapse easily and is reliable.
    It should be compliant or equivalent to the following standards:
    a. National Institute of Occupational Safety and Health (NIOSH) N95, EN 149 FFP2, and
    b. Fluid resistant at a minimum of 80 mmHg based on the guideline of American Society for Testing & Materials (ASTM) F1862, International Organization of Standardization (ISO) 22609 or equivalent (US Food and Drug Administration, 2020).

Triple-layered Medical Mask

As the name itself suggests, it is a triple-layered mask which is fluid-resistant and thus provides protection from the droplets and is disposable too. A triple-layered mask must be non-woven with a nose pin and ISI compliant with a filtering efficiency of 99% for 3-micron and larger particle size. It is recommended in low risk of exposure to COVID-19 or people working in non-COVID-19 areas/settings.

Goggles

They form an integral part of the protective equipment for face and should have a flexible frame making it fit tightly to the face and not allowing any particulate matter or droplets to enter the eyes (World Health Organization, 2020d). Usually, people working in high-risk area or exposure to COVID-19 need to wear goggles along with N95 masks.

The specifications and standards to be ensured for a mask include:

- Should have a good seal, transparent, made up of strong polymeric material, covering all sides with a good fitting.
- Preferably fog and scratch-resistant.
- An adjustable band that can firmly secure the position and does not lose out during the clinical activity.
- Should have an indirect vent to reduce fogging.
- It should preferably be reusable after adequate disinfection.

Gloves

The major source of getting infected after the droplet transmission is by physical contact, which is majorly through hands. Anybody who is dealing with moderate to high-risk areas (the areas where the infected or one with high risk are dealt with) has to ensure wearing gloves and also their proper disposal after use or else, they may also become a mode of transmission. However, maintenance of hand hygiene and PPE cannot be ignored even if someone is using gloves (alone) since the person may touch his face or other places after wearing the gloves.

Certain specifications and standards for gloves (non-sterile) include:

- Made up of Nitrile rubber (better resistance to chemicals than latex).
- Must be powder-free.
- Outer gloves should reach the mid-forearm (at least 280 mm total length).
- Available in different sizes.

Shoe Covers

The shoe covers are made of an impermeable material to cover the footwear and for personal protection which must be made of the same material as that of coverall and must cover the entire shoe and reach above the ankle. Shoe covers are recommended to people working in the high-risk areas or exposure to COVID-19.

Gowns or Coveralls

These are the full-body coverings generally made of polymers that ensure the safety of the body of the healthcare workers and provide a barrier to reduce or even eliminate the droplet contamination. It generally covers the whole body from head to feet and ensures complete protection if appropriately used. However, there might be some gaps at the backside of the gowns or coveralls, which may also cause contamination but ensuring a proper covering and doffing can minimize this risk. They can basically protect a person from the biologically contaminated particulate matter or solid (World Health Organization, 2020a).

The specification and standards for the coveralls and gowns include:

- Single-use and preferably light in colour to detect the contamination.
- Must be impermeable to blood and other body fluids and has an impermeability

pressure of at least 40 mmHg.
- Thumb/finger loops for anchoring the sleeves.

Must be equivalent, exceed or complaint with the following standard:

ISO 16603 Class-3 Exposure Pressure

The rationale of the use of PPEs as per the guidelines by Ministry of Health and Family Welfare, Government of India & World Health Organization, are stated below in Table **2** (EMR Division Ministry of Health and Family Welfare (Government of India), 2020b, 2020a; World Health Organization, 2020d, 2020c).

Table 2. The rationale for the use of personal protective equipment.

Sr. No.	Designated areas/Personnel	Level of Risk	PPE Recommended
Point of Entry			
1	Health desk, Immigration & Customs counters, Temperature checking, Security	Low	Triple-Layered Medical Mask Gloves.
2	Isolation, Holding Facility.	Moderate to High.	N-95 Mask Gloves Full PPE in the Isolation ward.
3	Sanitary staff	Moderate	N-95 Mask Gloves.
Hospital Setting **Out-Patient Department (OPD)**			
1	Triage, Screening area, Temperature recording station, Holding area, Doctor's chamber and Sanitary staff	Moderate	N-95 Mask Gloves.
2	Accompanying children and elderly people	Low	Triple-layered Medical Mask.
In-Patient Department (IPD)			
1	Individual isolation rooms and Sanitary staff	Moderate	N-95 Mask Gloves.
2	ICU, Treatment areas	High	Full PPE recommended.
Emergency Department			
1	Emergency cases, Attending SARI (Severe Acute Respiratory Infections) patients	Moderate to High	N-95 Mask, Gloves or Full PPE recommended.
Ambulatory and Ancillary Services			
1	Emergency transfer of SARI patients	High	Full PPE recommended.
2	Driving the ambulance	Low to Moderate	N-95 Mask Gloves.
3	Laboratory testing/radiologist	High	Full PPE recommended.

(Table 2) cont.....

Sr. No.	Designated areas/Personnel	Level of Risk	PPE Recommended
4	Sanitation, Laundry, Mortuary	Moderate	N-95 Mask Gloves.

Sr. No.	Designated areas/Personnel	Level of Risk	PPE Recommended
Community Health Workers			
1	Accredited Social Health Activists, Auxiliary Nurse Midwives, NGO workers, Supervisory doctors imparting field education	Low to Moderate	N-95 Mask Gloves
Quarantine Centre/Facility			
1	Persons being quarantined, Support staff	Low	Triple-Layered Mask
2	Healthcare staff	Moderate	N-95 Mask Gloves
Home Quarantine			
1	Person being quarantined and designated family member	Low	Triple-Layered Mask Gloves
General Public			
1	Individuals, Offices with no public dealing	Low	Triple-Layered Mask or Equivalent to Cover their Face whenever out
2	Offices with public dealing and Shops	Moderate	N-95 Mask or Triple Layered Mask or clothed mask Gloves

Note: A person wearing PPE must not ignore the basic rules of hand hygiene and public distancing and must take extra care in every aspect to avoid getting infected and transmit the disease.

SANITIZATION AND DISINFECTION

Hand Hygiene

The coronavirus pandemic is known for transmission through two major modes which include the droplet transmission or through contact. Transmission through contact occurs when a healthy person comes in contact, *i.e.,* touches an infected person, surfaces, *etc.,* with his hands and may carry the virus which may further enter in the body through nose, mouth or eyes while performing the day to day activities. To prevent this possibility of getting infected, one must always maintain the hands clean (Lotfinejad *et al.*, 2020; World Health Organization, 2020b).

Now the question is, what and how can someone achieve or maintain this hand hygiene? Well, it's quite simple, but certain considerations have to be ensured to stay safe such as:

For Public

- One can wash his hands with soap and water for a minimum of 20-30 seconds ensuring the proper scrubbing of all the areas of palm, fingers, nails and crevices is recommended till the wrist, and then the soap is properly washed with water and ensure that the hands are dry.
- One can also consider the use of hand sanitizers, which should contain not less than 70% of isopropyl alcohol when cleaning with soap and water is not possible or hands are not visibly soiled. A person allergic to alcohol-based hand rub can maintain hand hygiene using soap and water.

Everybody must consider washing hands or sanitizing them at regular intervals, especially during the following activities, namely:

- Before preparing and eating food.
- Before and after coming in contact with any person outside the house.
- After visiting a public place like an office, hospital, sports complexes *etc.*
- Before and after treating a wound or cut.
- After using public devices, others' phones and also touching surfaces such as lift buttons, doorknobs, public transport *etc.* (Fathizadeh *et al.*, 2020).
- After coughing or sneezing or vomiting.
- Before touching the face while outdoors.

Prevention of COVID-19 Among Frontline Healthcare Workers

As the frontline working force including the healthcare professionals, sanitization workers, law enforcement departments *etc.* are more susceptible to acquire the infection being in direct contact with the infected or in contact with a lot of people every day. Hence, it is very necessary for them to take care of hand hygiene importantly (Lotfinejad *et al.*, 2020). This can be done by the use of disposable hand gloves and repeatedly sanitizing the hands with a recommended sanitizer that has the alcohol content not less than 70%. Frontline workers not only have to take care of their hands but should also consider disinfecting their clothes and whole body once they relieve from their everyday duty to ensure maximum safety (World Health Organization, 2020a).

Cleaning of Vegetables-Fruits

Vegetables and fruits are an essential part of daily life and are very necessary to be consumed for maintaining sound health. But, in pandemic situations like COVID-19, there are chances of contamination of the fruits and vegetable surfaces as well, and to overcome this, certain steps have to be followed, such as:

- One should wash his hands efficiently before and after handling fruits/vegetables
- Initially, they can be classified into two types, *i.e.,* 1) Raw fruits & vegetables, and 2) Green leafy vegetables
- For the fruits and vegetables whose outer covering is removed before consumption, they can be soaked in clean water with some amount of salt or baking soda or potassium permanganate added to it and cleaned properly followed by washing them under a tap of clean running water with the application of a mild scrub or a brush for this activity, wherever applicable.
- In case of the green leafy vegetables, soaking them for 15 minutes in one part of vinegar and three parts of water or water added with a spoon of salt followed by thorough washing under running water is recommended.

Note:

- One should not use detergents or any disinfectants to clean edible substances as their consumption be harmful to our body.
- Purchase only fresh fruits and vegetables.
- Purchase prepacked fruits and vegetables, preferably which may have less contact with human hands or secretions.
- Avoid eating uncooked vegetables or improperly cleaned fruits and vegetables.
- Consumption of raw or stale meat must be avoided.

Safe Handling of Currency and Paper Documents

The paper currency notes tend to carry several microorganisms as they go hand by hand to several individuals and places, making them a potential carrier for bacteria and viruses. Hence, one must ensure proper hand hygiene as discussed above before and after handling currency, as there are possibilities of carrying the droplets over them (Oosterhoff and Palmer, 2020). Shifting towards cashless payment methods wherever possible is advised to reduce the chance of exposure.

Recently, a laboratory of Defense Research Development Organization (DRDO), India has developed a device which can sanitize items like paper currency, mobile phones, wallets, laptops *etc.* with the help of UV-C rays (predominantly 254 nm) which is an effective method to be adopted (Roza *et al.*, 1985). Few countries which have polymer-based water-proof currency have an additional advantage of the ease of sanitizing them, making it safer for use (IANS, 2020). Further, all the routine office procedures could be shifted to digital mode to reduce the handling of paper surfaces which moves between people and risk the exposure. Besides, the movement towards digital method further increases the efficiency, timeliness and transparency.

Cough or Respiratory Etiquettes

Individual responsibility plays a major role in efficient handling of such dreadful pandemic and containing the spread of disease, especially in practicing the cough or respiratory etiquettes.

Precautions to be Taken While Coughing/Sneezing or Any Physical Contact

It is strictly advisable that a person should cover the mouth and nose with a mask always. Irrespective of use of mask, it is advisable to cover the mouth with his elbow while sneezing or coughing and to sanitize the hands after it with an alcohol-based sanitizer.

Spitting or Littering in Public

Spitting in public areas or on roads is strictly unadvisable as well as prohibited in several places or punishable under law. Spitting in places can increase the risk of infection as the virus may remain in an open area for a longer period of time (PTI, 2020).

Disinfection of Public Places

Disinfection and sanitization of public places is another measure that has to be performed effectively to check the spread of coronavirus. There are certain standard procedures and chemicals that have to be used for the disinfection of these surfaces to ensure no viable form of virus stays there to spread the infection (Oosterhoff and Palmer, 2020).

Certain guidelines for effective disinfection of surfaces are given below:

- The surfaces of offices, rooms, hospitals must be mopped using phenol or 1% sodium hypochlorite solution or a bleaching agent at least twice daily.
- The frequently touched areas such as the tables, chairs, machines *etc.*, must be

cleaned using the same solution as mentioned in Table **3** below.

- Metallic surfaces such as lifts, doors knobs, handles, locks, and keys must be cleaned using 70% alcohol because using a bleaching agent or so could result in the rusting of these items.
- All the used products and disposable wastes must also be treated with 1% sodium hypochlorite solution preferably.
- Extra care must be taken for the cleaning of restrooms and all its surfaces and must be done at regular intervals with the aid of soaps, phenolic solutions, 1% sodium hypochlorite solution or using a bleaching agent (Xiao and Torok, 2020).
- There should be arrangements for disinfection of toilet seats present in public places. Closed flushing of the toilets must be practiced avoiding the generation of aerosols.

Table 3. Preparation and chlorine content of various disinfectants.

Sr. No.	Product	Preparation	Chlorine Content
1	Sodium hypochlorite	1 part in 4 parts of water	5%
2	Sodium dichloro-isocyanurate	17 g in 1000 ml of water	60%
3	Chloramine (powder)	80 g in 1000 ml of water	25%
4	Bleaching powder	7 g in 1000 ml of water	70%

Disposal and Disinfection of PPEs

As the PPEs are used as a barrier from the virus and is used when the risk is high; thus, the chances of them getting contaminated by the virus are also high. These contaminated kits cannot be disposed of as such and are needed to be treated with a disinfectant before disposal. For the disinfection, any phenolic solution or 1% sodium hypochlorite solution can be used.

Donning of PPE kits is recommended after proper sanitization of hands followed by the stepwise wearing of all the coverings from head to toe sequentially. Doffing of PPE kits requires utmost care and attention as there is a huge risk of contracting the virus. The steps for removal of PPE kits are shown in Fig. (**1**) below (World Health Organization, 2007).

WATER TREATMENT AND WASTE MANAGEMENT

Management of Water and Faecal Waste

Till date, there has been no significant evidence that the virus can be transmitted through sewage water, but studies have found viral fragments in the human excreta. Efficient wastewater treatment and disposal are essential to ensure that it will not pose any threat to nature or human beings. The general water treatment measures include the retention method, which is carried out for days (20 days), if sufficient and a final disinfection step may be considered to ensure better safety. Considering the safety requirements for the staff working in the respective water treatment plants, use of PPEs like heavy-duty gloves, masks, face shields, boots, goggles *etc.* must be practiced (World Health Organization, 2020e).

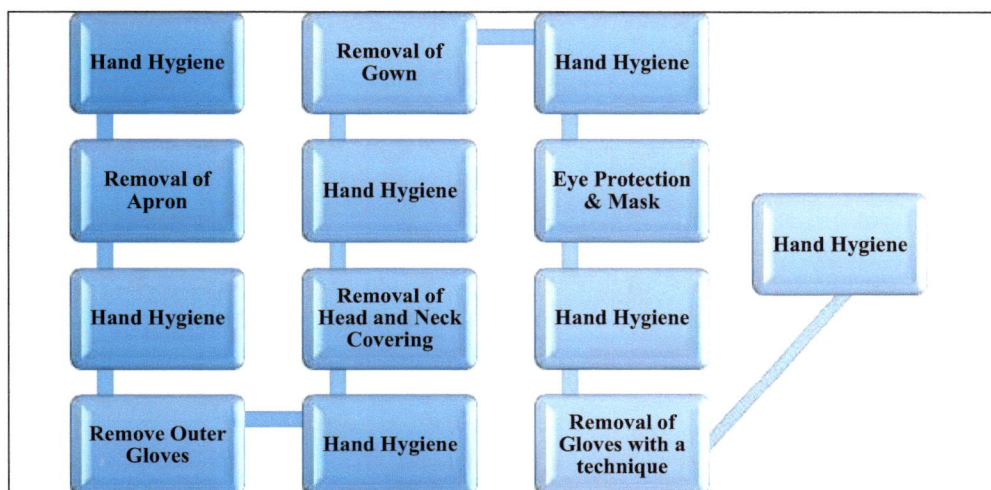

Fig. (1). Steps to doffing or removal of personal protective equipment.

Safety of Water Supplies

The basic measures that are taken for the treatment of water are enough to destroy coronavirus as they have sensitivity towards chlorination and the amount of residual chlorine ≥ 0.5 mg/L with 30 minutes of contact time at a pH of < 8 (World Health Organization, 2020e). Ultraviolet irradiation can also add up as a feature of extra safety to eradicate the chance of any viable form of virus remaining in water to render it unfit for consumption.

SOCIAL MEASURES

Physical Distancing

Through physical distancing (or also known as social distancing), *i.e.*, maintaining a possible safe distance and avoiding the large gatherings, the contact of an infected person and susceptible person is minimized. Hence, it lowers the chances of the spread of infection. It can also be called a non-technical infection control and preventive measure to check on the spread of the virus (Kissler *et al.*, 2020).

A thumb rule to ensure physical distancing is to maintain a distance of at least 1 meter (preferably 2 meters) from any individual. However, the more is the distance, and the lower are the chances of contracting the virus (Greenstone and Nigam, 2020). One can take advantage of technology to stay connected with their social groups, even while practicing physical distancing.

Application of door/home delivery, wherever possible, must be encouraged for the purchase of groceries, medications *etc.* If an individual is visiting any shop or a store, they must practice physical distancing.

Encouraging work from home can be another solution to avoid closed group gatherings and risk of exposures. Meetings and teaching must be conducted *via* video conferencing, or other online modes which can prevent large gatherings and yet fulfil the needs (Center for Disease Control, 2020; Ministry of Health and Family Welfare (Government of India), 2020a). The myths and facts related to social preventive measures during COVID-19 is described in Table **4**.

Table 4. Myths and facts related to social measures for preventing COVID-19.

Sr. No.	Myth	Fact
1	The practice of physical distancing can completely clear the risk of coronavirus transmission	Physical distancing can significantly reduce the risk by breaking the chain of transmission, but it cannot provide complete protection. For which, it should be augmented with proper use of mask, maintenance of hand hygiene and cough etiquette for near-complete protection.
2	Physical distancing is only for the elderly or people with high risk	Physical distancing is applicable for everyone irrespective of age, gender, or other social/demographic groups of the classification.
3	Only people being tested positive must ensure public distancing	Physical distancing should be practiced by everyone irrespective of the status of COVID-19 results as asymptomatic patients and patients in the incubation period will be in the community.
4	All human interactions need to be stopped	It is not practically possible, and the very purpose is to ensure there is no physical/close contact, but activities with a safer distance can be carried out.
5	If face is covered with a mask, there is no need for public distancing	Use of mask or maintenance of physical distancing alone will not provide complete protection from infection. All the four good practice (proper use of mask, maintenance of physical distancing, hand hygiene and cough etiquette) need to be practiced together always for reducing the risk of exposure.

Quarantine and Isolation

Quarantine is a practice of restricting the movement of an individual or a group of individuals for a particular period at a particular place who are potentially exposed to infection. This ensures early detection of infection among exposed individuals and reduces the chances of transmission through restricting the contact of a susceptible person with exposed person. Isolation can be simply termed as the separation of an infected patient from healthy/susceptible population to prevent further transmission of infection. Quarantine is traditionally employed among people who have a travel history from a place which is a hotspot for the disease or has come in contact with a person who has been diagnosed with the disease. This is basically done to break the chain of transmission (Nussbaumer-Streit *et al.*, 2020). This can be broadly classified into two types, *i.e.,* home quarantine and institutional quarantine, which is decided by the authorities dealing with the situation at the point taking several factors into consideration.

Home Quarantine

It is nothing but the restriction of movement of a person at his home itself for a period of 14 days (incubation period of the virus is 2-14 days) and taking care of necessary precautions like:

- Staying in a separate room and isolated from other family members especially the elderly, children and the ones with comorbidities.
- Avoid sharing of household items with other people at home.
- Using a mask all the time and also take proper care of its disposal like treating it with disinfectants before discarding.
- Only one person (caretaker) of the family is advised to serve the quarantined person with necessities, and that too without direct physical contact with practicing all the necessary precautions and visitors should never be allowed.
- If any symptoms of the disease are observed, then it must be immediately brought to the notice of responsible authorities.
- All the surfaces, including the objects used, must be disinfected or adequately and appropriately cleaned.
- Everyone in the house must practice hand hygiene measures and try to practice physical distancing as much as possible.
- They have to regularly update the health workers or in the given mobile application regarding their health status and presence of new symptoms.

Institutional Quarantine

Institutional quarantine is practiced especially for individuals who don't have adequate facilities like a separate room in their house and other amenities for practicing quarantine (Hu *et al.*, 2020). There are certain considerations needed to be taken care of for the efficient and purposeful functioning of a quarantine centre like:

Infrastructural Facilities

- The institute must be well maintained, has proper water supply, drainage facility and electricity.
- Well maintained beds with a distance of at least 2 meters from each other with a proper washroom facility.
- Basic amenities like fans, lights *etc.* must be ensured.

Staff Guidelines

- The entry into the institute must be restricted and strictly monitored, and also a logbook should be maintained for the movement of staff in and out of the facility
- An active medical team must evaluate all the individuals residing in the facility for any symptoms periodically (daily or twice daily)
- The staff dealing with the institutional tasks must ensure wearing proper personal protective equipment and its disposal

Utility Guidelines

- Basic needs such as food, water, housekeeping and laundry must be taken care of efficiently
- Disinfection of surfaces and washrooms must be done regularly
- Used clothes, masks or other daily use items must be washed/ disinfected/disposed efficiently

The myths and facts related to quarantine are given in Table **5**.

Table 5. Myths and facts related to Quarantine.

Sr. No	Myth	Fact
1	One can maintain close contact with other people in quarantine	A person under quarantine should not be visited by anyone except the fixed caregiver. During caregiving also, a physical distance of at least 1 meter must be practiced.

(Table 5) cont.....

Sr. No	Myth	Fact
2	One can meet people if home quarantined	Until the completion of the quarantine period, no one should be allowed to meet the quarantined person other than the fixed caregiver.
3	One can start a common lifestyle after the 14-day period	Individual tested negative at the end of the quarantine period can live a normal lifestyle. However, they have to follow all the precautions like use of face mask, practice physical distancing, hand hygiene and cough etiquette all the time post quarantine.

Lockdown and Travel Restrictions

A lockdown can be explained as a seizure of several non-essential and everyday activities in a particular area, state or country ensuring people stay at their home, thus resulting in better physical distancing, lesser gatherings and movements which will help to control the spread of the disease to an appreciable extent. As of now, to stop the spread of novel coronavirus, lockdowns and travel bans have become the frontline measures for the public and also containment of the disease.

Worldwide travel restrictions and bans have been observed to contain the spread of this deadly virus, which has proven to be an effective step towards prevention. Important myths and facts related to lockdowns and travel bans have been stated in Table **6** below.

Table 6. Myths and facts related to lockdown and travel restrictions.

Sr. No.	Myth	Fact
1	Normal life will return immediately after lockdown	The normal activities of life will resume gradually in a phased manner to check for an increasing number of cases or movement of people.
2	There is only one form of lockdown	The spectrum of lockdown can range from restriction for local or international travel to restriction of all non-essential activities to restriction of all activities. The severity of the situation decides the enforcement of a particular type of lockdown.
3	Lockdowns are the only measures to prevent COVID-19	Lockdown is not the only measure to prevent COVID-19. Measures like quarantine, early identification of cases and testing, isolation, and treatment of the patient are important measures which should go in parallel to lockdown. Further, enforcement of the use of the mask in public places, practicing physical distancing, hand hygiene and cough etiquettes are important individual level practices for prevention of COVID-19.
4	Wearing a mask and having a sanitizer is enough for safe travel	Use of mask and maintaining hand hygiene are good practices. In addition, physical distancing and avoiding unnecessary touching of objects/surfaces need to be practiced for enhanced prevention.

Zonal Classification of the Geography

Based on the number of cases reported and active cases from an area, it is classified as a red, orange or green zone based on the number of cases reported in the past 21 days, active cases and its doubling rate by the states/union territory. Further, the district authorities can demarcate it as containment zone, buffer zone and non-containment zone based on the spread of active cases and its contacts. Except for medical emergencies and essential supplies, all activities are restricted within the containment zone with a clear demarcation of entry and exit points for those movements. Importantly, active case finding through household surveys and testing will be the key strategy in this zone. Buffer zones are the areas delineated immediately around the containment zone. This is the immediate next attention area as it is the next closest area to active cases/contacts with restriction of movements to a certain extent. In non-containment zones, all normal activities are allowed as per the notification from time to time by the respective states/union territories (Thacker, 2020).

PROPHYLAXIS FOR COVID-19

COVID-19 is a disease for which an effective and safe therapy or a vaccine is yet to be discovered. In such conditions, one can rely on certain healthy practices and consume functional foods that can boost the immunity of the body and promote sound health.

Dietary Recommendations for the Prevention of COVID-19

It is always better to improve the immunity against a pathogen rather than consuming medications to treat the severity of symptoms. Certain functional foods and ingredients may help to a certain extent to improve immunity. However, an effective and proven dietary prophylaxis against COVID-19 yet to be identified.

Certain guidelines of healthy practices and foods have been issued by the Ministry of AYUSH, Government of India in accordance with the Ayurveda, Unani, Siddha and Homeopathy (AYUSH) system of medicine (traditional/ancient medicinal system of India) and are briefly discussed below (Patwardhan *et al.*, 2020).

General Measures

• Regular practice of yoga, meditation *etc.*, for at least 30 minutes a day can

relieve stress and promote physical, and psychological wellness.
- Drinking warm water.
- Use of spices like turmeric (known for the beneficial activities of curcumin), cumin, garlic, coriander, and ashwagandha which promote good health with the valuable phytoconstituents present therein, has been recommended (Golechha, 2020).

Medicinal Plant Measures/Procedures

- Consumption of herbal tea or decoction with ingredients such as basil leaves, cinnamon, black pepper, ginger, raisins *etc.*, which have also been proven to have beneficial effects with their chemical constituents and a glass of milk to which a spoon of turmeric powder is added.
- Consumption of fruits, especially citrus fruits, lemon juices *etc.*, which are rich in vitamin C are beneficial for immune functions
- Use of clove (Eugenol which is known for its anti-microbial activity), steam inhalation of the extracts of caraway seeds and mint to ease cough and sore throat.
- Simple ayurvedic procedures such as application of pure coconut oil in both nostrils or oil pulling therapy (swishing mouth with sesame/coconut oil for 2-3 minutes and spitting out followed by water rinsing) can also help ease the conditions of cough *etc.*
- All such measures have been practiced in India as part of its own medicinal system (Ayurveda) and have also proven beneficial both practically and scientifically (Ministry of AYUSH (Government of India), 2020; Tillu *et al.*, 2020). However, it needs to be proven against COVID-19 prevention, some of which are under study.

Medical Prophylaxis for Healthcare Workers and Contacts of a Positive Patient

- Being the frontline warriors (Healthcare workers), they are the ones who are in direct contact with the infected persons and are at a verge of getting infected easily, and use of personal protective equipment may not be sufficient due to underestimation of the risk of exposure and accidental exposures due to various operational issues while handling a COVID-19 positive patient.
- Governments of several countries like the USA and India have advised the healthcare workers to consume hydroxychloroquine (HCQ) tablets prophylactically on the basis of available pre-clinical and ongoing clinical data looking into the successful treatment of patients treated with it (Murthy, Gomersall and Fowler, 2020; Rathi *et al.*, 2020).

- As per Indian Council of Medical Research (ICMR), the prophylactic dose of HCQ for asymptomatic healthcare professionals is 400 mg dose twice a day on the first day and a single dose of 400 mg per week for seven weeks with meals. The duration of the regime for the asymptomatic household contacts has been restricted to three weeks (Ministry of Health and Family Welfare (Government of India), 2020b). However, use of this chemoprophylactic measure with the consumption of HCQ may be associated with certain cardiac side-effects which should be evaluated before starting the medication (Principi and Esposito, 2020).

There are a number of myths associated with various dietary recommendations or related to prophylaxis, and the common ones are tabulated below in Table **7**.

Table 7. Myths and facts related to dietary or medical prophylaxis against COVID-19 (Ministry of Health and Family Welfare (Government of India), 2020c).

Sr. No.	Myth	Fact
1	Adding black pepper to food can prevent COVID-19	Black pepper may improve general immunity. However, its effectiveness against COVID-19 needs to be proved.
2	Tobacco smoking clears the coronavirus from throat and lung due to its smoke	Not at all. Tobacco smoking reduces the lung function and causes/aggravates the inflammation which may result in severe disease
3	Tobacco chewing or smokeless tobacco use will kill the coronavirus due to the antiviral effects of the tobacco or its ingredient	Not at all. As chewing tobacco or the ingredients in the smokeless tobacco form causes or aggravates the inflammation, it may cause severe COVID-19.
4	Introducing or ingesting alcohol or disinfectant can kill the virus	Consuming such alcohol and disinfectant can cause severe damage to the gastrointestinal lining such as lesions, perforations and can be lethal in high concentration/quantity.
5	Exposing yourself to a higher temperature will prevent the infection	Exposure to sunlight or higher temperature will not prevent the infection.
6	Drinking more of hot drinks can stop COVID-19	No cool or hot drinks can stop the spread of the virus, and the practice of this may also harm the body.
7	Use of UV light on the skin can kill the virus	UV radiation should not be used to disinfect hands or other body parts as it may cause harm.
8	One should consume hydroxychloroquine to prevent COVID-19	Self-medication without a doctor's supervision is always dangerous and may cause death.

REGULAR SCREENING

Screening is an important disease containment strategy. High risk or population screening is needed based on the local epidemiological situation. Primarily, screening includes symptomatic screening or thermal screening. Recently, rapid antigen-based screening testing kits are also added in the list. Since these are screening tools with varying sensitivity and specificity, a confirmatory test is needed for providing clinical care to the patient (Gostic *et al.*, 2020). There is a number of digital applications like Arogya Setu or others for regular assessment of risk and closeness to confirmed COVID-19 cases which can be used by anyone after installation.

The person in quarantine (home or facility) will be checked for increased body temperature or symptoms suggestive of COVID-19 on a regular interval by the healthcare worker/self/using Arogya Setu or other applications. The patient must immediately contact the concerned authorities and act based on the symptoms or screen positivity (Paules, Marston and Fauci, 2020). The person must also be advised always to cover the face with a mask and follow all the quarantine guidelines (Augusta Health, 2020).

PRECAUTIONS FOR TRAVEL

The mandatory precautionary measures during travel include the use of mask, maintenance of hand hygiene and physical distancing and practice of cough etiquettes. Following these measures can lower the risk of infection. However, it will not eliminate the chances of spread.

As per guidelines given by WHO:

- Screening of the passengers while entering and exiting is important, and if the temperature happens to be more than 38°C with or without cough, then the person needs to be evaluated for the same.
- One must always carry a hand sanitizer and should take care of hand hygiene frequently.
- Travelling is not recommended for the geriatric and pediatric population.
- The passenger must maintain a distance of at least 1 meter, *i.e.,* physical distancing.
- Persons from the containment zone and under quarantine are strictly prohibited from travelling.
- Home quarantine for 14 days is advised to ensure that there is no spread of the virus in the port of arrival with or without linked with testing.

CONCLUSION

COVID-19 outbreak was recognized in early January 2020 in Wuhan city of China and later on declared as a pandemic by WHO. Till date, it has affected more than 200 countries. Prevention from the infection at all setting is important due to the availability of no/poor information about the exact origin of this virus, and non-availability of effective and proven treatment. Since the major route of transmission is through respiratory droplets emitted through coughing, sneezing, and through contact of fomites from surfaces, cloths or objects, use of face mask, maintenance of hand hygiene and physical distance (at least 1 metre) becomes an essential tool to prevent the spread. In light of the current scenario, authors wish to conclude with recommending the adoption of preventive measures by each member of the society which further will help to prevent other infectious diseases in the population.

LIST OF ABBREVIATIONS

ACE-2	Angiotensin-Converting Enzyme-2
ASTM	American Society for Testing & Materials
AYUSH	Ayurveda, Unani, Siddha and Homeopathy
CHW	Community Health Worker
COVID-19	Coronavirus Disease 2019
DRDO	Defense Research Development Organization
FFP	Filtering Face Piece
GoI	Government of India
HCQ	Hydroxychloroquine
ICMR	Indian Council of Medical Research
ILI	Influenza-Like Illness
IPD	Inpatient Department
ISO	International Organization of Standardization
MERS-CoV	Middle East Respiratory Syndrome Coronavirus
MoHFW	Ministry of Health and Family Welfare
nCoV	Novel Coronavirus
NGO	Non-governmental Organization
NIOSH	National Institute of Occupational Safety and Health
OPD	Outpatient Department
PPE	Personal Protective Equipment
RNA	Ribonucleic Acid
SARI	Severe Acute Respiratory Illness
SARS-CoV-2	Severe Acute Respiratory Syndrome Coronavirus 2
UV-C	Ultraviolet C

WHO   World Health Organization

CONSENT FOR PUBLICATION

Not applicable.

CONFLICT OF INTEREST

The author declares no conflict of interest, financial or otherwise.

ACKNOWLEDGEMENTS

Declared none.

REFERENCES

Augusta Health (2020) *The Difference Between COVID-19 Screening and Testing, Health Focused.* Available at: https://www.augustahealth.com/health-focused/the-difference-between-covid-19-screening-and-testing

Bai, Y, Yao, L, Wei, T, Tian, F, Jin, D-Y, Chen, L & Wang, M (2020) Presumed asymptomatic carrier transmission of COVID-19. *JAMA,* 323, 1406-7.
[http://dx.doi.org/10.1001/jama.2020.2565] [PMID: 32083643]

Bode Science Center (2020) FFP classes, CENTER\ Glossary. Available at: https://www.bode-science-center.com/center/glossary/ffp-classes.html

Center for Disease Control (2020) *Social Distancing Keep a Safe Distance to Slow the Spread, Your Health* Available at: https://www.cdc.gov/coronavirus/2019-ncov/prevent-getting-sick/social-distancing.html

EMR Division Ministry of Health and Family Welfare (Government of India) (2020a) *Advisory for managing Health care workers working in COVID and Non-COVID areas of the hospital.* Available at: https://www.mohfw.gov.in/pdf/Advisory for managing Health care workers working in COVID and NonCOVID areas of the hospital.pdf.

EMR Division Ministry of Health and Family Welfare (Government of India) (2020b) *Novel Coronavirus Disease 2019 (COVID-19): Guidelines on rational use of Personal Protective Equipment.* Available at: https://www.mohfw.gov.in/pdf/GuidelinesonrationaluseofPersonalProtectiveEquipment.pdf

Fathizadeh, H, Maroufi, P, Momen-Heravi, M, Dao, S, Köse, Ş, Ganbarov, K, Pagliano, P, Esposito, S & Kafil, HS (2020) Protection and disinfection policies against SARS-CoV-2 (COVID-19). *Infez Med,* 28, 185-91.
[PMID: 32275260]

Fong, LY (2020) *Frequently asked questions and myth busters on COVID-19, Saraya.* Available at: https://worldwide.saraya.com/about/news/item/frequently-asked-questions-and-myth- busters- on-covid-19

Golechha, M (2020) Time to realise the true potential of Ayurveda against COVID-19. *Brain Behav Immun,* 87, 130-1.
[http://dx.doi.org/10.1016/j.bbi.2020.05.003] [PMID: 32389701]

Gostic, K, Gomez, AC, Mummah, RO, Kucharski, AJ & Lloyd-Smith, JO (2020) Estimated effectiveness of symptom and risk screening to prevent the spread of COVID-19. *eLife,* 9, e55570.
[http://dx.doi.org/10.7554/eLife.55570] [PMID: 32091395]

Greenstone, M & Nigam, V (2020) 'Does social distancing matter?', *University of Chicago, Becker Friedman Institute for Economics Working Paper.* Chicago, p. 20.

[http://dx.doi.org/10.2139/ssrn.3561244]

Guo, YR, Cao, QD, Hong, ZS, Tan, YY, Chen, SD, Jin, HJ, Tan, KS, Wang, DY & Yan, Y (2020) The origin, transmission and clinical therapies on coronavirus disease 2019 (COVID-19) outbreak - an update on the status. *Milit Med Res,* 7, 11.
[http://dx.doi.org/10.1186/s40779-020-00240-0] [PMID: 32169119]

Gupta, A (2020) *COVID-19 Prevention: Face shield safer, more effective than masks against coronavirus, say experts, Health.* Available at: https://www.timesnownews.com/health/article/covid-19-prevention-f-ce-shield-safer-more-effective-than-masks-against-coronavirus-say-experts/597682

Hu, Zhiliang, Song, C, Xu, C, Jin, G, Chen, Y, Xu, X, Ma, H, Chen, W, Lin, Y, Zheng, Y, Wang, J, Hu, Z, Yi, Y & Shen, H (2020) Clinical characteristics of 24 asymptomatic infections with COVID-19 screened among close contacts in Nanjing, China. *Sci China Life Sci,* 63, 706-11.
[http://dx.doi.org/10.1007/s11427-020-1661-4] [PMID: 32146694]

IANS (2020) *Sanitizing phones, currency notes: DRDO develops devices, onmanorama.* Hyderabad. Available at: https://english.manoramaonline.com/lifestyle/ health/2020/05/11/ sanitizing-phones-curren-y-notes-drdo-devices.html

Kissler, S M, Tedijanto, C, Lipsitch, M & Grad, Y (2020) Social distancing strategies for curbing the COVID-19 epidemic', *medRxiv,* Preprint (Not peer reviewed), p. 21.
[http://dx.doi.org/10.1101/2020.03.22.20041079]

Lotfinejad, N, Peters, A & Pittet, D (2020) Hand hygiene and the novel coronavirus pandemic: the role of healthcare workers. *J Hosp Infect,* 105, 776-7.
[http://dx.doi.org/10.1016/j.jhin.2020.03.017] [PMID: 32201339]

Ministry of AYUSH (Government of India) (2020) *Ayurveda's immunity boosting measures for self care during COVID 19 crisis.* Available at: https://www.mohfw.gov.in/pdf/ImmunityBoostingAYUSHAdvisory.pdf

Ministry of Health and Family Welfare (Government of India) (2020) *Advisory on Social Distancing Measure in view of spread of COVID-19 disease.* Available at: https://www.mohfw.gov.in/pdf/ Social DistancingAdvisorybyMOHFW.pdf

Ministry of Health and Family Welfare (Government of India) (2020) *Advisory on the use of hydroxy-chloroquine as prophylaxis for SARS-CoV-2 infection.* Available at: https://www.mohfw.gov.in/ pdf/AdvisoryontheuseofHydroxy chloroquinasprophylaxisforSARSCoV2infection.pdf

Ministry of Health and Family Welfare (Government of India) (2020) *Role of Frontline Workers in Prevention and Management of Corona Virus.* Available at: https://www.mohfw.gov.in/pdf/Preventionand ManagementofCOVID19FLWEnglish.pdf

Murthy, S, Gomersall, CD & Fowler, RA (2020) Care for critically ill patients with COVID-19. *JAMA,* 323, 1499-500.
[http://dx.doi.org/10.1001/jama.2020.3633] [PMID: 32159735]

Nussbaumer-Streit, B, Mayr, V, Dobrescu, AI, Chapman, A, Persad, E, Klerings, I, Wagner, G, Siebert, U, Christof, C, Zachariah, C & Gartlehner, G (2020) Quarantine alone or in combination with other public health measures to control COVID-19: a rapid review. *Cochrane Database Syst Rev,* 4, CD013574.
[http://dx.doi.org/10.1002/14651858.CD013574] [PMID: 32267544]

Oosterhoff, B & Palmer, CA Psychological correlates of news monitoring, social distancing, disinfecting, and hoarding behaviors among US adolescents during the COVID-19 pandemic. *PsyArXiv Preprints,* 20.
[http://dx.doi.org/10.13140/RG.2.2.22362.49602]

Patwardhan, B, Chavan-Gautam, P, Gautam, M, Tillu, G, Chopra, A, Gairola, S & Jadhav, S (2020) Ayurveda rasayana in prophylaxis of covid-19. *Curr Sci,* 118, 1158-60.

Paules, CI, Marston, HD & Fauci, AS (2020) Coronavirus infections-more than just the common cold. *JAMA,* 323, 707-8.

[http://dx.doi.org/10.1001/jama.2020.0757] [PMID: 31971553]

Principi, N & Esposito, S (2020) Chloroquine or hydroxychloroquine for prophylaxis of COVID-19. *Lancet Infect Dis,* 20, 1118.
[http://dx.doi.org/10.1016/S1473-3099(20)30296-6] [PMID: 32311322]

PTI. (2020). *COVID-19: Prohibit use, spitting of smokeless tobacco in public places, health ministry tells states, The Economic Times Industry E-paper.* New Delhi, India. Available at: https://economictimes. indiatimes.com/industry/cons-products/tobacco/covid-19-prohibit-use-spitting-of-smokeless-t-bacco-in-public-places-health-ministry- tells-states/ articleshow/ 75091929.cms? from=mdr.

Rathi, S, Ish, P, Kalantri, A & Kalantri, S (2020) Hydroxychloroquine prophylaxis for COVID-19 contacts in India', *The Lancet Infectious Diseases,* p. 1.
[http://dx.doi.org/10.1016/S1473-3099(20)30313-3]

Robertson, P (2020) Comparison of Mask Standards, Ratings, and Filtration Effectiveness, SMART AIR. Available at: https://smartairfilters.com/en/blog/comparison-mask-standards-rating-effectiveness/#:~:text=In

Roza, L, van der Schans, GP & Lohman, PHM (1985) The induction and repair of DNA damage and its influence on cell death in primary human fibroblasts exposed to UV-A or UV-C irradiation. *Mutat Res,* 146, 89-98.
[http://dx.doi.org/10.1016/0167-8817(85)90059-8] [PMID: 4000150]

Sohrabi, C, Alsafi, Z, O'Neill, N, Khan, M, Kerwan, A, Al-Jabir, A, Iosifidis, C & Agha, R (2020) World Health Organization declares global emergency: A review of the 2019 novel coronavirus (COVID-19). *Int J Surg,* 76, 71-6.
[http://dx.doi.org/10.1016/j.ijsu.2020.02.034] [PMID: 32112977]

Thacker, T (2020). *Centre issues state-wise division of Covid-19 red, orange & green zones, The Economic Times\ Industry E-paper.* New Delhi, India. Available at: https://economictimes.indiatimes.com/news/politics-and-nation/ centre-issues-state-wise-division-of-covid-19-red-orange-green-zones/articleshow/ 75486277.cms

Tillu, G, Chaturvedi, S, Chopra, A & Patwardhan, B (2020) Public health approach of ayurveda and yoga for COVID-19 Prophylaxis. *J Altern Complement Med,* 26, 360-4.
[http://dx.doi.org/10.1089/acm.2020.0129] [PMID: 32310670]

US Food and Drug Administration (2020) *N95 Respirators, Surgical Masks, and Face Masks, Medical Devices.* Available at: https://www.fda.gov/medical-devices/personal-protective-equipment-infection-control/n95-respir ators-surgical-masks-and-face-masks

World Health Organization (2007). Steps to put on personal protective equipment (PPE) including coverall, Infographic. Available at: https://www.who.int/publications/i/item/steps-to-put-on-personal-protective-equipment-(-ppe)-including-coverall

World Health Organization (2020a) *Infection Prevention and Control during Health Care when COVID-19 is Suspected: Interim Guidance.* World Health Organization, Geneva, Switzerland.

World Health Organization (2020b) *Modes of Transmission of Virus Causing COVID-19: Implications for IPC Precaution Recommendations: Scientific Brief.* World Health Organization, Geneva, Switzerland.

World Health Organization (2020c). *Protocol for Assessment of Potential Risk Factors for Coronavirus Disease 2019 (COVID-19) among Health Workers in a Health Care Setting.* Geneva, Switzerland.

World Health Organization (2020d) *Rational Use of Personal Protective Equipment for Coronavirus Disease (COVID-19): Interim Guidance.* World Health Organization, Geneva, Switzerland.

World Health Organization (2020e) *Water, Sanitation, Hygiene, and Waste Management for the COVID-19 Virus: Interim Guidance.*

Xiao, Y & Torok, ME (2020) Taking the right measures to control COVID-19. *Lancet Infect Dis,* 20, 523-4.
[http://dx.doi.org/10.1016/S1473-3099(20)30152-3] [PMID: 32145766]

CHAPTER 2

Current Treatment Methods for Coronavirus Disease-19

Kuldeep Kumar[1], Sonal[1], Pankaj Bhatia[1], Dhandeep Singh[1], Amteshwar S. Jaggi[1] and Nirmal Singh[1,*]

[1] Department of Pharmaceutical Sciences and Drug Research, Punjabi University Patiala, Patiala, India

Abstract: The coronavirus disease (COVID-19) pandemic outbreak has created health havoc all over the world. Till now, no definite treatment has been found to combat the COVID-19 outbreak, probably due to a poor understanding of the molecular mechanism of this infection. As it's a health devastating situation, so due to lack of proper time for research, clinicians all over the world are exploring the already approved drug such as lopinavir, ritonavir, chloroquine (CQ), hydroxychloroquine (HCQ), azithromycin (AZ), remdesivir, favipiravir, ribavirin, nitozoxanide, interferon-α (IFN), arbidol, corticosteroids, ivermectin, teicoplanin, herbal drugs, *etc.* for anti-viral activity. Previous studies suggest that these drugs act by different mechanisms such as prevention of entry and fusion of the virus with host cell by blocking angiotensin-converting enzyme-2 (ACE-2) receptor and increasing endosomal pH respectively, inhibition of RNA polymerase and protease enzyme, inhibition of inflammatory pathway by blocking toll-like receptors (TLR's), inhibition of RNA synthesis, interference of glycosylation of cellular receptor, suppression of immune response, *etc.* Besides these drugs, few humanized monoclonal antibodies such as tocilizumab and sarilumab are also shown to be effective against COVID-19 by blocking interleukin-6 (IL-6) receptors. In addition to these drugs, convalescent plasma therapy is also being used to treat COVID-19 patients. Focus is on the development of a vaccine for COVID-19 at the earliest and indeed, many vaccines are in various stages of the development process, with some under clinical trials. This review gives an exhaustive view of current therapeutic strategies for the management of COVID-19.

Keywords: ACE-2, Arbidol, Azithromycin, COVID-19, Corticosteroids, Favipiravir, Hydroxychloroquine, IL-6, Immune response, Interferon-α, Ivermectin, Lopinavir, Monoclonal antibodies, Plasma therapy, Protease, Remdesivir, Ribavirin, Ritonavir, RNA polymerase, TLR's, Tocilizumab.

* **Corresponding author Nirmal Singh:** Department of Pharmaceutical Sciences and Drug Research, Punjabi University Patiala, Patiala, India; Tel: 91-9815129884; E-mail: nirmal_puru@rediffmail.com

Neeraj Mittal, Sanjay Kumar Bhadada, O. P. Katare and Varun Garg (Eds.)
All rights reserved-© 2021 Bentham Science Publishers

INTRODUCTION

The coronavirus disease (COVID-19), also referred as severe acute respiratory syndrome coronavirus-2 (SARS-CoV-2), has been the major health outbreak nowadays. This virus was firstly detected from Wuhan city of China in December, 2019, and now it has been spread worldwide (more than 190 countries) (Wang *et al.*, 2020). Till the end of May 2020, over 6 million human beings are reported to be affected and nearly half a million deaths have been reported due to COVID-19. Health machinery all over the world is trying its very best to combat this pandemic and facing a real challenge to tide over this crisis. Till today, no definite treatment has been found to combat this COVID-19 outbreak. Besides probationary drug therapy, some preventive, supportive, and precautionary measures such as self-isolation, social distancing, avoid unnecessary travel and crowded places are being advised and exercised to prevent the spread of this devastating infection (Chen *et al.*, 2020). Due to lack of time and a health emergency, clinicians are exploring the already approved drug for anti-viral activity (Savarino *et al.*, 2006; Rolain *et al.*, 2007; Mullard, 2012; Yan *et al.*, 2013; Agostini *et al.*, 2018; Bleibtreu *et al.*, 2018; Colson *et al.*, 2020; Cao *et al.*, 2020). In the wake of this, a number of drugs such as lopinavir, ritonavir (Cao *et al.*, 2020), chloroquine (CQ), hydroxychloroquine (HCQ) (Savarino *et al.*, 2006; Yan *et al.*, 2013), remdesivir (Agostini *et al.*, 2018), favipiravir, ribavirin, interferons (IFN's), corticosteroids, oseltamivir (Bleibtreu *et al.*, 2018), *etc.* have been tested on COVID-19 infected patients and are in current practice but with variable success. Critical insight into various treatment methods currently being employed to manage COVID-19 infection is being given in this review.

OVERVIEW OF VARIOUS TREATMENT STRATEGIES FOR COVID-19

Hydroxychloroquine

Cinchona bark and its derived constituents are considered as the primary treatment for malaria (Ruiz-Irastorza and Khamashta, 2008). CQ, a 9-aminoquinoline, has been used as the most effective anti-malarial compound (Wellems and Plowe, 2001). HCQ (7-Chloro-4-[4-(N-ethyl-Nb-hydroxy-methylamino)-1-methylbutylamino]quinoline sulfate) is a hydroxyl analogue of CQ that is a more safe and efficacious molecule (Sperber *et al.*, 1995). HCQ is a widely used clinical agent not only in the treatment of malaria but also for many other disorders such as fungal infections (Byrd and Horwitz, 1991; Henriet *et al.*, 2013), rheumatoid arthritis (RA) (Rainsford *et al.*, 2015), systemic lupus erythematosus (SLE) (Jessop *et al.*, 2001; Rainsford *et al.*, 2015), sjogran's syndrome (Oxholm *et al.*, 1998) and polymorphic light eruption (PLE) (Pareek *et al.*, 2008). In addition to the above disorders, HCQ is also demonstrated to possess anti-viral activity and has been used clinically for the treatment of several viral infections such as human immunodeficiency virus-1 (HIV-1) (Chiang *et al.*, 1996), Zika virus (ZIKV) (Kumar *et al.*, 2018), dengue virus (DENV) (Wang *et al.*, 2014) and severe acute respiratory syndrome coronavirus (SARS-Co-V) (Vincent *et al.*, 2005). HCQ has efficient absorption after oral administration with peak plasma concentration reaching after 2-3.5 hours and it has an elimination half-life around 22-45 days (Tett *et al.*, 1989; Lim *et al.*, 2009).

HCQ in Treatment of COVID-19

HCQ has become a molecule of the moment because of its utility in managing COVID-19 infection. Many *in-vitro* and controlled and uncontrolled clinical trials have substantiated the activity of HCQ against COVID-19 (Gautret *et al.*, 2020; Liu *et al.*, 2020; Yao *et al.*, 2020). These *in-vitro* reports are further supported by many clinical trial studies carried out, and being conducted in different countries such as China, U.S, Europe, *etc.* (Gao and Yang, 2020; NCT04261517; NCT04307693). Therefore, HCQ has seen variable success in these clinical trials. In a non-randomized, open-label clinical trial conducted out in France, 20 patients of COVID-19 were administered with HCQ at the dose of 200 mg three times daily (TID) and were compared with another group of patients who received supportive care. It was concluded that all patients well tolerated the HCQ and showed fast clearance of virus (Gautret *et al.*, 2020). Moreover, another study conducted in China reported that HCQ at the dose of 400 mg daily did not show any clinical benefits in mild COVID-19 patients (Chen *et al.*, 2020). Another parallel study from China conducted on more than 100 patients of COVID-19 gave evidence of less severe pneumonia, improvement in lung imaging and decreased disease duration in comparison to control group patients after receiving HCQ (Gao and Yang, 2020) and it was also documented that the treatment was safe. This study gave confidence to the experts in China to recommend HCQ at the dose of 500 mg twice daily for 10 days to mild, moderate, and severe patients of COVID-19 (Zhonghua *et al.*, 2020).

Probable Mechanism of HCQ in Treatment of COVID-19

It is being hypothesized that HCQ acts by inhibiting the replication of viral nucleic acid, glycosylation of viral proteins, assembly and transport of virus and release of virus molecule to achieve its anti-viral activity (Fox, 1993; Wang *et al.*, 2015; Kumar *et al.*, 2018) (Fig. **1**). It is suggested that HCQ has an immuno-modulatory effect, which further helps in decreasing the elevated level of cytokines, interleukin-6 (IL-6), and IL-10, which are primary contributors to multi-organ failure and death in COVID-19 patients (Chen *et al.*, 2020; Huang *et al.*, 2020). It is also being considered from the previous history of HCQ for inhibiting SARS-CoV that it can act by increasing endosomal pH, which is a key step of virus and host cell fusion (Mauthe *et al.*, 2018). HCQ is a weak diprotic basic, lipophilic and lysosomotropic drug that can cross the cell membrane easily and accumulates in the acidic vesicles (endosomes, lysosomes, golgi apparatus) of the cytoplasm. These acidic vesicles contain a number of hydrolytic enzymes that are activated by the acidic pH of these vesicles. HCQ accumulates in the lysosomes, thereby increasing the internal pH of lysosomes from their normal pH level of 4.7-4.8 to 6 (Mindell, 2012). The increased pH of lysosomes by HCQ further leads to expansion and vacuolization of lysosomes followed by inhibition of normal lysosomal functioning such as the release of an enzyme, recycling of receptor, cellular signalling, and plasma membrane repair eventually resulting in interference of normal functioning of the immune system (Hurst *et al.*, 1988; Kaufmann and Krise, 2007).

On the other side, it is also suggested that HCQ interferes in post-translational modifications of newly synthesized proteins in host cells infected by virus molecules. In addition to this, HCQ can sometimes inhibit endoplasmic vesicular enzymes such as proteases and glycosyltransferases that further inhibit post-translational modification of a viral envelope glycoproteins and also maturation of virus molecule (Randolph *et al.*, 1990).

Moreover, it is reported that CQ/HCQ also acts by increasing the zinc ions influx into the cytoplasm of host cells by acting as an ionophoric agent. After entry of the virus into host cells, zinc ion inhibits the polymerization of the virus molecule by inhibiting RNA dependent RNA polymerase (RdRp) enzyme. Sometimes virus gets mutated inside the host cells even than zinc ions inhibit the multiplication of virus molecules into the host cells. In any case, if the virus molecule somehow escapes from the zinc ion trapping mechanism, then the virus gets released from the cytoplasm of the host cells into intercellular space, interstitial matrix and will try to infect/target the healthy cells of the host. In this case, CQ/HCQ inhibits the re-attachment of the virus molecule with host cells by inducing some conformational changes in angiotensin-converting enzyme-2 (ACE-2) receptors that further mediates the binding of virus molecule with host cells (Vincent *et al.*, 2005; Zhu *et al.*, 2020).

Although, HCQ currently is one of the main drug interventions for the clinical management of COVID-19 cases. It has some adverse effects of concern, including QT prolongation with ventricular dysrhythmia, haematological disorders and impairment of hepatic and renal function (Cortegiani *et al.*, 2020). Instead of this, the use of HCQ is contraindicated in patients with retinopathy, QT prolongation in ECG, history of allergy to HCQ, deficiency of glucose-6-phosphate, and pregnant and breastfeeding ladies (Gautret *et al.*, 2020).

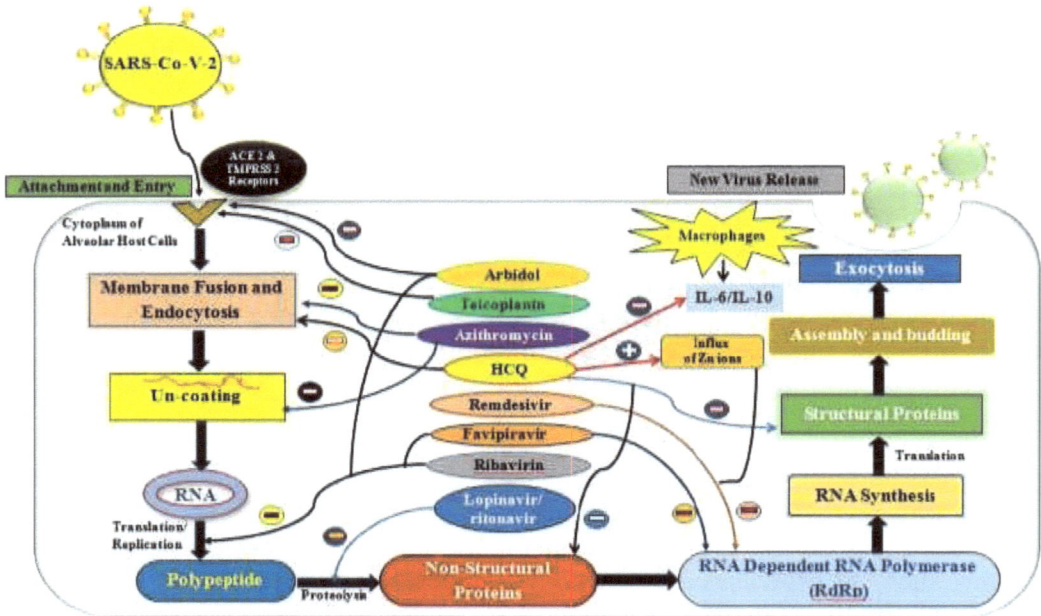

Fig. (1). Mechanism of action of various drugs at different steps of the virus life cycle into host cells. ACE-2: angiotensin-converting enzyme; HCQ: hydroxychloroquine; IL: interleukins; RNA: ribonucleic acid; RdRp: RNA dependent RNA polymerase; SARS-Co-V-2: severe acute respiratory syndrome corona virus-2; Zn: zinc.

Remdesivir

Remdesivir is another drug molecule that has gained immense popularity for its usefulness in COVID-19. It has a broad-spectrum anti-viral activity and was originally developed to treat Ebola by the Gilead Pharma Industry of France (Warren *et al.*, 2016; Mulangu *et al.*, 2019). Recently, it is also observed to possess promising efficacy in the treatment of MERS Co-V and SARS Co-V infections (Sheahan *et al.*, 2017; de Wit *et al.*, 2020). Remdesivir is a prodrug that, after activation, acts by inhibiting RdRp. Pharmacokinetic (P/K) studies on cynomolgus monkey indicated that the first-pass effect of the drug exhibits its lower distribution rate and intravenous (*i.v.*) infusion of the drug at a dose of 10 mg/kg is rapidly decomposed into triphosphates metabolites. Intravenous administration of remdesivir at the dose of 150 mg/kg for 1 hour a day showed linear P/K for a period of 14 days. Furthermore, intravenous infusion of remdesivir in a phase-1 clinical trial showed good P/K's without showing any adverse effects on vital organs (Cao *et al.*, 2020).

Remdesivir in Treatment of COVID-19

Currently, remdesivir is the second most discussed molecule after HCQ for its use in COVID-19 infection. Various pre-clinical and clinical studies have been carried and are being carried out to evaluate its efficacy in COVID-19 (Hillaker *et al.*, 2020; Holshue *et al.*, 2020). A study conducted in the USA, reported that remdesivir treatment *via i.v.* injection for 7 days produces promising results in the treatment of patients with COVID-19 (Holshue *et al.*, 2020). A clinical trial case report also depicts that remdesivir with a loading dose of 200 mg followed by 100 mg *i.v.* for the next 9 days shows promising result in 40- year- old COVID-19 patients. In addition to this, it has also been noticed that late initiation of remdesivir therapy is also effective in SARS Co-V-2 as compared to other anti-viral drugs like acyclovir and osmeltmivir (Hillaker *et al.*, 2020). One more observational cohort study on 200 patients is being conducting to evaluate the therapeutic effect of remdesivir in COVID-19 (NCT04365725).

Probable Mechanism of Action of Remdesivir in Treatment of COVID-19

Remdesivir is believed to act by interrupting viral RNA replication. When a virus infects host cells, the positive-sense RNA genome gets translated into host cells and produces viral poly-proteins which are essential for viral survival. In the next step, protein gets cleaved by viral proteases and produces 16 yield non-structural proteins called nsp^2, which is responsible for viral replication and transcription. Furthermore, nsp^2 forms a multi-subunit complex containing enzymes RNA polymerases (a characteristic of RNA virus but not specific to host cell). Remdesivir is an RdRp inhibitor. As it is a nucleotide analogue, so it gets converted into an active form, which is nucleotide triphosphate into the host cell and competes with ATP (an active adenosine triphosphate necessary for maturation of nascent RNA) that further leads to the premature synthesis of RNA and finally halt the growth of RNA strand (Kirchdoerser, 2020). Constipation is the major side effect observed with remdesivir (Fig. **1**).

Lopinavir/Ritonavir

These are protease inhibitors comprising an important class of anti-viral drugs used to treat HIV infection (Chandwani and Shuter, 2008). A Combination of lopinavir and ritonavir offers some advantages in that ritonavir enhances plasma concentration of lopinavir *via* inhibition of *Cyt P450* to aid in a more pronounced effect (Soliman *et al.*, 2011). A Combination of both lopinavir and ritonavir has already been tested to treat severe acute respiratory syndrome (SARS) and the Middle East respiratory syndrome (MERS) infection (Chu *et al.*, 2004; Arabi *et al.*, 2018).

Lopinavir/Ritonavir in Treatment of COVID-19

Some recent clinical studies have given the evidence that these drugs may be employed as a promising therapeutic agent to curb COVID-19 (Cao *et al.*, 2020; Lim *et al.*, 2020; Ye *et al.*, 2020). A study conducted in Korea concluded that lopinavir 200 mg/ritonavir 50 mg reduced β-coronavirus load and improved clinical symptoms (Lim *et al.*, 2020). Another study was conducted by Cao and colleagues on 199 patients of COVID-19. Among these, 99 patients were administered with lopinavir/ritonavir, and 100 patients were subjected to standard care. At the end of the study, it was concluded that no benefits were observed with the treatment beyond standard care (Cao *et al.*, 2020). One more study conducted in Ruian People's Hospital, China, on 19 patients and concluded that the treatment group with adjuvant therapy shows promising results in the treatment of COVID-19 without causing any side effects (Ye *et al.*, 2020).

Probable Mechanism of Action of Lopinavir/ritonavir in COVID-19

Lopinavir is a potent viral protease inhibitor but lopinavir/ritonavir co-formulation produces its anti-viral effect by inhibiting the action of 3-chymotrypsin like proteases enzyme that further mediates the processing of COVID-19 (Zhang *et al.*, 2020) (Fig. **1**).

Favipiravir

Favipiravir is a broad-spectrum anti-viral agent that has been approved by US-FDA to treat Ebola and Influenza (Nagata *et al.*, 2015). Favipiravir is a prodrug that belongs to the pyrazine carboxamide derivative category (Bocan *et al.*, 2019). It is phosphorylated and ribosylated by the hosts enzyme and gets converted into an active form Ibofuranosyl 5'triphosphate (Furuta *et al.*, 2017). Bioavailability of favipiravir is 97.6% and the apparent volume of distribution (V_d) is estimated at 15-20 L. It has 65% plasma protein binding specially with serum albumin. Favipiravir gets metabolized and undergoes hydroxylation by an enzyme aldehyde oxidase that converts it into inactive metabolite and excretes through urine.

Favipiravir in Treatment of COVID-19

Genome sequencing of Ebola and SARS Co-V-2 exhibits similarity therefore, it is believed that favipiravir can be used a promising therapeutic agent to treat COVID-19. Although, favipiravir is not approved by US-FDA for the treatment of COVID-19. National Medical Product Administration in China approved favipiravir for the treatment of SARS Co-V-2 infection (National Medical Product Administration, China). Several clinical trials have been carried out to substantiate the safety and efficacy of favipiravir in treatment of COVID-19 (ChiCTR2000029600; Cai *et al.*, 2020). The First clinical trial was conducted in China to evaluate the safety and efficacy of favipiravir and IFN in the treatment of

COVID-19 (ChiCTR2000029600). In this trial, 80 patients were selected and reported that the drug was employed as a target agent in COVID-19 without showing any adverse effects (Chen *et al.*, 2020). Another open labelled clinical trial also documented that favipiravir (1600 mg twice a day on day 1 and 600 mg twice daily on 2-14 days) plus IFN-α by aerosol inhalation (5 million U twice daily) produce a significant improvement rate in chest imaging and also reported faster viral clearance (Cai *et al.*, 2020). Two different dosage regimen of favipiravir *i.e.*1600 mg twice a day on day 1 followed by 600 mg thrice daily on day 2-14 (NCT04333589) and 1800 mg twice a day on day 1 followed by 600 mg thrice daily from day 2-14 (NCT04336904) have been exercised in clinical practice for COVID-19. Elevation of serum uric acid level, gastrointestinal discomfort, psychiatric symptoms and teratogenicity are few common side effects noticed with favipiravir.

Probable Mechanism of Action of Favipiravir in Treatment of COVID-19

Favipiravir competes with purine nucleosides and is incorporated into RNA of the virus. After incorporation into viral RNA, it disrupts the genome sequence of the viruses. In addition to this, favipiravir also inhibits viral replication due to inhibition of the RdRp enzyme (Furuta *et al.*, 2017) (Fig. **1**).

Azithromycin (AZ)

AZ (N-Methyl-11-aza-10-deoxoy-10-dihydro-erythromycin-A) belongs to the category of macrolide antibiotics which are broadly used in the treatment of several respiratory (bronchitis and pneumonia), enteric and genitor-urinary tract bacterial infections. AZ inhibits bacterial protein synthesis after binding with the 23S rRNA subunit of the 50S ribosomal unit (Bacharier *et al.*, 2015; Pfizer, 2020). AZ has rapid absorption after oral administration and long plasma half -life *i.e.* 68 hours (Pfizer, 2020) as well as a large volume of distribution (31L/kg) (Ishaqui *et al.*, 2020). Although, AZ is not a licensed drug which can be used as an anti-viral drug, however numerous *in-vitro* studies as well as clinical trials have been carried out to check its anti-viral efficacy against several viruses including COVID-19 (Kouznetsova *et al.*, 2014; Li *et al.*, 2019; Touret *et al.*, 2020).

AZ in COVID-19 Treatment

Recent *in-vitro* studies have been carried out to explore the effect of AZ in COVID-19 treatment (Andreania *et al.*, 2020; Touret *et al.*, 2020). Besides *in-vitro* studies, clinical studies have also been carried out to check the efficacy of AZ SARS-Co-V-2 infection. A recent study, carried out on 20 patients of severe COVID-19 in which AZ was administered at the dose of 500 mg on day 1, followed by 250 mg daily on day 2-5. It was observed that AZ has a synergistic effect if it is administered along with HCQ at a dose of 200 mg three times per day for 10 days (Gautret *et al.*, 2020).

Probable Mechanisms of AZ in COVID-19 Treatment

The exact mechanism of AZ for treating COVID-19 is still unexplored. However, from the record of previous studies of AZ for inhibiting other viruses, it is being hypothesized that it might act by increasing endosomal pH which is a key step of virus and host cell fusion (Fig. **1**). Being a weak basic drug, AZ can easily cross the cell membrane and accumulates in the acidic vesicles (endosomes, lysosomes, golgi apparatus) of the cytoplasm. When AZ accumulates in these acidic vesicles it increases the internal pH of vesicles. This increased pH by AZ further leads to expansion and vacuolization of vesicles followed by inhibition of normal functioning of these vesicles and can further inhibit endocytosis and viral replication (Tyteca *et al.*, 2002; Homolak and Kodvanj, 2020). In addition to this, it is also being predicted that AZ also inhibits the un-coating of enveloped viruses (Greber *et al.*, 1994). One another study has also proved that AZ maintains the normal functioning of epithelial cells and lungs by reducing the secretion of mucous (Cramer *et al.*, 2017). AZ shows similar effects and has similar P/K profile in elderly patients to that of young patients. However, the patients with mild to moderate renal impairment show a slight increase in mean C_{max} and area under the curve (AUC) after 1g dose administration of AZ. Moreover, patients with severe renal impairment show a significant surge in AUC and C_{max} in comparison to the patients with significant renal functioning, a point that needs to be taken in to consideration for prescribing AZ (Pfizer, 2020). Another major side effect associated with AZ is Torsades-de-Pointes.

Arbidol

Arbidol is an indole based anti-viral agent that already has been used in the treatment of influenza virus in China and Russia (Blaising *et al.*, 2014). Besides influenza, it has been used in the treatment of herpes simplex virus (HSV) (Li *et al.*, 2018), ZIKV (Haviernik *et al.*, 2018), and Ebola virus (Hulseberg *et al.*, 2019). It exerts its anti-viral effect through multiple pathways that help to inhibit the effect of the resistance of virus against the drug. Arbidol is rapidly absorbed after oral administration with an estimation of T_{max} *i.e.* 0.65-1.8 hours and C_{max} around 415-467 mg/ml (Liu *et al.*, 2009; Deng *et al.*, 2013). It gets metabolized by hepatic and intestinal microsomal enzymes through phase-1 pathways such as hydroxylation, sulfoxidation and N-demethylation followed by phase-2 conjugation (Song *et al.*, 2013; Deng *et al.*, 2013) and its plasma half -life is estimated as 25 hours (Deng *et al.*, 2013).

Arbidol in Treatment of COVID-19

Although, arbidol is not approved by US-FDA for the treatment of COVID-19, some pre-clinical and clinical studies have reported that it may be a very efficacious therapeutic molecule for COVID-19 (Deng *et al.*, 2020; Wang *et al.*, 2020). Arbidol has been included in the latest version of the guidelines issued by the National Health Commission (NHC) of the people's republic of China for the prevention, diagnosis, and treatment of novel coronavirus induced pneumonia at the recommended dose of 200 mg, 3 times/day for 10 days for adults (National Health Commission, China).

An *in-vitro* study claimed that arbidol is effective against COVID-19 at the concentration range of 10-30 µM (News: Abidol and darunavir can effectively inhibit corona virus (2020). A retrospective study conducted by Deng and colleagues reported that patients who received oral arbidol plus lopinavir/ritonavir showed improvement in clinical symptoms and reduced viral load as a compared to the patients who received lopinavir/ritonavir alone (Deng *et al.*, 2020). A randomized multi-centre controlled clinical trial of arbidol in the patients with COVID-19 is currently running in China (ChiCTR2000029573).

Besides this, one more study was conducted on 69 patients of COVID-19. In this study, it was reported that the administration of arbidol at the dose of 0.4 g, TID for 9 days improves the discharging rate from the hospital and also decreases the mortality rate of patients (Wang *et al.*, 2020). In addition, another study also reported that arbidol is more superior to the combination therapy of lopinavir/ritonavir (Zhu *et al.*, 2020).

Probable Mechanism of Action

It is hypothesized that arbidol inhibits the contact between the virus and host cell that further prevents the entry of the virus into host cells. It is also being predicted that arbidol also interferes with the late stages of virus cycle by interacting with lipids and proteins of the virus which are essential for the viral replication; probably arbidol binds with these essential components that further inhibit viral replication (Boriskin *et al.*, 2008) (Fig. **1**).

Ribavirin

Ribavirin is an analogue of guanosine and used in the treatment of several viral infections such as HCV, respiratory syncytial virus (RSV) and viral hemorrhagic fever (Martinez, 2020). It acts by interrupting the replication of DNA and RNA viruses into host cells (Chen *et al.*, 2020).

Ribavirin in COVID-19 Treatment

The anti-viral activity of ribavirin against SARS-Co-V is supported by an *in-vitro* study conducted by Chan and colleagues in 2015. They also calculated the anti-viral concentration of ribavirin against SARS-Co-V which was 50 µg/mL (Chan *et al.*, 2015).

To explore the efficacy of ribavirin in COVID-19 treatment, the government of China recommended the use of ribavirin in the diagnosis of pneumonia associated with COVID-19 based on Treatment Plan Edition-5. An oral loading dose of 4 g was administered followed by oral administration of 1.2 g after every 8 hours (Treatment Plan Edition 5, 2020). This schedule was further revised to 500 mg *i.v.* BID/TID (Treatment Plan Edition 5, revision edition, 2020). The outcome of these studies is not yet revealed (Huang *et al.*, 2020; Holshue *et al.*, 2020; Wang *et al.*, 2020). Besides this several new clinical studies have been announced to explore the efficacy of ribavirin in COVID-19 treatment (ChiCTR2000029387, 2020; NCT04276688; NCT04306497).

Probable Mechanism of Action in COVID-19 Treatment

Ribavirin shows anti-viral activity by inhibiting the polymerase activity followed by an interruption in the replication of the virus. Besides this polymerase inhibitory activity, ribavirin also acts by interfering RNA capping mechanism which further prevents RNA degradation. Also, ribavirin inhibits the generation of guanosine by inhibiting inosine monophosphate dehydrogenase enzyme naturally (Chen *et al.*, 2020) (Fig. **1**).

Ribavirin is reported to cause a reduction in haemoglobin which is very harmful to the patients of respiratory distress.

Teicoplanin

Teicoplanin is a glycopeptides antibiotic, broadly used in the treatment of gram-positive bacterial infections such as staphylococcal infections. In addition to bacterial infections, it is found to be effective in several viral infections such as Ebola, flavivirus, influenza, HIV, hepatitis C virus (HCV), and coronavirus *i.e.* MERS-Co-V and SARS-Co-V (Colson and Raoult, 2015; Pan *et al.*, 2015; Zhaou *et al.*, 2016).

Teicoplanin in COVID-19 Treatment

An *in-vitro* study, carried out by Zhang *et al.*, evident that teicoplanin can be used in the treatment of COVID-19. In the same study, it was also revealed that the concentration required to inhibit 50% viruses is 1.66 µM which is very less than the concentration reached in human blood (8.78 µM for a daily dose of 400 mg) (Zhang *et al.*, 2020). These results of preliminary studies further demand a randomized clinical trial.

Probable Mechanism of Action

Zhang and colleagues proposed that teicoplanin acts by inhibiting the initial step of the virus cell cycle. It acts by resisting the entry of the virus molecule into host cells *via* inhibition of the low pH cleavage of the viral spike protein by cathepsin L and cathepsin B in the late endosomes of host cells thereby preventing the release of genomic viral RNA and further halt the progress of virus replication cycle (Baron *et al.*, 2020; Zhang *et al.*, 2020) (Fig. **1**).

Ivermectin

Ivermectin is an anti-parasitic drug that has been approved by FDA and employed to treat many tropical parasites (Canga *et al.*, 2008). But, originally, it was developed to treat HIV. Ivermectin is a highly lipid-soluble drug and widely is distributed in the body (Krishna and Klotz, 1993). It has strong plasma protein binding and is not detected in cerebrospinal fluid (CSF) (Klotz, 1990). It is extensively metabolized by hepatic microsomal enzymes *Cyt P450* (Zeng *et al.*, 1998). Various pre-clinical studies have indicated its efficacy in treating tropical parasitic illness (Mastrangelo *et al.*, 2012; Lundberg *et al.*, 2013; Azeem *et al.*, 2015; Gotz *et al.*, 2016). The basic mechanism for its use as an anti-parasitic drug is that it binds with a high affinity to glutamate chloride ion channel of parasite and followed by enhancement of cell permeability that further leads to hyperpolarization and lyses of parasite cells.

Ivermectin in Treatment of COVID-19

In-vivo studies have given the evidence of the efficacy of ivermectin for the treatment of COVID-19 by using Vero-h SLAM cell lines. It mitigates the rate of infection 500 folds within 48 hrs of administration but does not show any further reduction in the severity of infection after an interval of 48 hrs (Caly *et al.*, 2020). In addition to this, a hypothesis given by Angela Patrì and Gabriella Fabbrocin purposed that concomitant administration of HCQ with ivermectin may produce a synergistic effect because both drugs do not exhibit any contradiction in combination. Moreover, HCQ already has been approved as a therapeutic agent for COVID-19 by US-FDA (Patrì and Fabbrocin, 2020). By considering the above facts, ivermectin may be a promising drug target for fighting against pandemic 2019. However, no clinical study has given any evidence for its usefulness in the treatment of COVID-19.

Probable Mechanism of Action in COVID-19

The basic mechanism behind its efficacy in COVID-19 is that it inhibits importins-α/β heterodimer which is a special type of karyopherins that transports viral protein into the nucleus of host cells. As protein entry is restricted then the virus could not be able to use host machinery for its replication and growth (Jans *et al.*, 2019). Ivermectin has reported rare side effects such as depression, ataxia and mydriasis.

Nitazoxanide

Nitazoxanide is a nitro-thiazole derivative which is de-acetylated *in-vivo* to tizoxanide. Nitazoxanide is used to treat protozoan infections (Rossignol, 2016). Besides, it has anti-bacterial and anti-viral properties. It has reported broad spectrum *in-vitro* anti-viral activity against influenza, parainfluenza, rotavirus, respiratory syncytial virus, and norovirus and is approved for the treatment of some human infections (Jasenosky *et al.*, 2019). Nitazoxanide is being investigated in the clinical trials (randomized controlled) for the management of influenza and other acute respiratory infections due to its broad spectrum anti-viral activity. Though, results are not encouraging or unavailable yet (Stahlmann and Lode, 2020).

Nitazoxanide in COVID-19 Treatment

It has recently been reported to demonstrate the potent *in-vitro* activity against SARS Co-V-2 (Choy *et al.*, 2020). Nitazoxanide acts by interfering the host-regulated pathways involved in the replication of virus molecule, amplifying cytoplasmic RNA sensing, and type-I IFN pathways (Rossignol, 2016). Nitazoxanide also up-regulates the innate anti-viral mechanisms by broadly amplifying cytoplasmic RNA sensing and type I IFN pathways. It also prevents the viral infection by up-regulating the precise host mechanisms that virus targets to bypass host cellular defence mechanisms (Jasenosky *et al.*, 2019). Indeed, the *in-vitro* activity of nitazoxanide against SARS-Co-V-2 is encouraging, still more data and clinical outcome are required to determine its role in the management of COVID-19 (Choy *et al.*, 2020).

Corticosteroids

Cytokine storm and inflammation are the two major hallmarks that are associated with the human coronavirus (SARS-Co-V-1, MERS-Co-V, and SARS-Co-V-2)

(Zhou *et al.*, 2014; Channappanavar and Perlman, 2017). In addition to anti-viral interventions, corticosteroids may be another supportive therapy that may suppress the aforementioned hallmarks of COVID-19. The idea behind the concept is the pharmacological nature of corticosteroids to treat lung infection and inflammation by suppressing the inflammatory genes that encode cytokines, cell adhesion molecules (Cruz-Topete *et al.*, 2015). Although, China National Health Commission released the fifth trial for prevention and diagnosis of COVID-19 that recommended the use of systemic corticosteroids at the dose of 1-2 mg/kg for 3-5 days as adjuvant therapy (http://www.nhc.gov.cn/yzygj/s7653p/202002/d4b895337e19445f8d728fcaf1e3e13a.shtml,2020).

Corticosteroids in the Treatment of COVID-19

The utility of corticosteroids in COVID-19 is like a double-edged sword which means some clinical evidence documented its promising results in the treatment of COVID-19 (Wang *et al.*, 2020; Zhao *et al.*, 2020), while other studies reported the controversial outcomes against the use of corticosteroids in COVID-19 treatment (Russell and Millar, 2020).

A retrospective study conducted in Wuhan Union Hospital depicts the early administration of corticosteroids at the dose of 1-2 mg/kg *i.v.* gives promising results by improving the severe condition of patients (returning to normal body temperature, improvement in SpO_2) (Cheng *et al.*, 2020; Fang *et al.*, 2020). In parallel to the first study's outcome, similar results were also observed when a high dose of corticosteroids with quinoline is administered for short term use (Yang *et al.*, 2020). The dosing schedule and side effects of various drugs used for the treatment of COVID-19 are summarized in Table **1**.

Table 1. Different drugs used for the treatment of COVID-19 along with their dosing schedule and side effects.

Sr. No.	Drug/Treatment	Dosing Schedule	Side Effects
1.	Hydroxychloroquine	200 mg; Three times a day for 10 days. 500 mg; Two times a day for 10 days.	QT prolongation, Ventricular dysrhythmia, Haematological disorders.
2.	Remdesivir	200 mg *i.v.* loading dose followed by 100 mg *i.v.* for next 9 days.	Constipation.
3.	Lopinavir/Ritonavir	Lopinavir- 200 mg Ritonavir- 50 mg	Diarrhoea, Stomach upset, Drowsiness, Bad taste of mouth, Troubled sleeping.

(Table 1) cont.....

Sr. No.	Drug/Treatment	Dosing Schedule	Side Effects
4.	Favipiravir	1600 mg Twice on day 1 followed by 600 mg Thrice daily from day 2-14. 1800 mg Twice on day 1 followed by 600 mg Thrice daily from day 2-14.	Elevation of serum uric acid level, GI discomfort, Teratogenicity.
5.	Azithromycin	500 mg on day 1 followed by 250 mg from day 2-5.	Torsades-de-pointes.
6.	Arbidol	200 mg Three times daily for 10 days. 400 mg Three times daily for 9 days.	No major side effects.
7.	Ribavirin	400 mg oral loading dose followed by 1200 mg after every 8 hours. 500 mg *i.v.* Twice daily.	Reduction in haemoglobin.
8.	Teicoplanin	400 mg daily.	Erythematous rashes.
9.	Ivermectin	Not defined	Depression, Ataxia, Mydriasis.
10.	Corticosteroids	1-2 mg/kg; *i.v.* for 3-5 days.	Swelling in lower legs, High blood pressure, Mood swing, Behavioural changes.

On the contrary, Russell and his colleagues summarized the outcomes of clinical studies conducted on SARS Co-V-2 patients and implied that a high dose of corticosteroids delayed viral clearance from the respiratory tract and also increase the chances of higher incidence of psychosis (Russell *et al.*, 2020).

In addition to this, another study reported that patients treated with oral corticosteroids (hydrocortisone and methyl prednisolone; *i.v.*) do not delay the viral clearance (Cheng *et al.*, 2020) but on the other side, a meta-analysis documented that corticosteroids may increase the mortality rate with severe adverse effects when administered in COVID-19 patients (Wang *et al.*, 2020). A recent study conducted by Henry Ford Hospital, USA concluded that the administration of corticosteroids worsens the condition of COVID-19 patients (NCT04374071).

As there are no fixed guidelines for the use of corticosteroid in COVID-19 and WHO also has not given any nod for its efficacy and safety (https://www. who.int/publications-detail/clinical-management-of-severe-acute-respiratory-inf-ection-when-novel-coronavirus-(ncov)-infection-is-suspected). However, it is suggested that there is need to follow some precautions while using corticosteroids in COVID-19 *i.e.* administration should be done at an early stage but not for long term use and administration should be avoided in severe ill-treated patients of COVID-19 (Liou *et al.*, 2020).

Immuno Modulating Agents-Interferons (IFN's)

When a virus invades the host cells, there is an activation of innate and adaptive immunity to protect host cells from the deleterious effects of the virus. But sometimes, due to misdirection and mutations in the virus, the immune system gets suppressed that contributes to enhanced viral replication in the host's cell. Based on this fact, non-conventional therapy which is immune modulation may be a novel approach to combat COVID-19.

IFN's are cytokines having anti-viral properties. Currently, there are three distinct types of IFN's *i.e.* INF-α, β, and γ are available (Price *et al.*, 2000; Samuel, 2001). IFN's are one of the innate immune-modulating agents that can be used in the treatment of COVID-19. Various clinical and pre-clinical trials have given the evidence and suggest that IFN's may be useful candidates to combat viral infections such as SARS-Co-V, MERS-Co-V, and SARS-Co-V-2 (Hensley *et al.*, 2004; Stockman *et al.*, 2006).

IFN's in Treatment of COVID-19

A pre-clinical study conducted on cynomolgus monkey showed that IFN-α protects primates against SARS-Co-V. Since the genome sequencing of SARS-Co-V is 80% homologous to SARS-Co-V-2 therefore, it is considered that IFN's can be used as a potential therapeutic agent for COVID-19. China also recommended the administration of 5 million IU of IFN-α *via* inhalation two times a day in combination with ribavarin (Dong *et al.*, 2020; Lu, 2020). Clinical trials have been registered to evaluate the efficacy and safety of IFN-α in combination with lopinavir/ritonavir (ChiCTR2000029387) and that of IFN-β1 with lopinavir/ritonavir and ribavarin (NCT04276688).

IFN-1 treatment has given conducible results through *in-vitro* as well as *in-vivo* studies against SARS Co-V and MERS Co-V in combination with or without lopinavir/ritonavir (Stockman *et al.*, 2006). However, IFN-1 subtype inhibits SARS Co-V (Hensley *et al.*, 2004) but IFN-β1 is more effective as compared to IFN-1 because IFN-β1 expresses more prominent activity in the lungs. It also up-regulates the CD73 in pulmonary cells that subsequently exhibits anti-inflammatory activity and inhibits acute respiratory syndrome (Chan *et al.*, 2015). Similarly, the *in-vivo* study of IFN-β with lopinavir/ritonavir against MERS Co-V and SARS Co-V reduced lung infection but did not inhibit viral replication (Sheahan *et al.*, 2020). The aforementioned pre-clinical study depicts that IFN-1 can reduce lung infection by inhibiting cytokine storm (a major hallmark of COVID-19).

Furthermore, a study also reported that human lung tissue infected with COVID-19 failed to induce expression of IFN (type 1, 2, 3) as compared to control tissue (Chu *et al.*, 2020). Similarly, it is also reported that mice lacking IFNδR1 are more prone to the infection of viruses and inflammation (Davidson *et al.*, 2016; Galani *et al.*, 2017). Hence, based on the above clinical and pre-clinical data, it is suggested that IFN's may be a promising therapeutic agent to combat COVID-19 infection.

Probable Mechanism of Action of IFN's in COVID-19

The exact mechanism of IFN's to exhibit their anti-viral activity is unclear but some of the reports suggest that IFN's promotes the activation of macrophages, that subsequently causes phagocytosis of the antigen and also block the replication of viruses (Ivashkiv and Donlin, 2014; Cao *et al.*, 2019) (Fig. **2**).

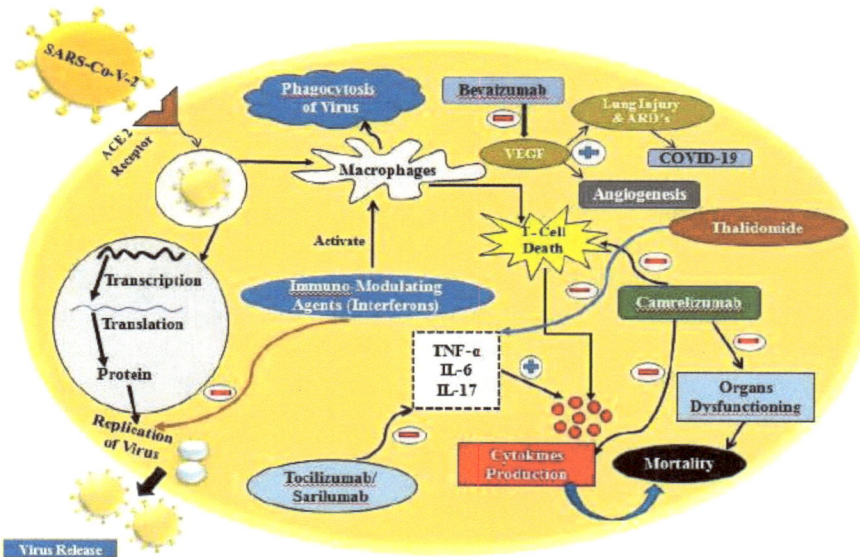

Fig. (2). Mechanism of action of different drugs at various steps of virus pathology into host cells. ACE-2: angiotensin-converting enzyme; ARD's: acute respiratory disorders; COVID-19: corona virus disease-19; IL: interleukins; SARS-Co-V-2: severe acute respiratory syndrome corona virus-2; TNF-α: tumour necrosis factor- α; VEGF: vascular endothelial growth factor.

Monoclonal Antibody Therapy

Monoclonal antibodies (mAb's) are a dynamic category of pharmaceuticals which are fortunate for the pharma industry and have a special attribute to treat a particular diseases (Meissner and Long, 2003; Berry *et al.*, 2010; Arabi *et al.*, 2015). They represent a major class of bio-therapeutics for passive immunotherapy to fight against all type of infections. In the recent years, many mAb's have been developed to fight against viruses and some are in pipeline also (Boyapati *et al.*, 2020; Shanmugaraj *et al.*, 2020).

Monoclonal antibodies can play a crucial role to curb COVID-19 infection. Evidence of *in-vitro* and *in-vivo* studies has suggested that mAb's targeting spike protein can be potentially effective against SARS-CoV-2. These can act directly by interrupting any stage of the viral lifecycle or may bind with the receptor proteins of the host cell surface so that virus could not use host's machinery and its growth gets halted. Pre-clinical studies suggest that various neutralizing antibodies are effective against SARS-Co-V infection of humans (Arabi *et al.*, 2015). The specific neutralizing mAb's either binds against receptor-binding domain (RBD) in spike protein or binds to ACE-2 receptors and further can effectively block the virus entry into host cells. Further, evidence indicates that neutralizing mAb binds to the ACE-2 RBD of the SARS S protein (Berry *et al.*, 2010), thus block the viral entry into host cells. Moreover, mechanistically co-operative binding of mAb's leads to conformational changes in the antigen which further alters the affinity of virus to get bind with host cell (Klonisch *et al.*, 1996). The mAb's has considered a passive immunotherapy to provide a quick response against viral infection. Brink and colleagues have suggested that passive transfer of polyclonal immune serum reduces pulmonary virus load in a mouse model of SARS-Co-V infection (Van Den Brink, 2005). Therefore, immuno-prophylaxis of SARS-Co-V infection with antibodies might be an effective SARS control strategy. Another strategy includes mAb's cocktail that may exhibit more potent anti-viral activity that could increase the effectiveness of the treatment and prevent the viral escape.

80R Immunoglobulin G1 (IgG1)

80R IgG1, a human mAb, has identified as a neutralizing antibody and plays an important role in immunity. It responses to the surface glycoproteins of enveloped viruses and has anti-viral activity against SARS-Co-V spike S protein. 80R IgG1 potentially neutralizes SARS-Co-V infection by efficiently inhibiting syncytia formation as it hinders the binding of the viral agent with the receptors (Sui *et al.*, 2004). 80R has been tested *in-vitro* and found to inhibit virus entry into host cells (Sui *et al.*, 2004). The passive administration of 80R human mAb's could provide an immediate response as a prophylaxis in the treatment of SARS-Co-V-2 infection (Mair-Jenkins *et al.*, 2015).

CR3014

Study suggests that the binding site of CR3014 and CR3022 mAb's is different from that of mAb 80R (Sui *et al.*, 2004). It has been evident by a study that CR3014 protects ferrets from SARS-Co-V-2 infection at 10 mg/kg dose by completely protecting the lung pathological markers that may further aggravate the severity in patients, and also abolished the shedding of the virus (Ter Meulen *et al.*, 2004). CR3014 has been reported to reduce replication of SARS-Co-V in the lungs of infected ferrets, abolished shedding of SARS-Co-V in pharyngeal secretions, and completely prevented the development of virus-induced macroscopic lung pathology (Van Den Brink *et al.*, 2005).

Effect of SARS-Co-V-2 can be abolished by human mAb's, which target the RBD of the virus. The mixture of both human mAb's CR3014 and CR3022 by its interaction with RBD has reported producing a synergistic effect in the neutralization of SARS-Co-V. The study has suggested that a combination of CR3014 and CR3022 have potential to provide adequate protection against not only SARS-Co-V strains but also against other SARS-Co-V like viruses originate from other animals. The combination of two non-competing human mAb's CR3014 and CR3022 potentially activates the immune response and increase the aura of shielding effect against viruses (Ter Meulen *et al.*, 2006).

Monoclonal Antibody Therapy in COVID-19 Treatment

Indeed, cytokine storms had been reported in many diseases including infections and rheumatic diseases. Macrophage activation syndrome (MAS) refers to acute inflammation caused by cytokine storm (Schulert and Grom *et al.*, 2015). The fact that the biological agents neutralizing IL-6 and IL-1 are highly effective treatments for systemic juvenile idiopathic arthritis, a rheumatic disease strongly associated with MAS also arise a ray of hope that suggests that the same therapy could be beneficial for delaying cytokine storm in inflammation associated with COVID-19 (Jiang *et al.*, 2020). Two mAb's that targets IL-6 signalling *viz.* tocilizumab and sarilumab have been approved for the treatment of rheumatoid arthritis (Boyapati *et al.*, 2020).

Tocilizumab

Tocilizumab is a potent immunosuppressive agent. It is a recombinant, humanized anti-human IL-6 receptor mAb's which was originally made to treat RA and has found to inhibit signal transduction pathways associated with severe inflammation (Xu *et al.*, 2020). The study has suggested the benefits of tocilizumab in controlling cytokine release syndrome in COVID-19 patients (Chen *et al.*, 2020). Tocilizumab works by inhibiting IL-6 receptor thereby reduce cytokine release syndrome-like features in severe patients of COVID-19 (Fig. **2**). Scientists and physicians in China suspect that IL-6 may play a crucial role in the treatment of COVID-19. Furthermore, healthcare professionals from China and Italy have already started the clinical trials to access the potential of drug tocilizumab in COVID-19 patients with severe symptoms (Chen *et al.*, 2020). Recently, interleukin-6 receptor (IL-6R) mAb (tocilizumab)-directed COVID-19 therapy clinical trial has been conducting in China (NCT04356937) and it has been involved into COVID-19 management guidelines generated in China by considering the concept of cytokine storm in COVID-19 pneumonia (Zhang *et al.*, 2020). More importantly, humans have a very high tolerance for tocilizumab. Thus, tocilizumab may be an effective treatment strategy in patients with severe cases of COVID-19. A tocilizumab trial in the US and Canada in patients with severe COVID-19 pneumonia is underway (NCT04320615).

Sarilumab

It acts in similar manner as like tocilizumab (Fig. **2**). IL-6 release may be responsible for cytokine storm and also used as a prognostic marker to evaluate the progression of COVID-19 diseases and patients with high IL-6 may be likely to benefit from sarilumab. A clinical trial already has been reported that patients with high IL-6 levels are effectively responding to sarilumab (Boyapati *et al.*, 2020).

Limitations and Suggestions Regarding mAb's

Although, several mAb's showed promising results in neutralizing SARS-Co-V infection, large-scale production of mAb's requires wide ranging of labour. Moreover, it is very expensive and time consuming process which outweighs the mAb's clinical use against the emerging pathogen.

With the recent advancement production of mAb's at lower production costs could be possible. In today's scenario the sequences of mAb's that are effective against SARS-Co-V are cloned in a satisfactory expression systems such as mammalian, yeast or plant, and recombinant mAb's would be tested against SARS-Co-V-2. Plant cloned system has a great advantage that it rapidly reproduce the mAb's in a less time at the nominal cost which is considered to be a major advantage of expression system during the pandemic situations. A Low dose combination of mAb's maybe a good strategy to fight against the SARS-CoV-2 outbreak.

Triple Therapy

This is another approach that has been exercised to contain COVID-19 infection.

Triple therapy involves combined administration of IFN-β1b, lopinavir/ritonavir, and ribavarin. A multi-centred open-label randomized clinical trial has given the evidence of efficacy and safety of triple therapy to tackle COVID-19. Inclusive criteria of the study were characterized by the patient's age, minimum should be 18, and the patient should be confirmed with COVID-19 infection (Hung *et al.*, 2020). The trial comprised the administration of oral lopinavir 400 mg, ritonavir 100 mg for every 12 hours *via* a nasogastric tube; ribavarin 400 mg every 12 hours, and one to three doses of IFN-β1b on alternate days continuously for 14 days. Lopinavir/ritonavir of the same dose was administered to the control group and outcome was conquered by shortening the duration of viral load, hospital stays with nasopharyngeal swab negative (NCT04276688).

Miscellaneous Drugs

Besides the drugs discussed above for COVID-19, many other drugs are supposed to exhibit therapeutic efficacy in COVID-19 infection with disparate mechanisms. These drugs mainly act by targeting the pathogenesis of COVID-19 instead of inhibiting the replication of the virus.

A drug like PD-1 inhibitor camrelizumab, primarily used for the treatment of relapsed or refractory classical hodgkin's lymphoma (Markham and Keam, 2019). A study has reported that the drug also inhibits the apoptosis of T-cell, cytokines production, and organ dysfunctioning (Fig. **2**) (Zhu *et al.*, 2020). As it is well proven that T-cell death, cytokines production and organ dysfunctioning are the major pathological hallmarks that lead the mortality of COVID-19 patients. Based on the aforementioned information, it is believed that camrelizumab may be used as a potential agent in the treatment of COVID-19. Substantiating this mechanism, a clinical study is conducted to evaluate its efficacy with severe pneumonia patients associated with lymphocytopenia (NCT04268537).

Another drug is bevaizumab that has been approved for the treatment of metastatic colon cancer (Heinzerling and Huerta *et al.*, 2006) and exhibits its therapeutic effects by inhibiting the vascular endothelial growth factor (VEGF) (Fig. **2**) (Ferrara *et al.*, 2004) which is a key promoter of angiogenesis (US-FDA, 2008, EMA 2008). A study has revealed that VEGF plays an important role in lung injury and acute respiratory disorders (ARD'S) which are directly related to the pathology of COVID-19 (Baratt *et al.*, 2014). Based on these facts, bevaizumab is presently clinical trial in patients with COVID-19 under trial name BEST-RCT and BEST-CP (NCT04305106 and NCT04275414).

TNF-α is the primary factor that aggravates the pathogenesis of COVID-19 which is suppressed by the drug thalidomide (Fig. **2**) (Mazzoccoli *et al.*, 2012). Considering this fact, thalidomide is also under the clinical trial (NCT04273529).

Now a day, thalidomide is being used in the treatment of interstitial pulmonary fibrosis, lung damage, and myeloma (Horton *et al.*, 2012).

SARS Co-V-2 vaccine which is developed by Shang and colleagues is in the clinical trial phase (NCT0428346). In addition to this, University of Pittsburgh School of Medicine also evolved the vaccine which was tested on mice. Antibodies produced by the SARS Co-V-2 vaccine were able to neutralize the virus (NCT0428346). An mRNA vaccine already has been administered to a person in the USA for treating COVID-19 (Cohen, 2020).

As we know that SARS Co-V-2 penetrates the cell membrane and gets activated by two proteins such as ACE-2 and TMPRSS2. Based on this fact, drugs like camostat mesylate and nafamosate which are synthetic candidates and can inhibit the aforementioned proteins further may prevent the emergence of COVID-19 (Hoffmann *et al.*, 2020; Zhou *et al.*, 2015). To evaluate the efficacy of these drugs, a randomized placebo clinical trial is being conducted on 180 patients (NCT04321096).

Herbal Drugs for COVID-19

In addition to various synthetic and semi-synthetic drugs discussed above, many natural compounds were also tested and tried for the management of COVID-19 infection. Most of the studies are reported with Chinese herbal drugs. Recent pre-clinical, clinical and *in-silico* data has given the evidence that Chinese herbal candidates like glycyrrhizin, scutellarin, baicalin, and hesperetin show their promising results in SARS COV-2 (Cinatl *et al.*, 2003; Pilcher, 2003; Chen *et al.*, 2020).

Glycyrrhizin

Glycyrrhizin a constituent of liquorice roots (*glycyrrhiza radix*) has earlier been reported to exert a beneficial effect in the treatment of SARS Co-V-1 (Pilcher, 2003). Besides the coronavirus, glycyrrhizin also has been used in the treatment of chronic hepatitis (Chen *et al.*, 2020). An *in-vitro* study also depicts that drug has anti-SARS activity with fewer side effects (Cinatl *et al.*, 2003). In addition to this, the clinical study indicated that glycyrrhizin produces conducible results against two strains of the virus (FFM-1, FFM2) in patients suffering from SARS who were admitted to the health care centre in Germany. It was reported that glycyrrhizin acts by inhibiting the replication of viruses and also by inhibiting adsorption and penetration of viruses into the host cells (Cinatl *et al.*, 2003). Besides these mechanisms, glycyrrhizin also up-regulates the expression of nitric acid in macrophages followed by inhibition of replication of viruses belongs to the flaviviridae family (Jeong and Kim, 2002).

Glycyrrhizin in COVID-19

This drug has a low selectivity index but it is a potent inhibitor of replication of viruses. Results of a docking study showed that glycyrrhizin binds with ACE-2 receptor with an estimated ΔG 9Kcl/mol which is an important entry point for SARS Co-V-2 into host cells (Chen and DU, 2020).

Hesperetin

Hesperetin, a bio flavonoid compound that has been found in plants *citrus aurantinum* and *citrus reticulate pericarpium*. It is a well known Chinese medicine that exhibits its dose-dependent effects and attenuates the cleavage activity of 3C-like proteases of SARS-Co-V in cell-based assays (Lin *et al.*, 2005). It also inhibits ACE-2 with an estimated value ΔG -8.3Kcal/mol, which is sufficient to evaluate its efficacy in COVID-19 (Chen *et al.*, 2020). However, there is no clinical trial evidence that delineates its efficacy in the treatment of COVID-19. Also, the *in-silico* experiment gives us hope about its efficacy in the treatment of pandemic 2019 in the future. Moreover, additional experimental studies are needed to prove its usefulness in COVID-19.

Baicalin

Baicalin is obtained from Chinese medicinal plant *Scutellaria Bericalensis Georgi* and has been reported to exert beneficial effects in oxidative stress, inflammation, and apoptosis (Chen *et al.*, 2017; Ishfaq *et al.*, 2019). Since, genomic sequencing revealed the information that almost 80% of the SARS viral genome is homologues to the genome of COVID-19. Baicalin has already proved its efficacy against SARS. Therefore, based on this fact, baicalin came under consideration as a probable therapeutic agent in the intervention of COVID-19. Moreover, the *in-silico* experiment conducted by Chen and co-workers gives the promising value of ΔG that shows its efficacy against COVID-19 (Chen *et al.*, 2020). Baicalin activity against SARS in fRhk cell lines is reported with promising results (Chen *et al.*, 2015). Also, this drug inhibits ACE-2 with an IC_{50} value of 2.24 µM and docking results also indicate that it can bind with ACE-2 with a ΔG -8.46Kcal/mol which is sufficient value for depicting its conducible results in the treatment of COVID-19 (Chen and Du, 2020).

Scutellarin

Scutellarin is another Chinese compound that is obtained from *Erigeran Brevis Capus*. Pharmacologically, the drug has a broad spectrum of effects in the treatment of inflammation and oxidative stress (Wang and Ma, 2018). An *in-vivo* study conducted by Wang and colleagues, showed that the drug inhibits the expression and activity of ACE-2 in brain tissue with an estimated IC_{50} (48.13±4.98 µM) value against SARS (Wang *et al.*, 2016). However, no *in-vivo* study has been conducted to report that this drug can inhibit ACE-2 but the *in-silico* study showed that scutellarin has the potential to treat COVID-19 with an estimated value ∆G (-14.98Kcal/mol) (Chen and Du, 2020).

Plasma Therapy

Convalescent plasma therapy is not a new concept, it's an old one, and has a similar mechanism of action based on the concept of immunization by vaccines as described by Edward Jenner. In this therapy, blood is collected from patients who have recovered from infectious illness and then transfused to patients who are currently diagnosed with COVID-19 illness. The concept behind this therapy is the production of antibodies that fights against infection. Convalescent plasma therapy has been successfully employed already, as a targeted therapy to treat influenza virus (H_1N_1), SARS-Co-V-1 epidemic, and MERS-Co-V epidemic (Hung *et al.*, 2011; Dodd, 2012). A meta-analysis done by Mair-Jenkins and his colleagues concluded that infusion of plasma attenuated the complications shown by patients suffering from a severe acute respiratory infection (Mair-Jenkins *et al.*, 2015). Moreover, the *in-vitro* trial also showed the efficacy of treatment and concluded that antibody production is responsible for blocking new infections and also for clearance of infected cells (Lu *et al.*, 2016).

Plasma Therapy in the Treatment of COVID-19

Several clinical studies have given the encouraging results for the treatment of COVID-19 (Shen *et al.*, 2020; Duan *et al.*, 2020). A recent clinical study conducted on 5 confirmed patients of COVID-19, has reported improvement in the symptoms of patients within 12 days after transfusion of convalescent plasma without showing any adverse effects (Shen *et al.*, 2020). Another study carried out on 10 patients of COVID-19, also given promising results without causing any severe adverse effects in the hospital (Duan *et al.*, 2020). To observe the efficacy of convalescent plasma therapy, the Italian National Board also gave a nod for treatment with convalescent plasma therapy but the board defined some mandatory conditions for donors which should be followed before donating plasma (Franchini *et al.*, 2020).

Besides advantages, convalescent plasma therapy also faces some challenges that are questionable regarding its efficacy (Zhao and He, 2020). Research on SARS-

Co-V confirmed that this therapy is more effective at an earlier stage and may aggravate hyper immune attacks. Convalescent plasma therapy can increase the chances of chills, fever, and anaphylactic shock. Besides this, the optimum volume of serum and optimal duration for administering convalescent plasma is required. Also, the risk of transfusion-transmitted infections can increase with this therapy (World Health Organization, 2020).

Potential of Stem Cell Therapy in COVID-19

Stem cell therapy has a special contribution to the field of regenerative medicines. This concept was given by Ernest McCulloch and James Till in 1960. Stem cells especially mesenchymal cells may also exhibit a pivotal role in the COVID-19 pandemic (Shetty, 2020). Mesenchymal cells are derived from the umbilical cord, placenta, and other tissues.

The concept behind the use of mesenchymal cells in the COVID-19 pandemic is the immune regulatory activity of cells that further inhibits ARD'S by activation of the paracrine mechanism (Fujita *et al.*, 2018). Moreover, mesenchymal stem cells also customize the attributes of both innate as well as adaptive immune cells *via* inhibiting the release of cytokines, IFN's from natural killer (NK) cells, and T-cells (Aggarwal and Pittenger, 2005). In addition to this, they also enhance the activity of phagocytes that directly activates the secretion of anti-microbial peptides and proteins (Krasnodembskaya *et al.*, 2010; Sutton *et al.*, 2016).

A clinical trial is conducted in China on four patients of COVID-19 and the study depicts that patients got recovered and discharged from hospital after administration of mesenchymal stem cell therapy. Multiple trials are under process to substantiate the efficacy of mesenchymal stem cell therapy in COVID-19 infection (NCT0425 2118, NCT04269525, NCT04273646, NCT04293692).

BCG Vaccine

Vaccination is one of the options which would be helpful to curb COVID-19 pandemic. However, the development of vaccines instantly is a tedious and time-consuming task. Therefore, researchers move towards pre-existing vaccine molecules and have started clinical trials on the molecules. BCG vaccine is one the candidate that garnered the interest of researchers to combat pandemic COVID-19. Albert Calmette and Camille Guerin had developed BCG vaccine in the 20th century and now used in the prevention of tuberculosis (Brewer and Colditz, 1995).

The idea behind the use of the BCG vaccine in COVID-19 is based upon two considerations. First, the countries which had already discontinued their universal vaccination policies of BCG vaccine in neonates are more prone to COVID-19, for instance, United States, Italy, Netherland. After exploring the epidemiological data, Miller and colleagues found that the aforementioned countries had completely discontinued their vaccine policy and are more prone to risk for COVID-19 as compared to other countries like Japan, India. Second, the effect of the BCG vaccine is non-specific and provides heterologous immunity that further strongly activates innate and adaptive immunity. Strong innate immunity (trained immunity) on second exposure to a pathogen (in case of COVID-19) leads to some transcriptional and epigenetic reprogramming of human monocytes and may show its effect in treating COVID-19, as shown in yellow fever vaccine (Arts *et al.*, 2018).

Two clinical trials on the BCG vaccine to combat the COVID-19 pandemic are under process (NCT04327206; NCTO4328441). Until clinical trial will complete, it is necessary to adhere to WHO's recommendation because of limited supply of BCG vaccine and haphazard use may jeopardize the situation in the case where it is needed to prevent the children from infection (https://www.who.int/news-room/commentaries/detail/bacille-calmette-gu%C3%A9rin-(bcg)-vaccination-and-COVID-19).

VARIOUS REGULATORY GUIDELINES GIVEN BY NIH (NATIONAL INSTITUTE OF HEALTH) FOR TREATMENT OF COVID-19

There are some specific recommendations issued by NIH related to drugs that have been used in COVID-19:

1. If HCQ is used for treatment, then the clinician should track the patients for adverse effects especially QT interval prolongation.
2. The use of a combination of HCQ and AZ is highly prohibited because of toxicities.
3. Neither combination of lopinavir/ritonavir (Kaletra) is recommended due to unfavourable pharmacodynamics and unfavourable trial results.
4. Guidelines have also recommended the use of ACE inhibitors or angiotensin receptor blockers (ARB) for pandemic 2020, but advised to take only by the patients who are taking drugs for cardiovascular and other diseases.
5. There is no guideline in favour of or in opposition to the regular use of extracorporeal membrane oxygenation for patients of COVID-19 with refractory hypoxemia.
6. Data is also insufficient or not giving promising results for convalescent plasma therapy in COVID-19. Moreover, regulatory guidelines are neither in favour nor against for the use of IL-6 and IL-1 antagonist such as tocilizumab and anavarin.

7. The panel does not allowed the use of IFN's and Janus kinase (JAK) inhibitors such as baricitinub, because of the ineffective outcome of IFN in MERS and SARS and immunosuppressive effect reflected by drug baricitinub.

8. Panelist of NIH are against the regular use of corticosteroid in COVID-19 patients who are mechanically ventilated, but also recommends its use at a lower dose, who are experiencing refractory shock and corticosteroid or NSAID use should not be discontinued to patients of COVID-19 who are taking medication in pre-existing conditions.

9. Data are also inadequate to recommend the use of drug remdesivir in COVID-19, originally developed to treat Ebola and MERS by Gilead Sciences.

CONCLUSION

Since its outbreak, COVID-19 has become a matter of concern globally and there is a drastic elevation of mortality graph. Understanding regarding the exact cause and transmission of the virus is in the nascent stage hence, posing a difficult situation and big challenge for researchers to develop a new molecule *i.e.* vaccine in a shorter period. In the current scenario, therefore the best strategy for treating COVID-19 is to move towards existing molecules that already have been used as an intervention target in SARS, MERS (homologous to COVID-19), and other viral infections with diverse mechanisms at different steps of viral life cycle into host cells. In this chapter, we have discussed the existing molecules as a conducible target in the treatment of COVID-19. Indeed, current treatment strategies discussed above have been moderately successful to curb COVID-19 infection but off course vaccine for COVID-19 which would be the ultimate solution to eradicate the COVID-19 pandemic is still missing. Researchers across the globe are working hard to develop COVID-19 vaccine; hopefully, a successful outcome is on the anvil very soon.

LIST OF ABBREVIATIONS

ACE-2	Angiotensin converting enzyme-2
ARB	Angiotensin receptor blocker
ARD	Acute respiratory disorder
AUC	Area under curve
AZ	Azithromycin
COVID-19	Corona virus diseases-19
CQ	Chloroquine
CSF	Cerebrospinal fluid
DENV	Dengue virus
HCQ	Hydroxychloroquine

HCV	Hepatitis-C-virus
HIV-1	Human immunodeficiency virus-1
HSV	Herpes simplex virus
IFN	Interferon
IL	Interleukin
JAK	Janus kinases
mAb's	Monoclonal antibodies
MAS	Macrophage activation syndrome
MERS Co-V	Middle east respiratory syndrome corona virus
NHC	National health commission
NK	Natural killer
P/K	Pharmacokinetic
PLE	Polymorphic light eruption
RA	Rheumatoid arthritis
RBD	Receptor binding domain
RdRp	RNA dependent RNA polymerase
RSV	Respiratory syncytial virus
SARS-Co-V-2	Severe acute respiratory syndrome corona virus
SLE	Systemic lupus erythematosus
TID	Three times daily
Vd	Volume of distribution
ZIKV	Zika Virus

AUTHORS CONTRIBUTION

Kuldeep Kumar, Sonal and Pankaj Bhatia carried out the relevant literature research and prepared the primary draft; Dr. Nirmal Singh prepared the final draft of the chapter; Dr. Dhandeep Singh and Dr. Amteshwar S. Jaggi co-conceptualized and provided valuable inputs in finalizing the chapter.

CONSENT FOR PUBLICATION

Not applicable.

CONFLICT OF INTEREST

The author declares no conflict of interest, financial or otherwise.

ACKNOWLEDGEMENTS

Authors are thankful to Department of Pharmaceutical Sciences & Drug Research, Punjabi University Patiala for providing the technical support.

REFERENCES

Aggarwal, S & Pittenger, MF (2005) Human mesenchymal stem cells modulate allogeneic immune cell responses. *Blood,* 105, 1815-22.
[http://dx.doi.org/10.1182/blood-2004-04-1559] [PMID: 15494428]

Agostini, ML, Andres, EL, Sims, AC, Graham, RL, Sheahan, TP, Lu, X, Smith, EC, Case, JB, Feng, JY, Jordan, R, Ray, AS, Cihlar, T, Siegel, D, Mackman, RL, Clarke, MO, Baric, RS & Denison, MR (2018) Coronavirus susceptibility to the antiviral remdesivir (GS-5734) is mediated by the viral polymerase and the proofreading exoribonuclease. *MBio,* 9, e00221-18.
[http://dx.doi.org/10.1128/mBio.00221-18] [PMID: 29511076]

Anand, K, Ziebuhr, J, Wadhwani, P, Mesters, JR & Hilgenfeld, R (2003) Coronavirus main proteinase (3CLpro) structure: basis for design of anti-SARS drugs. *Science,* 300, 1763-7.
[http://dx.doi.org/10.1126/science.1085658] [PMID: 12746549]

Andreani, J, Bideau, M, Duflot, I, Jardot, P, Rolland, C, Boxberger, M, Wurtz, N, Rolain, JM, Colson, P, La Scola, B & Raoult, D (2020) *In vitro* testing of combined hydroxychloroquine and azithromycin on SARS-CoV-2 shows synergistic effect. *Microb Pathog,* 145, 104228.
[http://dx.doi.org/10.1016/j.micpath.2020.104228] [PMID: 32344177]

Arabi, Y, Balkhy, H, Hajeer, AH, Bouchama, A, Hayden, FG, Al-Omari, A, Al-Hameed, FM, Taha, Y, Shindo, N, Whitehead, J, Merson, L, AlJohani, S, Al-Khairy, K, Carson, G, Luke, TC, Hensley, L, Al-Dawood, A, Al-Qahtani, S, Modjarrad, K, Sadat, M, Rohde, G, Leport, C & Fowler, R (2015) Feasibility, safety, clinical, and laboratory effects of convalescent plasma therapy for patients with Middle East respiratory syndrome coronavirus infection: a study protocol. *Springerplus,* 4, 709.
[http://dx.doi.org/10.1186/s40064-015-1490-9] [PMID: 26618098]

Arabi, YM, Alothman, A, Balkhy, HH, Al-Dawood, A, AlJohani, S, Al Harbi, S, Kojan, S, Al Jeraisy, M, Deeb, AM, Assiri, AM, Al-Hameed, F, AlSaedi, A, Mandourah, Y, Almekhlafi, GA, Sherbeeni, NM, Elzein, FE, Memon, J, Taha, Y, Almotairi, A, Maghrabi, KA, Qushmaq, I, Al Bshabshe, A, Kharaba, A, Shalhoub, S, Jose, J, Fowler, RA, Hayden, FG & Hussein, MA (2018) Treatment of middle east respiratory syndrome with a combination of lopinavir-ritonavir and interferon-β1b (MIRACLE trial): study protocol for a randomized controlled trial. *Trials,* 19, 81.
[http://dx.doi.org/10.1186/s13063-017-2427-0] [PMID: 29382391]

Arts RJW, Moorlag SJCFM, Novakovic B, Li Y, Wang SY, Oosting M, Kumar V, Xavier RJ, Wijmenga C, Joosten LAB, Reusken CBEM, Benn CS, Aaby P, Koopmans MP, Stunnenberg HG, van Crevel R, Netea MG (2018) BCG Vaccination Protects against Experimental Viral Infection in Humans through the Induction of Cytokines Associated with Trained Immunity. Cell Host Microbe, 23, 89-100.e5. doi: 10.1016/j.chom.2017.12.010. PMID: 29324233.

Azeem, S, Ashraf, M, Rasheed, MA, Anjum, AA & Hameed, R (2015) Evaluation of cytotoxicity and antiviral activity of ivermectin against Newcastle disease virus. *Pak J Pharm Sci,* 28, 597-602.
[PMID: 25730813]

Bacharier, LB, Guilbert, TW, Mauger, DT, Boehmer, S, Beigelman, A, Fitzpatrick, AM, Jackson, DJ, Baxi, SN, Benson, M, Burnham, CD, Cabana, M, Castro, M, Chmiel, JF, Covar, R, Daines, M, Gaffin, JM, Gentile, DA, Holguin, F, Israel, E, Kelly, HW, Lazarus, SC, Lemanske, RF, Jr, Ly, N, Meade, K, Morgan, W, Moy, J, Olin, T, Peters, SP, Phipatanakul, W, Pongracic, JA, Raissy, HH, Ross, K, Sheehan, WJ, Sorkness, C, Szefler, SJ, Teague, WG, Thyne, S & Martinez, FD (2015) Early administration of azithromycin and prevention of severe lower respiratory tract illnesses in preschool children with a history of such illnesses: A randomized clinical trial. *JAMA,* 314, 2034-44.

[http://dx.doi.org/10.1001/jama.2015.13896] [PMID: 26575060]

Baron, SA, Devaux, C, Colson, P, Raoult, D & Rolain, JM (2020) Teicoplanin: an alternative drug for the treatment of COVID-19? *Int J Antimicrob Agents,* 55, 105944.
[http://dx.doi.org/10.1016/j.ijantimicag.2020.105944] [PMID: 32179150]

Barratt, S, Medford, AR & Millar, AB (2014) Vascular endothelial growth factor in acute lung injury and acute respiratory distress syndrome. *Respiration,* 87, 329-42.
[http://dx.doi.org/10.1159/000356034] [PMID: 24356493]

Berry, JD, Hay, K, Rini, JM, Yu, M, Wang, L, Plummer, FA, Corbett, CR & Andonov, A (2010) Neutralizing epitopes of the SARS-CoV S-protein cluster independent of repertoire, antigen structure or mAb technology. *MAbs,* 2, 53-66.
[http://dx.doi.org/10.4161/mabs.2.1.10788] [PMID: 20168090]

Blaising, J, Polyak, SJ & Pécheur, EI (2014) Arbidol as a broad-spectrum antiviral: an update. *Antiviral Res,* 107, 84-94.
[http://dx.doi.org/10.1016/j.antiviral.2014.04.006] [PMID: 24769245]

Bleibtreu, A, Jaureguiberry, S, Houhou, N, Boutolleau, D, Guillot, H, Vallois, D, Lucet, JC, Robert, J, Mourvillier, B, Delemazure, J, Jaspard, M, Lescure, FX, Rioux, C, Caumes, E & Yazdanapanah, Y (2018) Clinical management of respiratory syndrome in patients hospitalized for suspected Middle East respiratory syndrome coronavirus infection in the Paris area from 2013 to 2016. *BMC Infect Dis,* 18, 331.
[http://dx.doi.org/10.1186/s12879-018-3223-5] [PMID: 30012113]

Bocan, TM, Basuli, F, Stafford, RG, Brown, JL, Zhang, X, Duplantier, AJ & Swenson, RE (2019) Synthesis of [18F] Favipiravir and biodistribution in C3H/HeN mice as assessed by positron emission tomography. *Sci Rep,* 9, 1785.
[http://dx.doi.org/10.1038/s41598-018-37866-z] [PMID: 30741966]

Boriskin, YS, Leneva, IA, Pécheur, EI & Polyak, SJ (2008) Arbidol: a broad-spectrum antiviral compound that blocks viral fusion. *Curr Med Chem,* 15, 997-1005.
[http://dx.doi.org/10.2174/092986708784049658] [PMID: 18393857]

Boyapati, A, Schwartzman, S, Msihid, J, Choy, E, Genovese, MC, Burmester, GR, Lam, G, Kimura, T, Sadeh, J, Weinreich, DM, Yancopoulos, GD & Graham, NMH (2020) High serum interleukin-6 is associated with severe progression of rheumatoid arthritis and increased treatment response differentiating sarilumab from adalimumab or methotrexate in a post hoc analysis. *Arthritis Rheumatol,* 72, 1456-66.
[http://dx.doi.org/10.1002/art.41299] [PMID: 32343882]

Brewer TF, Colditz GA (1995) Bacille Calmette-Guérin vaccination for the prevention of tuberculosis in health care workers. Clin Infect Dis. 1995 Jan;20(1):136-42.
[http://dx.doi.org/10.1093/clinids/20.1.136] [PMID: 7727639]

Byrd, TF & Horwitz, MA (1991) Chloroquine inhibits the intracellular multiplication of *Legionella pneumophila* by limiting the availability of iron. A potential new mechanism for the therapeutic effect of chloroquine against intracellular pathogens. *J Clin Invest,* 88, 351-7.
[http://dx.doi.org/10.1172/JCI115301] [PMID: 2056129]

Cai, Q, Yang, M, Liu, D, Chen, J, Shu, D, Xia, J, Liao, X, Gu, Y, Cai, Q, Yang, Y, Shen, C, Li, X, Peng, L, Huang, D, Zhang, J, Zhang, S, Wang, F, Liu, J, Chen, L, Chen, S, Wang, Z, Zhang, Z, Cao, R, Zhong, W, Liu, Y & Liu, L (2020) Experimental treatment with favipiravir for COVID-19: An open-label control study. *Engineering (Beijing),* 6, 1192-8.
[http://dx.doi.org/10.1016/j.eng.2020.03.007] [PMID: 32346491]

Caly, L, Druce, JD, Catton, MG, Jans, DA & Wagstaff, KM (2020) The FDA-approved drug ivermectin inhibits the replication of SARS-CoV-2 *in vitro. Antiviral Res,* 178, 104787.
[http://dx.doi.org/10.1016/j.antiviral.2020.104787] [PMID: 32251768]

Canga, AG, Prieto, AM, Liebana, MJ, Martínez, NF, Vega, MS & Vieitez, J (2008) The pharmacokinetics and interactions of ivermectin in humans--a mini-review. *Am Assoc Pharm Sci J,* 10, 42-6.

[http://dx.doi.org/10.1208/s12248-007-9000-9] [PMID: 18446504]

Cao, BY, Wang, Y, Wen, D, Liu, W, Wang, J, Fan, G, Ruan, L, Song, B, Cai, Y, Wei, M, Li, X, Xia, J, Chen, N, Xiang, J, Yu, T, Bai, T, Xie, X, Zhang, L, Li, C, Yuan, Y, Chen, H, Li, H, Huang, H, Tu, S, Gong, F, Liu, Y, Wei, Y, Dong, C, Zhou, F, Gu, X, Xu, J, Liu, Z, Zhang, Y, Li, H, Shang, L, Wang, K, Li, K, Zhou, X, Dong, X, Qu, Z, Lu, S, Hu, X, Ruan, S, Luo, S, Wu, J, Peng, L, Cheng, F, Pan, L, Zou, J, Jia, C, Wang, J, Liu, X, Wang, S, Wu, X, Ge, Q, He, J, Zhan, H, Qiu, F, Guo, L, Huang, C, Jaki, T, Hayden, FG, Horby, PW, Zhang, D & Wang, C (2020) A trial of lopinavir–ritonavir in adults hospitalized with severe COVID-19. *N Engl J Med*, 382, 1787-99.
[http://dx.doi.org/10.1056/NEJMoa2001282] [PMID: 32187464]

Cao, L, Ji, Y, Zeng, L, Liu, Q, Zhang, Z, Guo, S, Guo, X, Tong, Y, Zhao, X, Li, CM, Chen, Y & Guo, D (2019) P200 family protein IFI204 negatively regulates type I interferon responses by targeting IRF7 in nucleus. *PLoS Pathog*, 15, e1008079.
[http://dx.doi.org/10.1371/journal.ppat.1008079] [PMID: 31603949]

Chan, JFW, Yao, Y, Yeung, ML, Deng, W, Bao, L, Jia, L, Li, F, Xiao, C, Gao, H, Yu, P, Cai, JP, Chu, H, Zhou, J, Chen, H, Qin, C & Yuen, KY (2015) Treatment with lopinavir/ritonavir or interferon-β1b improves outcome of MERS-CoV infection in a nonhuman primate model of common marmoset. *J Infect Dis*, 212, 1904-13.
[http://dx.doi.org/10.1093/infdis/jiv392] [PMID: 26198719]

Chandwani, A & Shuter, J (2008) Lopinavir/ritonavir in the treatment of HIV-1 infection: a review. *Ther Clin Risk Manag*, 4, 1023-33.
[PMID: 19209283]

Channappanavar, R & Perlman, S (2017) Pathogenic human coronavirus infections: causes and consequences of cytokine storm and immunopathology. *Semin Immunopathol*, 39, 529-39.
[http://dx.doi.org/10.1007/s00281-017-0629-x] [PMID: 28466096]

Chen, J, Liu, D, Liu, L, Liu, P, Xu, Q, Xia, L, Ling, Y, Huang, D, Song, S, Zhang, D, Qian, Z, Li, T, Shen, T & Lu, H (2020) A pilot study of hydroxychloroquine in treatment of patients with common coronavirus disease-19 (COVID-19). *J Zhejiang Univ*, 49, 215-9. [Medical Science].
[PMID: 32391667]

Chen, L, Liu, HG, Liu, W, Liu, J, Liu, K & Shang, J (2020) Multicenter collaboration group of department of science and technology of guangdong province and health commission of guangdong province for chloroquine in the treatment of novel coronavirus pneumonia, 'Expert consensus on chloroquine phosphate for the treatment of novel coronavirus pneumonia. *Zhonghua Jie He He Hu Xi Za Zhi*, 43, 185-8.
[PMID: 32164085]

Chen, C, Huang, J, Cheng, Z, Wu, J, Chen, S, Zhang, Y, Chen, B, Lu, M, Luo, Y, Zhang, J, Yin, P & Wang, X (2020) Favipiravir *versus* arbidol for COVID-19: A randomized clinical trial. *bioRxiv*.
[http://dx.doi.org/10.1101/2020.03.17.20037432]

Chen, C, Qi, F, Shi, K, Li, Y, Li, J, Chen, Y, Pan, J, Zhou, T, Lin, X, Zhang, J, Luo, Y, Li, X & Xia, J (2020) Thalidomide combined with low-dose glucocorticoid in the treatment of COVID-19 pneumonia. *Preprints*, 2020, 2020020395.

Chen, F, Chan, KH, Jiang, Y, Kao, RY, Lu, HT, Fan, KW, Cheng, VCC, Tsui, WHW, Hung, IFN, Lee, TSW, Guan, Y, Peiris, JSM & Yuen, KY (2004) *In vitro* susceptibility of 10 clinical isolates of SARS coronavirus to selected antiviral compounds. *J Clin Virol*, 31, 69-75.
[http://dx.doi.org/10.1016/j.jcv.2004.03.003] [PMID: 15288617]

Chen, H & Du, Q (2020) Potential natural compounds for preventing 2019-nCoV infection. *Preprints*, 2020010358.
[http://dx.doi.org/10.20944/preprints202001.0358.v3]

Chen, HS, Qi, SH & Shen, JG (2017) One-compound-multi-target: Combination prospect of natural compounds with thrombolytic therapy in acute ischemic stroke. *Curr Neuropharmacol*, 15, 134-56.
[http://dx.doi.org/10.2174/1570159X14666160620102055] [PMID: 27334020]

Chen, L, Liu, HG, Liu, W, Liu, J, Liu, K, Shang, J, Deng, Y & Wei, S (2020) Analysis of clinical features of 29 patients with 2019 novel coronavirus pneumonia. *Zhonghua Jie He He Hu Xi Za Zhi,* 43, 203-8.
[PMID: 32164089]

Chen, N, Zhou, M, Dong, X, Qu, J, Gong, F, Han, Y, Qiu, Y, Wang, J, Liu, Y, Wei, Y, Xia, J, Yu, T, Zhang, X & Zhang, L (2020) Epidemiological and clinical characteristics of 99 cases of 2019 novel coronavirus pneumonia in Wuhan, China: a descriptive study. *Lancet,* 395, 507-13.
[http://dx.doi.org/10.1016/S0140-6736(20)30211-7] [PMID: 32007143]

Chiang, G, Sassaroli, M, Louie, M, Chen, H, Stecher, VJ & Sperber, K (1996) Inhibition of HIV-1 replication by hydroxychloroquine: mechanism of action and comparison with zidovudine. *Clin Ther,* 18, 1080-92.
[http://dx.doi.org/10.1016/S0149-2918(96)80063-4] [PMID: 9001825]

Cheng, W., Li, Y., Cui, L., Chen, Y., Shan, S., Xiao, D., Chen, X., Chen, Z., & Xu, A (2020) Efficacy and safety of corticosteroid treatment in patients with covid-19: a systematic review and meta-analysis. *Front Pharmacol,* 11, 571156.
[http://dx.doi.org/10.3389/fphar.2020.571156]

ChiCTR2000029387, 'Comparison of efficacy and safety of three antiviral regimens in patients with mild to moderate 2019-nCoV pneumonia: a randomized controlled trial'.

ChiCTR2000029387, http://www.chictr.org.cn/showprojen.aspx?proj=48782, Assessed on 30 April, 2020.

ChiCTR2000029600, http://www.chictr.org.cn/showprojen.aspx?proj=49042, Assessed on 30 April, 2020.

Choy, KT, Wong, AYL, Kaewpreedee, P, Sia, SF, Chen, D, Hui, KPY, Chu, DKW, Chan, MCW, Cheung, PPH, Huang, X, Peiris, M & Yen, HL (2020) Remdesivir, lopinavir, emetine, and homoharringtonine inhibit SARS-CoV-2 replication *in vitro. Antiviral Res,* 178, 104786.
[http://dx.doi.org/10.1016/j.antiviral.2020.104786] [PMID: 32251767]

Chu, CM, Cheng, VC, Hung, IF, Wong, MM, Chan, KH, Chan, KS, Kao, RY, Poon, LLM, Wong, CLP, Guan, Y, Peiris, JSM & Yuen, KY HKU/UCH SARS Study Group (2004) Role of lopinavir/ritonavir in the treatment of SARS: initial virological and clinical findings. *Thorax,* 59, 252-6.
[http://dx.doi.org/10.1136/thorax.2003.012658] [PMID: 14985565]

Chu, H, Chan, JF, Wang, Y, Yuen, TT, Chai, Y, Hou, Y, Shuai, H, Yang, D, Hu, B, Huang, X, Zhang, X, Cai, JP, Zhou, J, Yuan, S, Kok, KH, To, KK, Chan, IH, Zhang, AJ, Sit, KY, Au, WK & Yuen, KY (2020) Comparative replication and immune activation profiles of SARS-CoV-2 and SARS-CoV in human lungs: an *ex vivo* study with implications for the pathogenesis of COVID-19. *Clin Infect Dis,* 71, 1400-9.
[http://dx.doi.org/10.1093/cid/ciaa410] [PMID: 32270184]

Cinatl, J, Morgenstern, B, Bauer, G, Chandra, P, Rabenau, H & Doerr, HW (2003) Glycyrrhizin, an active component of liquorice roots, and replication of SARS-associated coronavirus. *Lancet,* 361, 2045-6.
[http://dx.doi.org/10.1016/S0140-6736(03)13615-X] [PMID: 12814717]

Clinical management of severe acute respiratory infection when COVID-19 is suspected. *Interim guidance by World Health Organization* Available at: https://www.who.int/publications-detail/clinical-management-of-severe-acute-respiratory-infection-when- novel-coronavirus-(ncov)-infection-is-suspected Assessed on 30 april, 2020.

Cohen, J (2020) Vaccine designers take first shots at COVID-19. *Science,* 368, 14-6.
[http://dx.doi.org/10.1126/science.368.6486.14] [PMID: 32241928]

Colson, P & Raoult, D (2016) Fighting viruses with antibiotics: an overlooked path. *Int J Antimicrob Agents,* 48, 349-52.
[http://dx.doi.org/10.1016/j.ijantimicag.2016.07.004] [PMID: 27546219]

Colson, P, Rolain, JM & Raoult, D (2020) Chloroquine for the 2019 novel coronavirus SARS-CoV-2. *Int J Antimicrob Agents,* 55, 105923.
[http://dx.doi.org/10.1016/j.ijantimicag.2020.105923] [PMID: 32070753]

Cortegiani, A, Ingoglia, G, Ippolito, M, Giarratano, A & Einav, S (2020) A systematic review on the efficacy

and safety of chloroquine for the treatment of COVID-19. *J Crit Care,* 57, 279-83.
[http://dx.doi.org/10.1016/j.jcrc.2020.03.005] [PMID: 32173110]

Cramer, CL, Patterson, A, Alchakaki, A & Soubani, AO (2017) Immunomodulatory indications of azithromycin in respiratory disease: a concise review for the clinician. *Postgrad Med,* 129, 493-9.
[http://dx.doi.org/10.1080/00325481.2017.1285677] [PMID: 28116959]

Cruz-Topete, D & Cidlowski, JA (2015) One hormone, two actions: anti- and pro-inflammatory effects of glucocorticoids. *Neuroimmunomodulation,* 22, 20-32.
[http://dx.doi.org/10.1159/000362724] [PMID: 25227506]

Cvetkovic, RS & Goa, KL (2003) Lopinavir/ritonavir: a review of its use in the management of HIV infection. *Drugs,* 63, 769-802.
[http://dx.doi.org/10.2165/00003495-200363080-00004] [PMID: 12662125]

Davidson, S, McCabe, TM, Crotta, S, Gad, HH, Hessel, EM, Beinke, S, Hartmann, R & Wack, A (2016) IFNλ is a potent anti-influenza therapeutic without the inflammatory side effects of IFNα treatment. *EMBO Mol Med,* 8, 1099-112.
[http://dx.doi.org/10.15252/emmm.201606413] [PMID: 27520969]

De Wit, E, Feldmann, F, Cronin, J, Jordan, R, Okumura, A, Thomas, T, Scott, D, Cihlar, T & Feldmann, H (2020) Prophylactic and therapeutic remdesivir (GS-5734) treatment in the rhesus macaque model of MERS-CoV infection. *Proc Natl Acad Sci USA,* 117, 6771-6.
[http://dx.doi.org/10.1073/pnas.1922083117] [PMID: 32054787]

Deng, L, Li, C, Zeng, Q, Liu, X, Li, X, Zhang, H, Hong, Z & Xia, J (2020) Arbidol combined with LPV/r *versus* LPV/r alone against Corona Virus Disease 2019: A retrospective cohort study. *J Infect,* 81, e1-5.
[http://dx.doi.org/10.1016/j.jinf.2020.03.002] [PMID: 32171872]

Deng, P, Zhong, D, Yu, K, Zhang, Y, Wang, T & Chen, X (2013) Pharmacokinetics, metabolism, and excretion of the antiviral drug arbidol in humans. *Antimicrob Agents Chemother,* 57, 1743-55.
[http://dx.doi.org/10.1128/AAC.02282-12] [PMID: 23357765]

Deng, YF, Aluko, RE, Jin, Q, Zhang, Y & Yuan, LJ (2012) Inhibitory activities of baicalin against renin and angiotensin-converting enzyme. *Pharm Biol,* 50, 401-6.
[http://dx.doi.org/10.3109/13880209.2011.608076] [PMID: 22136493]

Dodd, RY (2012) Emerging pathogens and their implications for the blood supply and transfusion transmitted infections. *Br J Haematol,* 159, 135-42.
[http://dx.doi.org/10.1111/bjh.12031] [PMID: 22924410]

Dong, L, Hu, S & Gao, J (2020) Discovering drugs to treat coronavirus disease 2019 (COVID-19). *Drug Discov Ther,* 14, 58-60.
[http://dx.doi.org/10.5582/ddt.2020.01012] [PMID: 32147628]

Duan, K, Liu, B, Li, C, Zhang, H, Yu, T, Qu, J, Zhou, M, Chen, L, Meng, S, Hu, Y, Peng, C, Yuan, M, Huang, J, Wang, Z, Yu, J, Gao, X, Wang, D, Yu, X, Li, L, Zhang, J, Wu, X, Li, B, Xu, Y, Chen, W, Peng, Y, Hu, Y, Lin, L, Liu, X, Huang, S, Zhou, Z, Zhang, L, Wang, Y, Zhang, Z, Deng, K, Xia, Z, Gong, Q, Zhang, W, Zheng, X, Liu, Y, Yang, H, Zhou, D, Yu, D, Hou, J, Shi, Z, Chen, S, Chen, Z, Zhang, X & Yang, X (2020) Effectiveness of convalescent plasma therapy in severe COVID-19 patients. *Proc Natl Acad Sci USA,* 117, 9490-6.
[http://dx.doi.org/10.1073/pnas.2004168117] [PMID: 32253318]

Ferrara, N, Hillan, KJ, Gerber, HP & Novotny, W (2004) Discovery and development of bevacizumab, an anti-VEGF antibody for treating cancer. *Nat Rev Drug Discov,* 3, 391-400.
[http://dx.doi.org/10.1038/nrd1381] [PMID: 15136787]

Fox, RI (1993) Mechanism of action of hydroxychloroquine as an antirheumatic drug. *Semin Arthritis Rheum,* 23 (Suppl. 1), 82-91.
[http://dx.doi.org/10.1016/S0049-0172(10)80012-5] [PMID: 8278823]

Franchini, M, Marano, G, Velati, C, Pati, I, Upella, S & Liumbruno, GM (2020) Operational protocol for

donation of anti-COVID-19 convalescent plasma in Italy. *Vox Sang,* 116, 136-7.
[http://dx.doi.org/10.1111/vox.12940] [PMID: 32324899]

Fujita, Y, Kadota, T, Araya, J, Ochiya, T & Kuwano, K (2018) Clinical application of mesenchymal stem cell-derived extracellular vesicle-based therapeutics for inflammatory lung diseases. *J Clin Med,* 7, 355.
[http://dx.doi.org/10.3390/jcm7100355] [PMID: 30322213]

Furuta, Y, Komeno, T & Nakamura, T (2017) Favipiravir (T-705), a broad spectrum inhibitor of viral RNA polymerase. *Proc Jpn Acad, Ser B, Phys Biol Sci,* 93, 449-63.
[http://dx.doi.org/10.2183/pjab.93.027] [PMID: 28769016]

Galani, IE, Triantafyllia, V, Eleminiadou, EE, Koltsida, O, Stavropoulos, A, Manioudaki, M, Thanos, D, Doyle, SE, Kotenko, SV, Thanopoulou, K & Andreakos, E (2017) Interferon-λ mediates non-redundant front-line antiviral protection against influenza virus infection without compromising host fitness. *Immunity,* 46, 875-890.e6.
[http://dx.doi.org/10.1016/j.immuni.2017.04.025] [PMID: 28514692]

Gao, J, Tian, Z & Yang, X (2020) Breakthrough: Chloroquine phosphate has shown apparent efficacy in treatment of COVID-19 associated pneumonia in clinical studies. *Biosci Trends,* 14, 72-3.
[http://dx.doi.org/10.5582/bst.2020.01047] [PMID: 32074550]

Gautret, P, Lagier, JC, Parola, P, Hoang, VT, Meddeb, L, Mailhe, M, Doudier, B, Courjon, J, Giordanengo, V, Vieira, VE, Tissot Dupont, H, Honoré, S, Colson, P, Chabrière, E, La Scola, B, Rolain, JM, Brouqui, P & Raoult, D (2020) Hydroxychloroquine and azithromycin as a treatment of COVID-19: results of an open-label non-randomized clinical trial. *Int J Antimicrob Agents,* 56, 105949.
[http://dx.doi.org/10.1016/j.ijantimicag.2020.105949] [PMID: 32205204]

Goa, KL, McTavish, D & Clissold, SP (1991) Ivermectin. *Drugs,* 42, 640-58.
[http://dx.doi.org/10.2165/00003495-199142040-00007] [PMID: 1723366]

Gotz, V, Magar, L, Dornfeld, D, Giese, S, Pohlmann, A & Höper, D (2016) Corrigendum: Influenza A viruses escape from MxA restriction at the expense of efficient nuclear vRNP import. *Sci Rep,* 6, 25428.
[http://dx.doi.org/10.1038/srep25428] [PMID: 27156930]

Greber, UF, Singh, I & Helenius, A (1994) Mechanisms of virus uncoating. *Trends Microbiol,* 2, 52-6.
[http://dx.doi.org/10.1016/0966-842X(94)90126-0] [PMID: 8162442]

Haviernik, J, Stefanik, M, Fojtikova, M, Kali, S, Tordo, N, Rudolf, I, Hubálek, Z, Eyer, L & Ruzek, D (2018) Arbidol (Umifenovir): A broad-spectrum antiviral drug that Inhibits medically important arthropod-borne flaviviruses. *Viruses,* 10, 184.
[http://dx.doi.org/10.3390/v10040184]

Heinzerling, JH & Huerta, S (2006) Bowel perforation from bevacizumab for the treatment of metastatic colon cancer: incidence, etiology, and management. *Curr Surg,* 63, 334-7.
[http://dx.doi.org/10.1016/j.cursur.2006.06.002] [PMID: 16971205]

Henriet, SS, Jans, J, Simonetti, E, Kwon-Chung, KJ, Rijs, AJ, Hermans, PW, Holland, SM, de Jonge, MI & Warris, A (2013) Chloroquine modulates the fungal immune response in phagocytic cells from patients with chronic granulomatous disease. *J Infect Dis,* 207, 1932-9.
[http://dx.doi.org/10.1093/infdis/jit103] [PMID: 23482646]

Hensley, LE, Fritz, LE, Jahrling, PB, Karp, CL, Huggins, JW & Geisbert, TW (2004) Interferon-β 1a and SARS coronavirus replication. *Emerg Infect Dis,* 10, 317-9.
[http://dx.doi.org/10.3201/eid1002.030482] [PMID: 15030704]

Hillaker, E, Belfer, JJ, Bondici, A, Murad, H & Dumkow, LE (2020) Delayed initiation of remdesivir in a COVID-19 positive patient pharmacotherapy. *Pharmacotherapy,* 40, 592-8.
[http://dx.doi.org/10.1002/phar.2403] [PMID: 32281114]

Hoffmann, M, Kleine-Weber, H, Schroeder, S, Krüger, N, Herrler, T & Erichsen, S (2020) 'SARS-CoV-2 cell entry depends on ACE 2 and TMPRSS2 and is blocked by a clinically proven protease inhibitor', *Cell,* S0092-8674 (20), p. 30229-4.

Holshue, ML, DeBolt, C, Lindquist, S, Lofy, KH, Wiesman, J, Bruce, H, Spitters, C, Ericson, K, Wilkerson, S, Tural, A, Diaz, G, Cohn, A, Fox, L, Patel, A, Gerber, SI, Kim, L, Tong, S, Lu, X, Lindstrom, S, Pallansch, MA, Weldon, WC, Biggs, HM, Uyeki, TM & Pillai, SK (2020) First case of 2019 novel coronavirus in the United States. *N Engl J Med,* 382, 929-36.
[http://dx.doi.org/10.1056/NEJMoa2001191] [PMID: 32004427]

Homolak, J & Kodvanj, I (2020) Widely available lysosome targeting agents should be considered as a potential therapy for COVID-19. *Preprints.*
[http://dx.doi.org/1020944/preprints2020030345v2]

Horton, MR, Santopietro, V, Mathew, L, Horton, KM, Polito, AJ, Liu, MC, Danoff, SK & Lechtzin, N (2012) Thalidomide for the treatment of cough in idiopathic pulmonary fibrosis: a randomized trial. *Ann Intern Med,* 157, 398-406.
[http://dx.doi.org/10.7326/0003-4819-157-6-201209180-00003] [PMID: 22986377]

Huang, C, Wang, Y, Li, X, Ren, L, Zhao, J, Hu, Y, Zhang, L, Fan, G, Xu, J, Gu, X, Cheng, Z, Yu, T, Xia, J, Wei, Y, Wu, W, Xie, X, Yin, W, Li, H, Liu, M, Xiao, Y, Gao, H, Guo, L, Xie, J, Wang, G, Jiang, R, Gao, Z, Jin, Q, Wang, J & Cao, B (2020) Clinical features of patients infected with 2019 novel coronavirus in Wuhan, China. *Lancet,* 395, 497-506.
[http://dx.doi.org/10.1016/S0140-6736(20)30183-5] [PMID: 31986264]

Hulseberg, CE, Fénéant, L, Szymańska-de Wijs, KM, Kessler, NP, Nelson, EA, Shoemaker, CJ, Schmaljohn, CS, Polyak, SJ & White, JM (2019) Arbidol and other low-molecular-weight drugs that inhibit lassa and ebola viruses. *J Virol,* 93, e02185-18.
[http://dx.doi.org/10.1128/JVI.02185-18] [PMID: 30700611]

Hung, IF, Lung, KC, Tso, EY, Liu, R, Chung, TW, Chu, MY, Ng, YY, Lo, J, Chan, J, Tam, AR, Shum, HP, Chan, V, Wu, AK, Sin, KM, Leung, WS, Law, WL, Lung, DC, Sin, S, Yeung, P, Yip, CC, Zhang, RR, Fung, AY, Yan, EY, Leung, KH, Ip, JD, Chu, AW, Chan, WM, Ng, AC, Lee, R, Fung, K, Yeung, A, Wu, TC, Chan, JW, Yan, WW, Chan, WM, Chan, JF, Lie, AK, Tsang, OT, Cheng, VC, Que, TL, Lau, CS, Chan, KH, To, KK & Yuen, KY (2020) Triple combination of interferon beta-1b, lopinavir-ritonavir, and ribavirin in the treatment of patients admitted to hospital with COVID-19: an open-label, randomised, phase 2 trial. *Lancet,* 395, 1695-704.
[http://dx.doi.org/10.1016/S0140-6736(20)31042-4] [PMID: 32401715]

Hung, IF, To, KK, Lee, CK, Lee, KL, Chan, K, Yan, WW, Liu, R, Watt, CL, Chan, WM, Lai, KY, Koo, CK, Buckley, T, Chow, FL, Wong, KK, Chan, HS, Ching, CK, Tang, BS, Lau, CC, Li, IW, Liu, SH, Chan, KH, Lin, CK & Yuen, KY (2011) Convalescent plasma treatment reduced mortality in patients with severe pandemic influenza A (H1N1) 2009 virus infection. *Clin Infect Dis,* 52, 447-56.
[http://dx.doi.org/10.1093/cid/ciq106] [PMID: 21248066]

Hurst, NP, French, JK, Gorjatschko, L & Betts, WH (1988) Chloroquine and hydroxychloroquine inhibit multiple sites in metabolic pathways leading to neutrophil superoxide release. *J Rheumatol,* 15, 23-7.
[PMID: 2832600]

Ishaqui, AA, Khan, AH, Sulaiman, SAS, Alsultan, MT, Khan, I & Naqvi, AA (2020) Assessment of efficacy of Oseltamivir-Azithromycin combination therapy in prevention of influenza-A (H1N1)pdm09 infection complications and rapidity of symptoms relief. *Expert Rev Respir Med,* 14, 533-41.
[http://dx.doi.org/10.1080/17476348.2020.1730180] [PMID: 32053044]

Ishfaq, M, Chen, C, Bao, J, Zhang, W, Wu, Z, Wang, J, Liu, Y, Tian, E, Hamid, S, Li, R, Ding, L & Li, J (2019) Baicalin ameliorates oxidative stress and apoptosis by restoring mitochondrial dynamics in the spleen of chickens via the opposite modulation of NF-κB and Nrf2/HO-1 signaling pathway during Mycoplasma gallisepticum infection. *Poult Sci,* 98, 6296-310.
[http://dx.doi.org/10.3382/ps/pez406] [PMID: 31376349]

Ivashkiv, LB & Donlin, LT (2014) Regulation of type I interferon responses. *Nat Rev Immunol,* 14, 36-49.
[http://dx.doi.org/10.1038/nri3581] [PMID: 24362405]

Jallouli, M, Galicier, L, Zahr, N, Aumaître, O, Francès, C, Le Guern, V, Lioté, F, Smail, A, Limal, N, Perard,

L, Desmurs-Clavel, H, Le Thi Huong, D, Asli, B, Kahn, JE, Pourrat, J, Sailler, L, Ackermann, F, Papo, T, Sacré, K, Fain, O, Stirnemann, J, Cacoub, P, Leroux, G, Cohen-Bittan, J, Sellam, J, Mariette, X, Blanchet, B, Hulot, JS, Amoura, Z, Piette, JC & Costedoat-Chalumeau, N Plaquenil Lupus Systemic Study Group (2015) Determinants of hydroxychloroquine blood concentration variations in systemic lupus erythematosus. *Arthritis Rheumatol,* 67, 2176-84.
[http://dx.doi.org/10.1002/art.39194] [PMID: 25989906]

Jans, DA, Martin, AJ & Wagstaff, KM (2019) Inhibitors of nuclear transport. *Curr Opin Cell Biol,* 58, 50-60.
[http://dx.doi.org/10.1016/j.ceb.2019.01.001] [PMID: 30826604]

Jasenosky, LD, Cadena, C, Mire, CE, Borisevich, V, Haridas, V, Ranjbar, S & Nambu, A (2019) The FDA-approved oral drug nitazoxanide amplifies host antiviral responses and inhibits Ebola virus. *iScience,* 19, 1279-90.

Jeong, HG & Kim, JY (2002) Induction of inducible nitric oxide synthase expression by 18beta-glycyrrhetinic acid in macrophages. *FEBS Lett,* 513, 208-12.
[http://dx.doi.org/10.1016/S0014-5793(02)02311-6] [PMID: 11904152]

Jessop, S, Whitelaw, D & Jordaan, F (2001) Drugs for discoid lupus erythematosus. *Cochrane Database Syst Rev,* 1, CD002954.
[PMID: 11279785]

Jiang S, Zhang X, Yang Y, Hotez PJ, Du L (2020) Neutralizing antibodies for the treatment of COVID-19. Nat Biomed Eng, 1134-1139.
[http://dx.doi.org/10.1038/s41551-020-00660-2] [PMID: 33293725]

Kaufmann, AM & Krise, JP (2007) Lysosomal sequestration of amine-containing drugs: analysis and therapeutic implications. *J Pharm Sci,* 96, 729-46.
[http://dx.doi.org/10.1002/jps.20792] [PMID: 17117426]

Kirchdoerfer, RN (2020) Halting coronavirus polymerase. J Biol Chem, 295, 4780-4781.
[http://dx.doi.org/10.1074/jbc.H120.013397] [PMID: 32277065]

Klonisch, T, Panayotou, G, Edwards, P, Jackson, AM, Berger, P, Delves, PJ, Lund, T & Roitt, IM (1996) Enhancement in antigen binding by a combination of synergy and antibody capture. *Immunology,* 89, 165-71.
[http://dx.doi.org/10.1046/j.1365-2567.1996.d01-722.x] [PMID: 8943709]

Klotz, U, Ogbuokiri, JE & Okonkwo, PO (1990) Ivermectin binds avidly to plasma proteins. *Eur J Clin Pharmacol,* 39, 607-8.
[http://dx.doi.org/10.1007/BF00316107] [PMID: 2095348]

Kouznetsova, J, Sun, W, Martínez-Romero, C, Tawa, G, Shinn, P, Chen, CZ, Schimmer, A, Sanderson, P, McKew, JC, Zheng, W & García-Sastre, A (2014) Identification of 53 compounds that block Ebola virus-like particle entry *via* a repurposing screen of approved drugs. *Emerg Microbes Infect,* 3, e84.
[http://dx.doi.org/10.1038/emi.2014.88] [PMID: 26038505]

Krasnodembskaya, A, Song, Y, Fang, X, Gupta, N, Serikov, V, Lee, JW & Matthay, MA (2010) Antibacterial effect of human mesenchymal stem cells is mediated in part from secretion of the antimicrobial peptide LL-37. *Stem Cells,* 28, 2229-38.
[http://dx.doi.org/10.1002/stem.544] [PMID: 20945332]

Krishna, DR & Klotz, U (1993) Determination of ivermectin in human plasma by high-performance liquid chromatography. *Arzneimittelforschung,* 43, 609-11.
[PMID: 8329009]

Kumar, A, Liang, B, Aarthy, M, Singh, SK, Garg, N, Mysorekar, IU & Giri, R (2018) Hydroxychloroquine inhibits zika virus NS2B-NS3 protease. *ACS Omega,* 3, 18132-41.
[http://dx.doi.org/10.1021/acsomega.8b01002] [PMID: 30613818]

Li, C, Zu, S, Deng, YQ, Li, D, Parvatiyar, K, Quanquin, N, Shang, J, Sun, N, Su, J, Liu, Z, Wang, M, Aliyari, SR, Li, XF, Jung, JU, Qin, FXF, Qin, CF & Cheng, G (2019) Azithromycin protects against zika virus infection by up-regulating virus-induced type I and III interferon responses. *Antimicrob Agents Chemother,*

63, 394-19.
[http://dx.doi.org/10.1128/AAC.00394-19]

Li, MK, Liu, YY, Wei, F, Shen, MX, Zhong, Y, Li, S, Chen, LJ, Ma, N, Liu, BY, Mao, YD, Li, N, Hou, W, Xiong, HR & Yang, ZQ (2018) Antiviral activity of arbidol hydrochloride against herpes simplex virus I *in vitro* and *in vivo*. *Int J Antimicrob Agents,* 51, 98-106.
[http://dx.doi.org/10.1016/j.ijantimicag.2017.09.001] [PMID: 28890393]

Lim, HS, Im, JS, Cho, JY, Bae, KS, Klein, TA, Yeom, JS, Kim, TS, Choi, JS, Jang, IJ & Park, JW (2009) Pharmacokinetics of hydroxychloroquine and its clinical implications in chemoprophylaxis against malaria caused by Plasmodium vivax. *Antimicrob Agents Chemother,* 53, 1468-75.
[http://dx.doi.org/10.1128/AAC.00339-08] [PMID: 19188392]

Lim, J, Jeon, S, Shin, HY, Kim, MJ, Seong, YM, Lee, WJ, Choe, KW, Kang, YM, Lee, B & Park, SJ (2020) Case of the index patient who caused tertiary transmission of coronavirus disease 2019 in Korea: The application of lopinavir/ritonavir for the treatment of COVID-19 pneumonia monitored by quantitative RT-PCR. *J Korean Med Sci,* 35, e79.

Lin, CW, Tsai, FJ, Tsai, CH, Lai, CC, Wan, L, Ho, TY, Hsieh, CC & Chao, PD (2005) Anti-SARS coronavirus 3C-like protease effects of Isatis indigotica root and plant-derived phenolic compounds. *Antiviral Res,* 68, 36-42.
[http://dx.doi.org/10.1016/j.antiviral.2005.07.002] [PMID: 16115693]

Liu, J, Cao, R, Xu, M, Wang, X, Zhang, H, Hu, H, Li, Y, Hu, Z, Zhong, W & Wang, M (2020) Hydroxychloroquine, a less toxic derivative of chloroquine, is effective in inhibiting SARS-CoV-2 infection *in vitro*. *Cell Discov,* 6, 16.
[http://dx.doi.org/10.1038/s41421-020-0156-0] [PMID: 32194981]

Liu, MY, Wang, S, Yao, WF, Wu, HZ, Meng, SN & Wei, MJ (2009) Pharmacokinetic properties and bioequivalence of two formulations of arbidol: an open-label, single-dose, randomized-sequence, two-period crossover study in healthy Chinese male volunteers. *Clin Ther,* 31, 784-92.
[http://dx.doi.org/10.1016/j.clinthera.2009.04.016] [PMID: 19446151]

Liou TG, Adler FR, Hatton ND (2020) The Uncertain Role of Corticosteroids in the Treatment of COVID-19. *JAMA Intern Med,* 181,139-140.
[http://dx.doi.org/10.1001/jamainternmed.2020.2438] [PMID: 32744622]

Lu, CL, Murakowski, DK, Bournazos, S, Schoofs, T, Sarkar, D, Halper-Stromberg, A, Horwitz, JA, Nogueira, L, Golijanin, J, Gazumyan, A, Ravetch, JV, Caskey, M, Chakraborty, AK & Nussenzweig, MC (2016) Enhanced clearance of HIV-1-infected cells by broadly neutralizing antibodies against HIV-1 *in vivo*. *Science,* 352, 1001-4.
[http://dx.doi.org/10.1126/science.aaf1279] [PMID: 27199430]

Lu, H (2020) Drug treatment options for the 2019-new coronavirus (2019-nCoV). *Biosci Trends,* 14, 69-71.
[http://dx.doi.org/10.5582/bst.2020.01020] [PMID: 31996494]

Lundberg, L, Pinkham, C, Baer, A, Amaya, M, Narayanan, A, Wagstaff, KM, Jans, DA & Kehn-Hall, K (2013) Nuclear import and export inhibitors alter capsid protein distribution in mammalian cells and reduce Venezuelan Equine Encephalitis Virus replication. *Antiviral Res,* 100, 662-72.
[http://dx.doi.org/10.1016/j.antiviral.2013.10.004] [PMID: 24161512]

Madelain, V, Nguyen, TH, Olivo, A, de Lamballerie, X, Guedj, J, Taburet, AM & Mentré, F (2016) Ebola virus infection: Review of the pharmacokinetic and pharmacodynamic properties of drugs considered for testing in human efficacy trials. *Clin Pharmacokinet,* 55, 907-23.
[http://dx.doi.org/10.1007/s40262-015-0364-1] [PMID: 26798032]

Mair-Jenkins, J, Saavedra-Campos, M, Baillie, JK, Cleary, P, Khaw, FM, Lim, WS, Makki, S, Rooney, KD, Nguyen-Van-Tam, JS & Beck, CR Convalescent Plasma Study Group (2015) The effectiveness of convalescent plasma and hyperimmune immunoglobulin for the treatment of severe acute respiratory infections of viral etiology: a systematic review and exploratory meta-analysis. *J Infect Dis,* 211, 80-90.
[http://dx.doi.org/10.1093/infdis/jiu396] [PMID: 25030060]

Marano, G, Vaglio, S, Pupella, S, Facco, G, Catalano, L, Liumbruno, GM & Grazzini, G (2016) Convalescent plasma: new evidence for an old therapeutic tool? *Blood Transfus,* 14, 152-7.
[PMID: 26674811]

Markham, A & Keam, SJ (2019) Camrelizumab: First Global Approval. *Drugs,* 79, 1355-61.
[http://dx.doi.org/10.1007/s40265-019-01167-0] [PMID: 31313098]

Martinez, MA (2020) Compounds with therapeutic potential against novel respiratory 2019 coronavirus. *Antimicrob Agents Chemother,* 64, e00399-20.
[http://dx.doi.org/10.1128/AAC.00399-20] [PMID: 32152082]

Mastrangelo, E, Pezzullo, M, De Burghgraeve, T, Kaptein, S, Pastorino, B, Dallmeier, K, de Lamballerie, X, Neyts, J, Hanson, AM, Frick, DN, Bolognesi, M & Milani, M (2012) Ivermectin is a potent inhibitor of flavivirus replication specifically targeting NS3 helicase activity: new prospects for an old drug. *J Antimicrob Chemother,* 67, 1884-94.
[http://dx.doi.org/10.1093/jac/dks147] [PMID: 22535622]

Mauthe, M, Orhon, I, Rocchi, C, Zhou, X, Luhr, M, Hijlkema, KJ, Coppes, RP, Engedal, N, Mari, M & Reggiori, F (2018) Chloroquine inhibits autophagic flux by decreasing autophagosome-lysosome fusion. *Autophagy,* 14, 1435-55.
[http://dx.doi.org/10.1080/15548627.2018.1474314] [PMID: 29940786]

Mazzoccoli, L, Cadoso, SH, Amarante, GW, de Souza, MV, Domingues, R, Machado, MA, de Almeida, MV & Teixeira, HC (2012) Novel thalidomide analogues from diamines inhibit pro-inflammatory cytokine production and CD80 expression while enhancing IL-10. *Biomed Pharmacother,* 66, 323-9.
[http://dx.doi.org/10.1016/j.biopha.2012.05.001] [PMID: 22770990]

Meissner, HC & Long, SS (2003) Revised indications for the use of palivizumab and respiratory syncytial virus immune globulin intravenous for the prevention of respiratory syncytial virus infections. *Pediatrics,* 112, 1447-52.
[http://dx.doi.org/10.1542/peds.112.6.1447] [PMID: 14654628]

Mindell, JA (2012) Lysosomal acidification mechanisms. *Annu Rev Physiol,* 74, 69-86.
[http://dx.doi.org/10.1146/annurev-physiol-012110-142317] [PMID: 22335796]

Morgenstern, B, Michaelis, M, Baer, PC, Doerr, HW & Cinatl, J, Jr (2005) Ribavirin and interferon-β synergistically inhibit SARS-associated coronavirus replication in animal and human cell lines. *Biochem Biophys Res Commun,* 326, 905-8.
[http://dx.doi.org/10.1016/j.bbrc.2004.11.128] [PMID: 15607755]

Mulangu, S, Dodd, LE, Davey, RT, Jr, Tshiani Mbaya, O, Proschan, M, Mukadi, D, Lusakibanza Manzo, M, Nzolo, D, Tshomba Oloma, A, Ibanda, A, Ali, R, Coulibaly, S, Levine, AC, Grais, R, Diaz, J, Lane, HC, Muyembe-Tamfum, JJ, Sivahera, B, Camara, M, Kojan, R, Walker, R, Dighero-Kemp, B, Cao, H, Mukumbayi, P, Mbala-Kingebeni, P, Ahuka, S, Albert, S, Bonnett, T, Crozier, I, Duvenhage, M, Proffitt, C, Teitelbaum, M, Moench, T, Aboulhab, J, Barrett, K, Cahill, K, Cone, K, Eckes, R, Hensley, L, Herpin, B, Higgs, E, Ledgerwood, J, Pierson, J, Smolskis, M, Sow, Y, Tierney, J, Sivapalasingam, S, Holman, W, Gettinger, N, Vallée, D & Nordwall, J PALM Writing Group; (2019) PALM Consortium Study Team (2019) A randomized, controlled trial of Ebola virus disease therapeutics. *N Engl J Med,* 381, 2293-303.
[http://dx.doi.org/10.1056/NEJMoa1910993] [PMID: 31774950]

Mullard, A (2012) Drug repurposing programmes get lift off. *Nat Rev Drug Discov,* 11, 505-6.
[http://dx.doi.org/10.1038/nrd3776] [PMID: 22743966]

Nagata, T, Lefor, AK, Hasegawa, M & Ishii, M (2015) Favipiravir: a new medication for the Ebola virus disease pandemic. *Disaster Med Public Health Prep,* 9, 79-81.
[http://dx.doi.org/10.1017/dmp.2014.151] [PMID: 25544306]

National Health Commission of the people's republic of China. The 5th trial version of diagnosis and treatment scheme for pneumonitis with 2019-nCoV infection (In Chinese). http://www.nhc.gov.cn/yzygj/s7653p/202002/d4b895337e19445f8d728fcaf1e3e13a.shtml (2020)

NCT04306497, https://clinicaltrials.gov/ct2/show/NCT04306497, Assessed on 30 April, 2020.

NCT04321096, https://clinicaltrials.gov/ct2/show/NCT04321096?term=camostat, Assessed on 30 April, 2020

NCT04273529, https://clinicaltrials.gov/ct2/show/record/NCT04273529, Accessed on 5 May, 2020.

NCT04268537, https://clinicaltrials.gov/ct2/show/NCT04268537, Assessed on 5 May, 2020

NCT04275414, https://clinicaltrials.gov/ct2/show/NCT04275414, Assessed on 5 May, 2020

NCT04252118, https://clinicaltrials.gov/ct2/show/NCT04252118, Assessed on 5 May, 2020

NCT04305106, https://clinicaltrials.gov/ct2/show/NCT04305106?cond=COVID-19&draw=10, Assessed on 5 May, 2020.

NCT04252118, https://clinicaltrials.gov/ct2/show/NCT04252118, Assessed on 30 April, 2020

NCT04293692, https://clinicaltrials.gov/ ct2/show/ NCT04293692? term=stem+ cells&cond= Corona+Virus+ Infection &draw=2&rank=7, Assessed on 5 May, 2020

NCT04269525, https://clinicaltrials.gov/ct2/show/NCT04269525?term=stem+cells&cond=Corona+Virus+Infection&draw=2, Assessed on 5 May, 2020

NCT04320615, https://clinicaltrials.gov/ct2/show/NCT04320615, Assessed on 5 May, 2020

NCT04276688, https://clinicaltrials.gov/ct2/show/NCT04276688, Assessed on 30 April, 2020.

NCT04333589 (NCT04336904), Assessed on 30 April, 2020. www.clinical trial.gov

NCT04336904, https://clinicaltrials.gov/ct2/show/NCT04336904, Assessed on 30 April, 2020.

NCT04365725, https://clinicaltrials.gov/ct2/show/NCT04365725, Assessed on 30 April, 2020.

NCT04374071, https://clinicaltrials.gov/ct2/show/NCT04374071, Assessed on 30 April, 2020.

News: Abidol and darunavir can effectively inhibit corona virus (2020) http://www.sd.chinanews.com/2/2020/0205/70145.html

Ottesen, EA & Campbell, WC (1994) Ivermectin in human medicine. *J Antimicrob Chemother,* 34, 195-203. [http://dx.doi.org/10.1093/jac/34.2.195] [PMID: 7814280]

Oxholm, P, Prause, JU & Schiødt, M (1998) Rational drug therapy recommendations for the treatment of patients with Sjögren's syndrome. *Drugs,* 56, 345-53. [http://dx.doi.org/10.2165/00003495-199856030-00004] [PMID: 9777311]

Pan, T, Zhou, N & Zhang, H (2015) Use of teicoplanin in anti-middle east respiratory syndrome corona virus', WO/2016/201692.

Pareek, A, Khopkar, U, Sacchidanand, S, Chandurkar, N & Naik, GS (2008) Comparative study of efficacy and safety of hydroxychloroquine and chloroquine in polymorphic light eruption: a randomized, double-blind, multicentric study. *Indian J Dermatol Venereol Leprol,* 74, 18-22. [http://dx.doi.org/10.4103/0378-6323.38401] [PMID: 18187817]

Patrì, A, Fabbrocini, G (2020) Hydroxychloroquine and ivermectin: A synergistic combination for COVID-19 chemoprophylaxis and treatment? *J Am Acad Dermatol*, 82, e221. doi:10.1016/j.jaad.2020.04.017. PMID: 32283237

Pfizer (2020), 'Zithromax-azithromycin dihydrate tablet, film coated Zithromaxazithromycin dihydrate powder, for suspension', *USP Product labeling.*

Pilcher, H (2003) Liquorice may tackle SARS. *Nature.* [http://dx.doi.org/10.1038/news030609-16]

Price, GE, Gaszewska-Mastarlarz, A & Moskophidis, D (2000) The role of alpha/beta and gamma interferons in development of immunity to influenza A virus in mice. *J Virol,* 74, 3996-4003.

[http://dx.doi.org/10.1128/JVI.74.9.3996-4003.2000] [PMID: 10756011]

Rainsford, KD, Parke, AL, Clifford-Rashotte, M, Kean, WF & Al-Bari, MAA (2015) Therapy and pharmacological properties of hydroxychloroquine and chloroquine in treatment of systemic lupus erythematosus, rheumatoid arthritis and related diseases. *Inflammopharmacology, 23*, 231-69.
[http://dx.doi.org/10.1007/s10787-015-0239-y] [PMID: 26246395]

Randolph, VB, Winkler, G & Stollar, V (1990) Acidotropic amines inhibit proteolytic processing of flavivirus prM protein. *Virology, 174*, 450-8.
[http://dx.doi.org/10.1016/0042-6822(90)90099-D] [PMID: 2154882]

Rolain, JM, Colson, P & Raoult, D (2007) Recycling of chloroquine and its hydroxyl analogue to face bacterial, fungal and viral infections in the 21st century. *Int J Antimicrob Agents, 30*, 297-308.
[http://dx.doi.org/10.1016/j.ijantimicag.2007.05.015] [PMID: 17629679]

Rossignol, JF (2016) Nitazoxanide, a new drug candidate for the treatment of Middle East respiratory syndrome coronavirus. *J Infect Public Health, 9*, 227-30.
[http://dx.doi.org/10.1016/j.jiph.2016.04.001] [PMID: 27095301]

Ruiz-Irastorza, G & Khamashta, MA (2008) Hydroxychloroquine: the cornerstone of lupus therapy. *Lupus, 17*, 271-3.
[http://dx.doi.org/10.1177/0961203307086643] [PMID: 18413405]

Russell, CD, Millar, JE & Baillie, JK (2020) Clinical evidence does not support corticosteroid treatment for 2019-nCoV lung injury. *Lancet, 395*, 473-5.
[http://dx.doi.org/10.1016/S0140-6736(20)30317-2] [PMID: 32043983]

Samuel, CE (2001) Antiviral actions of interferons. *Clin Microbiol Rev, 14*, 778-809.
[http://dx.doi.org/10.1128/CMR.14.4.778-809.2001] [PMID: 11585785]

Savarino, A, Di Trani, L, Donatelli, I, Cauda, R & Cassone, A (2006) New insights into the antiviral effects of chloroquine. *Lancet Infect Dis, 6*, 67-9.
[http://dx.doi.org/10.1016/S1473-3099(06)70361-9] [PMID: 16439323]

Schulert, GS & Grom, AA (2015) Pathogenesis of macrophage activation syndrome and potential for cytokine- directed therapies. *Annu Rev Med, 66*, 145-59.
[http://dx.doi.org/10.1146/annurev-med-061813-012806] [PMID: 25386930]

Shang, L, Zhao, J, Hu, Y, Du, R & Cao, B (2020) On the use of corticosteroids for 2019-nCoV pneumonia. *Lancet, 395*, 683-4.
[http://dx.doi.org/10.1016/S0140-6736(20)30361-5] [PMID: 32122468]

Shang, W, Yang, Y, Rao, Y & Rao, X (2020) The outbreak of SARS-CoV-2 pneumonia calls for viral vaccines. *NPJ Vaccines, 5*, 18.
[http://dx.doi.org/10.1038/s41541-020-0170-0]

Shanmugaraj, B, Siriwattananon, K, Wangkanont, K & Phoolcharoen, W (2020) Perspectives on monoclonal antibody therapy as potential therapeutic intervention for Coronavirus disease-19 (COVID-19). *Asian Pac J Allergy Immunol, 38*, 10-8.
[PMID: 32134278]

Sheahan, TP, Sims, AC, Graham, RL, Menachery, VD, Gralinski, LE, Case, JB, Leist, SR, Pyrc, K, Feng, JY, Trantcheva, I, Bannister, R, Park, Y, Babusis, D, Clarke, MO, Mackman, RL, Spahn, JE, Palmiotti, CA, Siegel, D, Ray, AS, Cihlar, T, Jordan, R, Denison, MR & Baric, RS (2017) Broad-spectrum antiviral GS-5734 inhibits both epidemic and zoonotic coronaviruses. *Sci Transl Med, 9*, eaal3653.
[http://dx.doi.org/10.1126/scitranslmed.aal3653] [PMID: 28659436]

Sheahan, TP, Sims, AC, Leist, SR, Schäfer, A, Won, J, Brown, AJ, Montgomery, SA, Hogg, A, Babusis, D, Clarke, MO, Spahn, JE, Bauer, L, Sellers, S, Porter, D, Feng, JY, Cihlar, T, Jordan, R, Denison, MR & Baric, RS (2020) Comparative therapeutic efficacy of remdesivir and combination lopinavir, ritonavir, and interferon beta against MERS-CoV. *Nat Commun, 11*, 222.
[http://dx.doi.org/10.1038/s41467-019-13940-6] [PMID: 31924756]

Shen, C, Wang, Z, Zhao, F, Yang, Y, Li, J, Yuan, J, Wang, F, Li, D, Yang, M, Xing, L, Wei, J, Xiao, H, Yang, Y, Qu, J, Qing, L, Chen, L, Xu, Z, Peng, L, Li, Y, Zheng, H, Chen, F, Huang, K, Jiang, Y, Liu, D, Zhang, Z, Liu, Y & Liu, L (2020) Treatment of 5 critically ill patients with COVID-19 with convalescent plasma. *JAMA,* 323, 1582-9.
[http://dx.doi.org/10.1001/jama.2020.4783] [PMID: 32219428]

Shetty, AK (2020) Mesenchymal stem cell infusion shows promise for combating coronavirus (COVID-19) induced pneumonia. *Aging Dis,* 11, 462-4.
[http://dx.doi.org/10.14336/AD.2020.0301] [PMID: 32257554]

Soliman, EZ, Lundgren, JD, Roediger, MP, Duprez, DA, Temesgen, Z, Bickel, M, Shlay, JC, Somboonwit, C, Reiss, P, Stein, JH & Neaton, JD INSIGHT SMART Study Group (2011) Boosted protease inhibitors and the electrocardiographic measures of QT and PR durations. *AIDS,* 25, 367-77.
[http://dx.doi.org/10.1097/QAD.0b013e328341dcc0] [PMID: 21150558]

Song, JH, Fang, ZZ, Zhu, LL, Cao, YF, Hu, CM, Ge, GB & Zhao, DW (2013) Glucuronidation of the broad-spectrum antiviral drug arbidol by UGT isoforms. *J Pharm Pharmacol,* 65, 521-7.
[http://dx.doi.org/10.1111/jphp.12014] [PMID: 23488780]

Sperber, K, Louie, M, Kraus, T, Proner, J, Sapira, E, Lin, S, Stecher, V & Mayer, L (1995) Hydroxychloroquine treatment of patients with human immunodeficiency virus type 1. *Clin Ther,* 17, 622-36.
[http://dx.doi.org/10.1016/0149-2918(95)80039-5] [PMID: 8565026]

Stahlmann, R & Lode, H (2020) Medication for COVID-19--an overview of approaches currently under study. *Deutsches Aerzteblatt Int,* 117, 213-9.
[http://dx.doi.org/10.3238/arztebl.2020.0213]

Stockman, LJ, Bellamy, R & Garner, P (2006) SARS: systematic review of treatment effects. *PLoS Med,* 3, e343.
[http://dx.doi.org/10.1371/journal.pmed.0030343] [PMID: 16968120]

Sui, J, Li, W, Murakami, A, Tamin, A, Matthews, LJ, Wong, SK, Moore, MJ, Tallarico, AS, Olurinde, M, Choe, H, Anderson, LJ, Bellini, WJ, Farzan, M & Marasco, WA (2004) Potent neutralization of severe acute respiratory syndrome (SARS) coronavirus by a human mAb to S1 protein that blocks receptor association. *Proc Natl Acad Sci USA,* 101, 2536-41.
[http://dx.doi.org/10.1073/pnas.0307140101] [PMID: 14983044]

Sui, J, Li, W, Roberts, A, Matthews, LJ, Murakami, A, Vogel, L, Wong, SK, Subbarao, K, Farzan, M & Marasco, WA (2005) Evaluation of human monoclonal antibody 80R for immunoprophylaxis of severe acute respiratory syndrome by an animal study, epitope mapping, and analysis of spike variants. *J Virol,* 79, 5900-6.
[http://dx.doi.org/10.1128/JVI.79.10.5900-5906.2005] [PMID: 15857975]

Sutton, MT, Fletcher, D, Ghosh, SK, Weinberg, A, van Heeckeren, R, Kaur, S, Sadeghi, Z, Hijaz, A, Reese, J, Lazarus, HM, Lennon, DP, Caplan, AI & Bonfield, TL (2016) Antimicrobial properties of mesenchymal stem cells: therapeutic potential for cystic fibrosis infection and treatment. *Stem Cells Int,* 2016, 5303048.
[http://dx.doi.org/10.1155/2016/5303048] [PMID: 26925108]

Ter Meulen, J, Bakker, AB, van den Brink, EN, Weverling, GJ, Martina, BE, Haagmans, BL, Kuiken, T, de Kruif, J, Preiser, W, Spaan, W, Gelderblom, HR, Goudsmit, J & Osterhaus, ADME (2004) Human monoclonal antibody as prophylaxis for SARS coronavirus infection in ferrets. *Lancet,* 363, 2139-41.
[http://dx.doi.org/10.1016/S0140-6736(04)16506-9] [PMID: 15220038]

Ter Meulen, J, van den Brink, EN, Poon, LL, Marissen, WE, Leung, CS, Cox, F, Cheung, CY, Bakker, AQ, Bogaards, JA, van Deventer, E, Preiser, W, Doerr, HW, Chow, VT, de Kruif, J, Peiris, JSM & Goudsmit, J (2006) Human monoclonal antibody combination against SARS coronavirus: synergy and coverage of escape mutants. *PLoS Med,* 3, e237.
[http://dx.doi.org/10.1371/journal.pmed.0030237] [PMID: 16796401]

Tett, SE, Cutler, DJ, Day, RO & Brown, KF (1989) Bioavailability of hydroxychloroquine tablets in healthy volunteers. *Br J Clin Pharmacol,* 27, 771-9.

[http://dx.doi.org/10.1111/j.1365-2125.1989.tb03439.x] [PMID: 2757893]

Touret, F, Gilles, M, Barral, K, Nougairède, A, Decroly, E, Lamballerie, X & Coutard, B (2020) *In-vitro* screening of a FDA approved chemical library reveals potential inhibitors of SARS-CoV-2 replication. *Sci Rep,* 10, 13093.
[http://dx.doi.org/10.1038/s41598-020-70143-6]

Treatment plan edition 5 revision edition (2020). http://www.gov.cn/ zhengce/ zhengceku/ 2020-02/09/ 5476407/ files/ 765d1e65b7d1443081053c29ad37fb07.pdf

Treatment plan edition 5 (2020). www.gov.cn/zhengce/ zhengceku/ 2020-02/05/ 5474791/files/de44557832ad4be- 1929091dcbcfca891.pdf

Tyteca, D, Van Der Smissen, P, Mettlen, M, Van Bambeke, F, Tulkens, PM, Mingeot-Leclercq, MP & Courtoy, PJ (2002) Azithromycin, a lysosomotropic antibiotic, has distinct effects on fluid-phase and receptor-mediated endocytosis, but does not impair phagocytosis in J774 macrophages. *Exp Cell Res,* 281, 86-100.
[http://dx.doi.org/10.1006/excr.2002.5613] [PMID: 12441132]

US-FDA (2008), U.S. Food and Drug Administration Center for drug evaluation and research. Final Labeling Text, BL125085 Supplement.

Van Den Brink, EN, Ter Meulen, J, Cox, F, Jongeneelen, MA, Thijsse, A, Throsby, M, Marissen, WE, Rood, PML, Bakker, ABH, Gelderblom, HR, Martina, BE, Osterhaus, AD, Preiser, W, Doerr, HW, de Kruif, J & Goudsmit, J (2005) Molecular and biological characterization of human monoclonal antibodies binding to the spike and nucleocapsid proteins of severe acute respiratory syndrome coronavirus. *J Virol,* 79, 1635-44.
[http://dx.doi.org/10.1128/JVI.79.3.1635-1644.2005] [PMID: 15650189]

Vincent, MJ, Bergeron, E, Benjannet, S, Erickson, BR, Rollin, PE, Ksiazek, TG, Seidah, NG & Nichol, ST (2005) Chloroquine is a potent inhibitor of SARS coronavirus infection and spread. *Virol J,* 2, 69.
[http://dx.doi.org/10.1186/1743-422X-2-69] [PMID: 16115318]

Wagstaff, KM, Sivakumaran, H, Heaton, SM, Harrich, D & Jans, DA (2012) Ivermectin is a specific inhibitor of importin α/β-mediated nuclear import able to inhibit replication of HIV-1 and dengue virus. *Biochem J,* 443, 851-6.
[http://dx.doi.org/10.1042/BJ20120150] [PMID: 22417684]

Wang, C, Horby, PW, Hayden, FG & Gao, GF (2020) A novel coronavirus outbreak of global health concern. *Lancet,* 395, 470-3.
[http://dx.doi.org/10.1016/S0140-6736(20)30185-9] [PMID: 31986257]

Wang, D, Hu, B, Hu, C, Zhu, F, Liu, X, Zhang, J, Wang, B, Xiang, H, Cheng, Z, Xiong, Y, Zhao, Y, Li, Y, Wang, X & Peng, Z (2020) Clinical characteristics of 138 hospitalized patients with 2019 novel coronavirus-infected pneumonia in Wuhan, China. *JAMA,* 323, 1061-9.
[http://dx.doi.org/10.1001/jama.2020.1585] [PMID: 32031570]

Wang, L & Ma, Q (2018) Clinical benefits and pharmacology of scutellarin: A comprehensive review. *Pharmacol Ther,* 190, 105-27.
[http://dx.doi.org/10.1016/j.pharmthera.2018.05.006] [PMID: 29742480]

Wang, LF, Lin, YS, Huang, NC, Yu, CY, Tsai, WL, Chen, JJ, Kubota, T, Matsuoka, M, Chen, SR, Yang, CS, Lu, RW, Lin, YL & Chang, TH (2015) Hydroxychloroquine-inhibited dengue virus is associated with host defense machinery. *J Interferon Cytokine Res,* 35, 143-56.
[http://dx.doi.org/10.1089/jir.2014.0038] [PMID: 25321315]

Wang, M, Cao, R, Zhang, L, Yang, X, Liu, J, Xu, M, Shi, Z, Hu, Z, Zhong, W & Xiao, G (2020) Remdesivir and chloroquine effectively inhibit the recently emerged novel coronavirus (2019-nCoV) *in vitro*. *Cell Res,* 30, 269-71.
[http://dx.doi.org/10.1038/s41422-020-0282-0] [PMID: 32020029]

Wang, W, Ma, X, Han, J, Zhou, M, Ren, H, Pan, Q, Zheng, C & Zheng, Q (2016) Neuroprotective effect of scutellarin on ischemic cerebral injury by down-regulating the expression of angiotensin-converting enzyme

and AT1 receptor. *PLoS One,* 11, e0146197.
[http://dx.doi.org/10.1371/journal.pone.0146197] [PMID: 26730961]

Wang, Y, Jiang, W, He, Q, Wang, C, Wang, B, Zhou, P, Dong, N & Tong, Q (2020) Early, low-dose and short-term application of corticosteroid treatment in patients with severe COVID-19 pneumonia: single-center experience from Wuhan. MedRxiv, China.

Wang, Z, Yang, B, Li, Q, Wen, L & Zhang, R (2020) Clinical features of 69 cases with coronavirus disease 2019 in Wuhan, China. *Clin Infect Dis,* 71, 769-77.
[http://dx.doi.org/10.1093/cid/ciaa272] [PMID: 32176772]

Warren, TK, Jordan, R, Lo, MK, Ray, AS, Mackman, RL, Soloveva, V, Siegel, D, Perron, M, Bannister, R, Hui, HC, Larson, N, Strickley, R, Wells, J, Stuthman, KS, Van Tongeren, SA, Garza, NL, Donnelly, G, Shurtleff, AC, Retterer, CJ, Gharaibeh, D, Zamani, R, Kenny, T, Eaton, BP, Grimes, E, Welch, LS, Gomba, L, Wilhelmsen, CL, Nichols, DK, Nuss, JE, Nagle, ER, Kugelman, JR, Palacios, G, Doerffler, E, Neville, S, Carra, E, Clarke, MO, Zhang, L, Lew, W, Ross, B, Wang, Q, Chun, K, Wolfe, L, Babusis, D, Park, Y, Stray, KM, Trancheva, I, Feng, JY, Barauskas, O, Xu, Y, Wong, P, Braun, MR, Flint, M, McMullan, LK, Chen, SS, Fearns, R, Swaminathan, S, Mayers, DL, Spiropoulou, CF, Lee, WA, Nichol, ST, Cihlar, T & Bavari, S (2016) Therapeutic efficacy of the small molecule GS-5734 against Ebola virus in rhesus monkeys. *Nature,* 531, 381-5.
[http://dx.doi.org/10.1038/nature17180] [PMID: 26934220]

Wellems, TE & Plowe, CV (2001) Chloroquine-resistant malaria. *J Infect Dis,* 184, 770-6.
[http://dx.doi.org/10.1086/322858] [PMID: 11517439]

World Health Organization (2014) Use of convalescent whole blood or plasma collected from patients recovered from Ebola virus disease for transfusion, as an empirical treatment during outbreaks.
https://apps.who.int/ iris/handle/10665/135591

Xiaowei, F, Qing, M, Tianjun, Y, Lei, L, Yinzhong, W, Fei, T, Geng, S & Pan, A (2020) Low-dose corticosteroid therapy does not delay viral clearance inpatients with COVID-19. *J Infect,* 81, 147-78.
[http://dx.doi.org/10.1016/j.jinf.2020.03.039]

Xiong, HR, Zhang, YH, Deng, K, Liu, Q, Liu, YY, Luo, F, Hou, W & Yang, ZQ (2016) Antiviral activity and mechanism of action of arbidol against Hantaan virus infection. *Trop J Pharm Res,* 15, 1439-45.
[http://dx.doi.org/10.4314/tjpr.v15i7.12]

Xu, X, Han, M, Li, T, Sun, W, Wang, D, Fu, B, Zhou, Y, Zheng, X, Yang, Y, Li, X, Zhang, X, Pan, A & Wei, H (2020) Effective treatment of severe COVID-19 patients with tocilizumab. *Proc Natl Acad Sci USA,* 117, 10970-5.
[http://dx.doi.org/10.1073/pnas.2005615117] [PMID: 32350134]

Yan, Y, Zou, Z, Sun, Y, Li, X, Xu, KF, Wei, Y, Jin, N & Jiang, C (2013) Anti-malaria drug chloroquine is highly effective in treating avian influenza A H5N1 virus infection in an animal model. *Cell Res,* 23, 300-2.
[http://dx.doi.org/10.1038/cr.2012.165] [PMID: 23208422]

Yang, Z, Liu, J, Zhou, Y, Zhao, X, Zhao, Q & Liu, J (2020) The effect of corticosteroid treatment on patients with coronavirus infection: a systematic review and meta-analysis. *J Infect,* 81, e13-20.
[http://dx.doi.org/10.1016/j.jinf.2020.03.062] [PMID: 32283144]

Yao, X, Ye, F, Zhang, M, Cui, C, Huang, B, Niu, P, Liu, X, Zhao, L, Dong, E, Song, C, Zhan, S, Lu, R, Li, H, Tan, W & Liu, D (2020) *In-vitro* antiviral activity and projection of optimized dosing design of hydroxychloroquine for the treatment of severe acute respiratory syndrome coronavirus-2 (SARS-Co-V-2). *Clin Infect Dis,* 71, 732-9.
[http://dx.doi.org/10.1093/cid/ciaa237] [PMID: 32150618]

Yates, DM & Wolstenholme, AJ (2004) An ivermectin-sensitive glutamate-gated chloride channel subunit from Dirofilaria immitis. *Int J Parasitol,* 34, 1075-81.
[http://dx.doi.org/10.1016/j.ijpara.2004.04.010] [PMID: 15313134]

Şimşek Yavuz, S & Ünal, S (2020) Antiviral treatment of COVID-19. *Turk J Med Sci,* 50, 611-9.

[http://dx.doi.org/10.3906/sag-2004-145] [PMID: 32293834]

Ye, XT, Luo, YL, Xia, SC, Sun, QF, Ding, JG, Zhou, Y, Chen, W, Wang, XF, Zhang, WW, Du, WJ, Ruan, ZW & Hong, L (2020) Clinical efficacy of lopinavir/ritonavir in the treatment of Coronavirus disease 2019. *Eur Rev Med Pharmacol Sci,* 24, 3390-6.
[PMID: 32271456]

Zeng, Z, Andrew, NW, Arison, BH, Luffer-Atlas, D & Wang, RW (1998) Identification of cytochrome P4503A4 as the major enzyme responsible for the metabolism of ivermectin by human liver microsomes. *Xenobiotica,* 28, 313-21.
[http://dx.doi.org/10.1080/004982598239597] [PMID: 9574819]

Zhang, J, Ma, X, Yu, F, Liu, J, Zou, F, Pan, T & Zhang, H (2020) Teicoplanin potently blocks the cell entry of 2019-nCo-V. *bioRxiv.*
[http://dx.doi.org/10.1101/2020.02.05.935387]

Zhang, L, Lin, D, Sun, X, Curth, U, Drosten, C, Sauerhering, L, Becker, S, Rox, K & Hilgenfeld, R (2020) Crystal structure of SARS-CoV-2 main protease provides a basis for design of improved α-ketoamide inhibitors. *Science,* 368, 409-12.
[http://dx.doi.org/10.1126/science.abb3405] [PMID: 32198291]

Zhang, Y, Zhong, Y, Pan, L & Dong, J (2020) Treat 2019 novel coronavirus (COVID-19) with IL-6 inhibitor: Are we already that far? *Drug Discov Ther,* 14, 100-2.
[http://dx.doi.org/10.5582/ddt.2020.03006] [PMID: 32378647]

Zhao, Q & He, Y (2020) Challenges of convalescent plasma therapy on COVID-19. *J Clin Virol,* 127, 104358.
[http://dx.doi.org/10.1016/j.jcv.2020.104358] [PMID: 32305026]

Zhou, J, Chu, H & Li, C (2014) Active MERS- CoV replication and aberrant induction of inflammatory cytokines and chemokines in human macrophages: implications for pathogenesis. *J Infect Dis,* 209, 1331-42.
[http://dx.doi.org/10.1093/infdis/jit504] [PMID: 24065148]

Zhou, N, Pan, T, Zhang, J, Li, Q, Zhang, X, Bai, C, Huang, F, Peng, T, Zhang, J, Liu, C, Tao, L & Zhang, H (2016) Glycopeptide antibiotics potently inhibit cathepsin-L in the late endosome/lysosome and block the entry of Ebola virus, middle east respiratory syndrome coronavirus (MERS-Co-V) and severe acute respiratory syndrome coronavirus (SARS-Co-V). *J Biol Chem,* 291, 9218-32.
[http://dx.doi.org/10.1074/jbc.M116.716100] [PMID: 26953343]

Zhou, W, Liu, Y, Tian, D, Wang, C, Wang, S, Cheng, J, Hu, M, Fang, M & Gao, Y (2020) Potential benefits of precise corticosteroids therapy for severe 2019-nCoV pneumonia. *Signal Transduct Target Ther,* 5, 18.
[http://dx.doi.org/10.1038/s41392-020-0127-9] [PMID: 32296012]

Zhu, L, Xu, X, Ma, K, Yang, J, Guan, H, Chen, S, Chen, Z & Chen, G (2020) Successful recovery of COVID-19 pneumonia in a renal transplant recipient with long-term immunosuppression. *Am J Transplant,* 20, 1859-63.
[http://dx.doi.org/10.1111/ajt.15869] [PMID: 32181990]

Zhu, N, Zhang, D, Wang, W, Li, X, Yang, B, Song, J, Zhao, X, Huang, B, Shi, W, Lu, R, Niu, P, Zhan, F, Ma, X, Wang, D, Xu, W, Wu, G, Gao, GF & Tan, W China Novel Coronavirus Investigating and Research Team (2020) A novel coronavirus from patients with pneumonia in China, 2019. *N Engl J Med,* 382, 727-33.
[http://dx.doi.org/10.1056/NEJMoa2001017] [PMID: 31978945]

Zhu, Z, Lu, Z, Xu, T, Chen, C, Yang, G, Zha, T, Lu, J & Xue, Y (2020) Arbidol monotherapy is superior to lopinavir/ritonavir in treating COVID-19. *J Infect,* 81, e21-3.
[http://dx.doi.org/10.1016/j.jinf.2020.03.060] [PMID: 32283143]

CHAPTER 3

COVID-19 and Mortality

Rimesh Pal[1] and **Sanjay Kumar Bhadada**[1,*]

[1] *Department of Endocrinology, Post Graduate Institute of Medical Education and Research Chandigarh-160012, India*

Abstract: The novel coronavirus disease (COVID-19) has scourged the world ever since its outbreak in December 2019 in Wuhan, China. The disease tends to be asymptomatic or mild in nearly 80% of the patients. However, around 5% of the patients tend to have critical disease complicated by acute respiratory distress syndrome (ARDS), shock and multiple organ failure. Mortality in COVID-19, as represented by the case-fatality rate (CFR), is around 6% (as of June 4, 2020). The CFR of COVID-19 is lower as compared to other coronavirus-related diseases like the Severe Acute Respiratory Syndrome (SARS) and the Middle East Respiratory Syndrome (MERS), however, it is likely to increase as we reach the end of the pandemic. The CFR also varies widely from one nation to another with the maximum mortality being hitherto reported from the European nations and the least from Singapore, Cambodia, Vietnam and Iceland. The common causes of death in COVID-19 include respiratory failure, consequently leading to ARDS, pulmonary thromboembolism, shock and multiple organ failure. Advancing age and presence of comorbid illness are consistently associated with an increased risk of death, while certain biochemical and hematological parameters, notably C-reactive protein, IL-6, cardiac troponin, D-dimer and absolute count can also help predict mortality in patients with COVID-19.

Keywords: ACE2, ARDS, Case-fatality rate, Comorbidities, COVID-19, Cytokine storm, D-dimer, Death, Diabetes mellitus, Hypertension, IL-6, Lymphopenia, Mortality, Mortality rate, Novel coronavirus disease, Old age, SARS-CoV-2, Shock, Thromboembolism, Troponin.

INTRODUCTION

An unprecedented outbreak of 'pneumonia of unknown cause' emerged in the Wuhan City of China in December 2019 (Pneumonia of unknown cause – China, 2020). The patients presented with clinical symptoms of fever, dry cough, dyspnea, and bilateral lung infiltrates on imaging. Cases were claimed to be all

---

* **Corresponding author Sanjay Kumar Bhadada:** Department of Endocrinology, Post Graduate Institute of Medical Education and Research Chandigarh-160012, India; E-mail: bhadadask@rediffmail.com

Neeraj Mittal, Sanjay Kumar Bhadada, O. P. Katare and Varun Garg (Eds.)

linked to the Wuhan's Seafood Wholesale Market, which trades in fish and a wide variety of live animal species, including poultry, bats, rats, marmots, and snakes. The causative pathogen was identified from throat swab samples collected from the patients and was subsequently named Severe Acute Respiratory Syndrome Coronavirus 2 (SARS-CoV-2). The disease was named novel coronavirus disease (COVID-19) by the World Health Organization (WHO). With the increase in the number of cases outside China, the WHO declared the outbreak of COVID-19 to be a Public Health Emergency of International Concern, posing a high risk to countries with vulnerable health systems on January 30, 2020. Subsequently, with the emergence of new epicenters in Italy and Iran, COVID-19 was declared a pandemic on March 11, 2020.

Ever since its outbreak, COVID-19 has scourged the world, affecting over 6.2 million people, inflicting more than 379000 casualties worldwide (Coronavirus disease (COVID-19) Situation Report – 135, 2020). Hitherto, the maximum number of cases has been reported from the United States of America, Brazil, Russia, the United Kingdom, Spain, Italy, India, Germany, Peru, Turkey, Iran and France (Coronavirus (COVID-19), 2020). The inherent ability of SARS-CoV-2 to withstand extremes of the ambient environment and its remarkable stability on inanimate objects and surfaces make it an ideal pathogen for human-to-human transmission. The basic reproductive number (R_0) of COVID-19, defined as the average number of secondary cases attributable to infection by an index case after that case is introduced into a susceptible population, is high, ranging from 1.5 to 6.68 with a mean of 3.28 (Liu *et al.,* 2020). The high R_0 of SARS-CoV-2 has accounted for the rapid increase in the number of COVID-19 cases worldwide. In addition, there have been instances of super-spreader events, in which an individual, who may or not be symptomatic, infects a large number of susceptible subjects (Coronavirus disease 2019 (COVID-19) Situation Report – 24, 2020.; Coronavirus disease 2019 (COVID-19) Situation Report – 36, 2020). In fact, the outbreak of COVID-19 in Wuhan might have been a super-spreader event as it had coincided with one of the world's largest mass gathering, the Chinese Spring Festival (Ebrahim and Memish, 2020).

Despite being highly contagious, more than 80% of patients with COVID-19 are either asymptomatic (no pneumonia) or have mild symptoms (mild pneumonia). Only 14% of patients develop the severe disease; the rest 5% develop critical disease manifesting as respiratory failure, septic shock, and/or multiple organ dysfunction or failure (Wu and McGoogan, 2020). Case-fatality rates in COVID-19 have been highly variable, ranging from as low as 0.5% to as high as 21.8% (Mortality Risk of COVID-19, 2020). Nevertheless, advancing age and the presence of underlying co-morbidities have been consistently associated with increased mortality in COVID-19. In addition, certain biochemical parameters have emerged as potential predictors of mortality in COVID-19.

Herein, we have discussed in detail the multiple aspects of mortality in relation to COVID-19.

REPRESENTING MORTALITY – MORTALITY RATE *VS.* CASE-FATALITY RATE

Often the terms mortality rate and case-fatality rates are used interchangeably. Although both the parameters are used to define death rates, the two are not synonymous. According to the *Dictionary of Epidemiology*, the mortality rate is defined as "an estimate of the portion of a population that dies during a specified period". Going by the definition, the mortality rate should be ideally expressed as the number of deaths occurring per 100000 population per year, rather than representing the figure as a percentage. On the other hand, the case-fatality rate (CFR) is defined as "the proportion of cases of a specified condition that are fatal within a specified time" (Spychalski *et al.,* 2020). Accordingly, most of the estimates of death expressed as a percentage are case-fatality rates rather than mortality rates. We have referred to CFR throughout the subsequent discussion unless otherwise specified.

FALLACIES IN ESTIMATING MORTALITY USING CASE-FATALITY RATE

Case-fatality rates amid an ongoing pandemic should be interpreted with caution. The CFR is affected by the total number of cases (the denominator) as much as it is affected by the actual number of deaths (the numerator). For example, in countries where massive population screening has been undertaken, as in Switzerland and South Korea, case-fatality rates are less than 1%, as the denominator includes a large number of mild/asymptomatic cases. However, in countries where only symptomatic patients or those requiring hospital admissions are being screened, as in Italy and Spain, case-fatality rates have exceeded 5%, because the denominator is much smaller (Vincent and Taccone, 2020). Besides, the CFR might be over or underestimated based on how a 'case' is defined. During an ongoing epidemic, cases might be defined either as total cases (every confirmed case) or as closed cases (only those who have recovered or died). Hence, the denominator for calculating CFR might be either of these numbers. In the initial phase of an epidemic, the number of closed cases is relatively small, and so the CFR calculated per closed cases is an overestimate. By contrast, when the CFR is calculated per total cases, the whole calculation becomes an underestimate. As an example, early in the course of COVID-19, even before it was declared a pandemic, the WHO had opined on March 3, 2020, that the global COVID-19 CFR was 3.4% (WHO Director-General's opening remarks at the media briefing on COVID-19 - March 3, 2020). As of June 4, 2020, the global CFR stands at 6.1% based on the WHO statistics (Coronavirus disease (COVID-19) Situation Report – 135, 2020). Nevertheless, irrespective of the method used (either total cases or closed cases), all calculations are biased in the initial part of an epidemic, and tend to merge once all the cases are closed (Spychalski *et al.*, 2020). Moreover, there exist reporting errors that become transparent towards the end of an epidemic. China had suddenly increased the death toll in Wuhan by 50% after the pandemic had subsided, stating that the newly reported 1290 COVID-19-related deaths were attributed to casualties that occurred at home at the beginning of the outbreak, as well as deaths that were wrongly reported by hospitals. Thus, once the pandemic ends and all the available statistics are reanalyzed, only then can the true CFR be estimated. Notwithstanding this fact, it seems that the CFR calculated per total cases is the least affected by reporting biases and remains the best tool to express the fatality of a disease, even though it might underestimate the figure in the initial phase of an outbreak (Spychalski *et al.*, 2020).

REPORTING COVID-19-RELATED DEATHS

A major barrier to the estimation of true CFR is the inaccurate reporting of COVID-19-related deaths ("Inaccurate Covid-19 death reporting can lower international health assistance," 2020). In addition, there have been allegations that certain nations are under-reporting or censoring COVID-19 death statistics ("Coronavirus: Europe 'wary of confronting China over deaths,'" 2020.; "Inaccurate Covid-19 death reporting can lower international health assistance," 2020; "Iran Uses Arrests, Censorship to Silence Critical COVID-19 Coverage," 2020). To bring uniformity in reporting, the WHO has introduced emergency "International Classification of Disease, Tenth Revision (ICD-10)" codes to help define and code COVID-19-related deaths. The ICD-10 codes presently recommended by the WHO for mortality coding have been summarized in Table **1** (Guidance for appropriate recording of COVID-19 related deaths in India, 2020). Of note, COVID-19 should be recorded as an underlying cause of death (UCOD) in patients with confirmed or suspected COVID-19. Often deaths in patients with COVID-19 are being attributed to underlying pre-existing comorbidities. Although underlying co-morbidities may increase the severity of COVID-19, these conditions should not replace COVID-19 as the UCOD. Such malpractice would naturally lead to under-reporting of COVID-19-related deaths and thereby skew the mortality statistics.

Table 1. Table showing ICD-10 codes presently recommended by the WHO for COVID-19-related mortality coding.

Test	Symptoms of COVID-19	Diagnosis	ICD-10 Code
Positive	None	Confirmed COVID-19	U07.1
Positive	Present	Confirmed COVID-19 documented as UCOD	U07.1
Positive	Present with co-morbid conditions	Confirmed COVID-19 documented as UCOD	U07.1
Negative	Present	Clinically-Epidemiologically diagnosed COVID-19	U07.2
Awaited	Present	Suspected COVID-19	U07.2
Inconclusive	Present	Probable COVID-19	U07.2

COMPARING CASE-FATALITY RATES OF COVID-19 WITH OTHER RELATED VIRAL DISEASES

Before the COVID-19 outbreak, the world had witnessed the outbreak of two coronavirus-related diseases, namely the Severe Acute Respiratory Syndrome (SARS) in 2003 and the Middle East Respiratory Syndrome (MERS) in 2012. A comparison of the CFR of the three coronavirus-related diseases (Coronavirus disease (COVID-19) Situation Report – 135, 2020; Middle East respiratory syndrome coronavirus (MERS-CoV); Summary of probable SARS cases with onset of illness from 1 November 2002 to 31 July 2003) and adult seasonal influenza (Disease Burden of Influenza; Faust and del Rio, 2020) has been summarized in Table **2**.

Table 2. Table showing case-fatality rates of COVID-19, SARS, MERS and adult seasonal influenza.

Disease	Case-fatality Rate
COVID-19	6.1% (as on June 4, 2020)
SARS	9.6%
MERS	34.4%
Seasonal influenza	< 0.1%

Apparently, the CFR of COVID-19 is less than that of SARS and MERS, however, considering the magnitude of the pandemic, the absolute number of deaths are much higher in COVID-19 than either SARS or MERS. The WHO had reported only 774 SARS-related deaths and only 878 deaths due to MERS (Middle East respiratory syndrome coronavirus (MERS-CoV); Summary of probable SARS cases with onset of illness from 1 November 2002 to 31 July

2003). On the contrary, COVID-19 has already claimed more than 379000 lives globally (Coronavirus disease (COVID-19) Situation Report – 135, 2020). As the pandemic wages on and case reporting becomes more uniform and efficient, it might be expected that the CFR of COVID-19 would approach that of SARS.

COMPARING COVID-19 CASE-FATALITY RATES AMONG VARIOUS NATIONS

The COVID-19 case-fatality rates differ widely from one nation to another. As of June 4, 2020, CFR as low as 0.5% has been reported from Iceland. On the other hand, Yemen presently has the highest CFR of 21.8% (Mortality Risk of COVID-19). Overall, the European nations have high case-fatality rates, being 19.1% in France, 14.3% in Italy, 14.2% in the United Kingdom, 13.6% in Hungary, 11.6% in Spain and 11.1% in Sweden. Although the absolute number of deaths has been the highest in the United States of America (USA), the CFR (5.8%) is not exorbitantly high as in most of the European nations. This can again be attributed to the large number of COVID-19 cases diagnosed in the USA with nearly 2 million cases being reported from the continent. Mexico, on the other hand, has a high CFR of 11.6%. As far as South America is concerned, the highest case-fatality rates have been reported from Equador (8.5%) and Brazil (5.6%). Most of the Asian nations have reported a reasonable CFR, ranging from 0% in Cambodia and Vietman, 0.07% in Singapore, 2.3% in South Korea, 2.8% in India, 5.5% in China to 6.0% in Indonesia. Surprisingly, Yemen has recently witnessed a surge in the number of COVID-19-related deaths, taking its CFR to 21.8%, however, the neighboring nations of Saudi Arabia and Oman have strikingly low CFR of 0.6% and 0.5%, respectively. Russia presently has a CFR of 1.2%; similarly, Australia and New Zealand have low case-fatality rates of 1.4% and 1.9%, respectively. Case-fatality rates in different parts of Africa are variable, being highest in Liberia (8.8%) and Chad (8.0%) with no deaths yet reported from Uganda (Mortality Risk of COVID-19).

Table 3. Table showing COVID-19-related case-fatality rates in different continents/nations (as of June 4, 2020).

Nation/Continent	Case-fatality Rate
Yemen	21.8%
France	19.1%
Italy	14.3%
United Kingdom	14.2%
Hungary	13.6%
Spain	11.6%

(Table 3) cont.....

Nation/Continent	Case-fatality Rate
Mexico	11.6%
Sweden	11.1%
Canada	8.0%
Romania	6.5%
Indonesia	6.0%
United States of America	5.8%
Brazil	5.6%
China	5.5%
Japan	5.3%
Iran	4.9%
Germany	4.7%
Egypt	3.8%
India	2.8%
South Korea	2.3%
South Africa	2.1%
Australia	1.4%
Russia	1.2%
Iceland	0.5%
Singapore	0.07%
Cambodia	0.0%
Vietnam	0.0%

CAUSES OF DEATH IN COVID-19

The SARS-CoV-2 primarily attacks the lungs, resulting in viral pneumonia in a susceptible individual. In patients with mild and moderate disease, pneumonia resolves with time; however, in patients with severe and critical COVID-19, life-threatening complications ensue. Although the virus *per se* has directly been implicated in the causation of myocarditis (Inciardi *et al.*, 2020; Siripanthong *et al.*, 2020), acute renal failure (Batlle *et al.*, 2020) and pancreatitis (Wang *et al.*, 2020), complications most often result from a "cytokine storm" induced by the virus (Coperchini *et al.*, 2020). Cytokine storm, also known as cytokine storm syndrome, is a state characterized by the uncontrolled release of immune cells and excessive and disproportionate release of pro-inflammatory cytokines into circulation (Tisoncik *et al.*, 2012). Although first described in association with graft-*versus*-host disease (Ferrara *et al.*, 1993), the term has since been linked to infectious pathogens, notably, cytomegalovirus, Epstein-Barr virus-associated hemophagocytic lymphohistiocytosis, group A streptococcus, influenza virus (specifically H5N1 avian influenza virus), variola virus, and severe acute respiratory syndrome coronavirus (SARS-CoV) (Tisoncik *et al.*, 2012).

The concept of cytokine storm originated from the observation that patients with COVID-19 requiring admission in an intensive care unit (ICU) had higher serum levels of CXCL10, CCL2 and TNFα as compared to those with the less severe disease not requiring intensive care. In addition, several studies have shown that the serum IL-6 levels are increased in patients with COVID-19 and correlate with disease severity (McGonagle *et al.*, 2020; Zhang *et al.*, 2020). Learning from prior experience, increased circulating levels of pro-inflammatory cytokines (*e.g*, IFNγ, IL-1β, IL-6, IL-12) and chemokines (CXCL10, and CCL2) had been associated with pulmonary inflammation and extensive lung involvement in SARS patients, similarly to what had happened in MERS-CoV infection (Channappanavar and Perlman, 2017). Thus, the release of large amounts of pro-inflammatory mediators precipitates and sustains the aberrant systemic inflammatory response. The cytokine storm is readily followed by the host immune system attacking the body, which in turn causes acute respiratory distress syndrome (ARDS) and multiple organ failure, culminating in death, at least in the most severe cases of SARS-CoV-2 infection (Xu *et al.*, 2020).

Respiratory failure, secondary to ARDS, obviously remains the main cause of mortality in COVID-19 (Ruan *et al.*, 2020), as was seen in previous viral pandemics, such as the Spanish flu (1918), SARS and MERS. About one-third of the worsened patients (Chen *et al.*, 2020; Zhou *et al.*, 2020) and up to 41.8% (Wu *et al.*, 2020a) suffer from complications of respiratory failure and ARDS. Besides, COVID-19 can sometimes be complicated by shock and multiple organ failure that can also lead to the demise of the patient (Chen *et al.*, 2020). Shock is most often a result of the cytokine storm and represents a form of vasoplegic shock. Shock in COVID-19 can also result from an increased intrathoracic pressure secondary to invasive ventilation that can impede cardiac filling (Pal, 2020). Besides, cardiac involvement and secondary bacterial/fungal infections can lead to shock in patients with COVID-19 (Vincent and Taccone, 2020; Zhou *et al.*, 2020). Bacterial and fungal infections are common complications of viral pneumonia. In influenza patients, bacterial co-infection occurs in around 0.5% of young individuals and 2.5% of older individuals (Chertow and Memoli, 2013). Every one in 4 H1N1 patients during the 2009 pandemic had a coexisting bacterial or fungi infection (MacIntyre *et al.*, 2018). According to a report, 20 of 90 SARS patients had secondary lower respiratory tract infections in 2003, which accounted for 70.6% of those critical SARS patients who underwent an invasive operation. The pathogens causing secondary infections were diverse: gram-negative bacilli were the most common but Candida was not uncommon (Zhou *et al.*, 2020). Bacterial and fungal co-infections or super-infections in COVID-19 patients have been inadequately investigated and reported thus far. Only a few articles have reported secondary infection, mostly without pathogen details. Besides, the complications resulting from bacterial or fungal infections in COVID-19 were not included in the prognosis analysis in most of the published papers. However, it should be kept in mind that most of the current infection control protocols aim to prevent the transmission and cross infection by SARS-CoV-2, thereby overlooking the prevention of bacterial or fungal secondary infections (Zhou *et al.*, 2020). As a matter of fact, in one Chinese study, secondary infections were found in 50% of the non-surviving COVID-19 patients (Zhou *et al.*, 2020).

Of late, pulmonary embolism (PE) has been implicated as a major cause of death in patients with COVID-19. Wichmann *et al.* reported the findings of 12 consecutive autopsies of patients with COVID-19. The authors reported a high incidence of PE with or without underlying deep vein thrombosis (DVT), in spite of the absence of a history of venous thromboembolism (VTE). Massive pulmonary embolism was the cause of death in one-third of the cases. Seventy-five percent were men and two-third of them were noted to have recent thrombosis in prostatic venous plexus (Wichmann *et al.*, 2020). In another autopsy study by Lax and colleagues, grossly visible pulmonary arterial thrombi were noted in all the 11 cases with associated infarcts in 9 cases (81%). During the hospital stay, most of the patients had received prophylactic anticoagulant therapy; thereby suggesting that pulmonary thrombi had formed despite anticoagulation (Lax *et al.*, 2020). Amongst non-autopsy studies, pulmonary thromboembolism has been reported on computerized tomography in patients with COVID-19 pneumonia with high as well as normal D-dimer levels (Danzi *et al.*, 2020; Scialpi *et al.*, 2020; Xie *et al.*, 2020). In a study by Klok *et al.*, computer tomography pulmonary angiogram (CTPA) and/or ultrasonography done based on clinical suspicion confirmed VTE in 27% and arterial thrombotic events in 3.7% of 184 COVID-19 patients admitted in ICU. Pulmonary embolism was the most frequent thrombotic complication (81%) (Klok *et al.*, 2020). An observational study had suggested that up to 5–10% of patients with COVID-19 who require mechanical ventilation have acute PE and/or DVT (Scialpi *et al.*, 2020). The pathophysiology of thrombotic events in COVID-19 patients involves direct endothelial cell injury by SARS-CoV-2 (Zhang *et al.*, 2020), hypercoagulability (Becker, 2020), hyperviscosity (Maier *et al.*, 2020) and traditional risk factors that include immobility inherent in a critically ill patient (Scialpi *et al.*, 2020). The common causes of death in patients with COVID-19 have been summarized in Table **4.**

Table 4. Table showing the common causes of death in patients with COVID-19.

Respiratory Failure (Acute Respiratory Distress Syndrome)
Thromboembolism
Shock (vasoplegic)
Multiple organ failure
Cardiogenic shock
Septic shock secondary to bacterial or fungal co-infection

PARAMETERS PREDICTING MORTALITY IN COVID-19

Various studies to date have pointed out at multiple factors that can predict mortality in patients with COVID-19. The factors can be broadly classified into two categories: clinical and laboratory. These have been summarized in Table **5**.

Table 5. Table summarizing the clinical and laboratory parameters predicting mortality and/or severe disease in patients with COVID-19.

Clinical Parameters	Laboratory Parameters
Age	C-reactive protein
Gender	Interleukin-6
Symptoms	D-dimer
Complications	Cardiac troponin
Comorbid illness	Creatinine
Smoking	Alanine transaminase
Secondary bacterial infections	Albumin
-	Blood urea nitrogen
-	Myoglobin
-	Lactate dehydrogenase
-	Ferritin
-	Total leukocyte count
-	Lymphocyte count
-	CD3+CD8+ T cell subset

Clinical Parameters

Age

Of all the clinical parameters, *advancing age* is consistently associated with mortality in COVID-19. Multivariate logistic regression analyses have shown that the age ≥ 65 years is associated with a 3.7-fold increased risk of death (Du *et al.*, 2020). Advancing age as a predictor of mortality has been consistently replicated in multiple studies (Jin *et al.*, 2020; Martins-Filho *et al.*, 2020; Ruan *et al.*, 2020; Zhou *et al.*, 2020). The same reason has been proposed as the cause of the strikingly high CFR in Italy as compared to China. Individuals aged 70 years or older represent 37.6% of cases in Italy and only 11.9% in China. In addition, a relevant number of cases in Italy are in people aged 90 years or older. Thus, the overall older age distribution in Italy relative to that in China may explain, in part, the higher average CFR in Italy (Onder *et al.*, 2020). On the contrary, children, adolescents and young adults have strikingly low case-fatality rates (as shown in Table **6**).

Table 6. Showing age-specific case-fatality rates in Italy and China (Onder *et al.*, 2020).

Age Groups (Years)	Case-fatality Rate in Italy (As of March 17, 2020)	Case-fatality Rate in China (As of February 11, 2020)
0-9	0%	0%
10-19	0%	0.2%
20-29	0%	0.2%
30-39	0.3%	0.2%
40-49	0.4%	0.4%
50-59	1.0%	1.3%
60-69	3.5%	3.6%
70-79	12.8%	8.0%
≥ 80	20.2%	14.8%

Statistics from other countries have shown a similar trend with data from the USA showing that patients aged 0-17 years account for only 0.06% of the COVID-19-related deaths while those 75 years or above account for 48.7% of the casualties (Age, Sex, Existing Conditions of COVID-19 Cases and Deaths). The high case-fatality rate in older adults reflects their poor immune system and the high prevalence of underlying co-morbidities (Pal and Bhadada, 2020a). Elderly patients have higher Pneumonia Severity Index score (PSI score) and involvement of multiple pulmonary lobes compared to young and middle-aged patients (Liu *et al.*, 2020).

Gender

Gender disparity in COVID-19-related mortality has been reported in a few studies (Jin *et al.*, 2020; Martins-Filho *et al.*, 2020). In a meta-analysis involving

852 patients (489 male and 363 female) with confirmed SARS-CoV-2 infection by real time-polymerase chain reaction, it was found that male gender was associated an increased risk for in-hospital death (relative risk 1.3, 95%CI 1.1 to 1.4) (Martins-Filho *et al.*, 2020). In another study by Jin *et al.*, it was found that while men and women had the same prevalence, men with COVID-19 were more at risk for worse outcomes and death, independent of age (Jin *et al.*, 2020). The reasons underlying high mortality in men are obscure; high circulating angiotensin-converting enzyme 2 (ACE2) in men have been proposed as a plausible reason (Jin *et al.*, 2020).

Symptoms

Presenting symptoms in patients with COVID-19 have been evaluated as potential predictors of subsequent mortality. Ruan *et al.* had compared initial symptoms in 150 patients with COVID-19 who had either died or had been discharged. Out of fever, cough, sputum production, dyspnea, fatigue, myalgia and hemoptysis, only dyspnea was found to be statistically more prevalent in patients who had died as compared to those who were discharged (87% *vs.* 62%, *P* value=0.001) (Ruan *et al.*, 2020). Similarly, the presence of dyspnea was found to increase the risk of in-hospital death by 1.8-folds to 2.6-folds (Martins-Filho *et al.*, 2020; J. Xie *et al.*, 2020). The presence of dyspnea suggests impending ARDS and hence portends a poor prognosis in patients with COVID-19. The early recognition of respiratory distress can make a difference in the final prognosis of the patients (Martins-Filho *et al.*, 2020).

Complications

Complications of SARS-CoV-2 infection that are commonly seen in critically ill patients, notably, ARDS (relative risk 7.4), acute cardiac injury (relative risk 6.9), acute kidney injury (relative risk 22.6), disseminated intravascular coagulation (DIC) (relative risk 27.1), and sepsis (relative risk 2.4) have been found to be risk factors for the COVID-19-related death. Xie *et al.* found that hypoxemia was independently associated with in-hospital mortality. An oxygen saturation (SpO$_2$) cut-off of 90.5% had 84.6% sensitivity and 97.2% specificity for prediction of survival. Higher SpO$_2$ levels after oxygen supplementation were associated with reduced mortality independent of age and sex (Xie *et al.*, 2020). Another Chinese study from Wuhan showed that a higher Sequential Organ Failure Assessment (SOFA) score at admission was an independent predictor of in-hospital death with an odds ratio of 5.65 (Zhou *et al.*, 2020). In another report from Wuhan, mortality was 62% among critically ill patients with COVID-19 and 81% among those requiring mechanical ventilation (Yang *et al.*, 2020). Thus, mortality is high among patients with COVID-19 who have severe disease and suffer from complications.

Comorbid Illness

Patients with underlying comorbidities are invariably at a high risk of mortality with COVID-19. The pre-existing comorbidities that have been consistently associated with poor outcomes in COVID-19 include hypertension, coronary heart disease, cerebrovascular disease, diabetes mellitus, obesity, chronic lung disease, chronic kidney disease and malignancy (Martins-Filho *et al.*, 2020; Pal and Bhadada, 2020a; Ruan *et al.*, 2020; Tian *et al.*, 2020). The effect size of individual comorbidities varies from one study to another. The presence of hypertension has been associated with a 1.5-fold to 2.5-fold increased risk of mortality in COVID-19. Underlying concurrent coronary heart disease (cardiovascular disease) and cerebrovascular disease have been shown to increase the chances of mortality by 3-fold to 3.8 fold and 3.3-fold, respectively. Likewise, the presence of diabetes mellitus has been associated with a 1.6-fold to 2-fold increased probability of dying with COVID-19 (Martins-Filho *et al.*, 2020; Tian *et al.*, 2020). Similarly, chronic lung disease (especially chronic obstructive pulmonary disease), chronic kidney disease and malignancy have been reported to be associated with mortality in COVID-19 (Guan *et al.*, 2020a; Martins-Filho *et al.*, 2020).

The association between hypertension, cardiovascular and cerebrovascular diseases and COVID-19-related mortality is probably mediated by the confounding effect of angiotensin-converting enzyme inhibitors (ACEi) and angiotensin-receptor blockers (ARBs), drugs that are widely used in this subset of patients (Pal and Bhadada, 2020a; Schiffrin *et al.*, 2020). The use of ACEi/ARBs is associated with the upregulation of angiotensin-converting enzyme 2 (ACE2), a monocarboxypeptidase that cleaves angiotensin-II and to a smaller extent angiotensin-I to angiotensin (1-7) and angiotensin (1-9), respectively (Pal and Bhansali, 2020). Unfortunately, the SARS-CoV-2 uses ACE2 as a receptor to gain entrance into the host pneumocytes. Thus, the upregulation of ACE2 with the use of ACEi/ARBs would prove to be counterproductive (Pal and Bhadada, 2020a). On the other hand, ACE2/angiotensin (1-7) system is known to exert a profound anti-inflammatory and anti-oxidant effect and thereby protect against inflammation-related lung injury. In this regard, upregulation of ACE2 by ACEi/ARBs would be expected to protect the lungs against ARDS (Pal and Bhansali, 2020; Schiffrin *et al.*, 2020). Whether ACEi/ARBs are actually beneficial or potentially nefarious in patients with COVID-19 is yet to be explored in large-scale studies.

The association between diabetes mellitus (DM) and increased mortality in COVID-19 is multipronged. Diabetes mellitus, especially uncontrolled DM is associated with a dysfunctional immune system. The innate immune system, the first line of defense against SARS-CoV-2 is compromised in people with DM (Geerlings and Hoepelman, 1999). Even short-term hyperglycemia has been shown to transiently stun the innate immune system (Jafar *et al.*, 2016). Moreover, DM is characterized by an exaggerated pro-inflammatory cytokine response, notably IL-1, IL-6 and TNFα, in the absence of an appropriate immunostimulation (Geerlings and Hoepelman, 1999); this is further exaggerated in response to a stimulus. This has been depicted in COVID-19 patients wherein serum levels of IL-6, C-reactive protein and ferritin were significantly higher in patients with DM than those without DM (Guo *et al.*, 2020). This suggests that people with diabetes are more susceptible to an inflammatory cytokine storm eventually leading to ARDS, shock and death in COVID-19 (Pal and Bhadada, 2020b). In addition, COVID-19 patients with DM also had higher D-dimer levels than those without DM (Guo *et al.*, 2020), perhaps signifying an over-activation of the hemostatic system. Amid an already underlying pro-thrombotic hypercoagulable state predisposed by the mere presence of DM, over-activation of the coagulation cascade in COVID-19 can lead to thromboembolic complications and eventual mortality (Pal and Bhadada, 2020b). Besides, DM is associated with reduced expression of ACE2 and low ACE2 expression might partly explain the increased incidence of severe lung injury and ARDS with COVID-19 (Pal and Bhansali, 2020; Tikellis and Thomas, 2012). Herein, also lies the confounding role of ACEi/ARBs that are also commonly prescribed because of their additional renoprotective effects in people with DM (Pal and Bhadada, 2020b; Pal and Bhansali, 2020). In addition, certain drugs used in the management of type 2 diabetes mellitus (T2DM), notably, liraglutide and pioglitazone have also been shown to upregulate ACE2 (Pal and Bhadada, 2020c). Although there exists little literature on people with type 1 diabetes mellitus (T1DM), the recently published CORONADO study has shown that people with T1DM and T2DM are equally at a high risk of endotracheal intubation for mechanical ventilation and/or death with 7 days of admission (primary outcome). The study also highlights the fact that death in people with DM is independently predicted by BMI, age, treated obstructive sleep apnoea, micro- and macrovascular complications. Surprisingly, long-term glucose control as reflected by HbA1c neither admission plasma glucose as not associated with the primary outcome on multivariate analysis (Cariou *et al.*, 2020).

Obesity has also been found to be associated with severe disease and mortality in COVID-19 (Dietz and Santos-Burgoa, 2020; Kassir, 2020; Pal and Banerjee, 2020). Adipose tissue express ACE2; with higher adipose tissue, more would be the overall ACE2 expression that would act as receptors for SARS-CoV-2

(Kassir, 2020). As in diabetes mellitus, even in basal state, obese patients have a higher concentration of several pro-inflammatory cytokines such as TNFα, IL-6 and MCP-1, produced by visceral and subcutaneous adipose tissue (Richard *et al.*, 2017). This could again predispose an obese individual to an exaggerated cytokine response in the presence of SARS-CoV-2, manifesting as severe disease, ARDS and finally, death (Pal and Banerjee, 2020).

In patients with chronic obstructive pulmonary disease (COPD), there is inactivation of the innate immune system and underexpression of pulmonary interferon-β, a cytokine involved in the defense against coronavirus (García-Valero *et al.*, 2019), thereby explaining the increased severity of COVID-19 in this subset of patients. Patients with underlying chronic kidney disease and malignancy are also immunocompromised, thereby explaining an increased propensity for severe disease and mortality in COVID-19 (Pal and Bhadada, 2020a).

Smoking

The association between smoking and COVID-19 is controversial. A systematic review and meta-analysis involving 11 case series with a total of 2002 cases had concluded that the pooled odds ratio of ongoing smoking and the development of severe COVID-19 was 1.98 (Zhao *et al.*, 2020). Another systematic review incorporating five studies had reported that the smokers were 1.4 times more likely (relative risk 1.4) to have severe symptoms of COVID-19 and approximately 2.4 times more likely to be admitted to an ICU, need mechanical ventilation or die compared to non-smokers (relative risk 2.4) (Vardavas and Nikitara, 2020). The plausible reason for this apparent adverse association between smoking and COVID-19 lies in the fact that smoking has been shown to upregulate ACE2 (Brake *et al.*, 2020). However, another meta-analysis involving 5 studies, totaling 1399 COVID-19 patients, 288 of whom (20.6%) had severe disease, did not find any significant association between active smoking and disease severity (Lippi and Henry, 2020).

Secondary Infections

Ruan *et al.* had shown that the prevalence of secondary infections was significantly higher in COVID-19 patients who had died as against those who had been discharged from the hospital (16% *vs.* 1%, *P* value=0.002). Secondary infections (bacterial or fungal) would increase the chances of septic shock and subsequent mortality.

Laboratory Parameters

An array of biochemical and hematological parameters has been associated with increased mortality in COVID-19. The biochemical markers are either indirect indicators of the severity of the underlying inflammation (as an example, C-reactive protein, erythrocyte sedimentation rate, IL-6, ferritin) or pointers towards underling end-organ damage (as an example, cardiac troponin, lactate dehydrogenase, creatinine, blood urea nitrogen, myoglobin, alanine transaminase) (Martins-Filho *et al.*, 2020; Ruan *et al.*, 2020; Tian *et al.*, 2020; Zhou *et al.*, 2020). Interleukin-6 needs a special mention. The cytokine has been implicated as one of the primary mediators of cytokine storm and hence, is elevated in patients with severe COVID-19. A meta-analysis of five studies reporting data on overall mortality and serum IL-6 in COVID-19 patients demonstrated that increasing mean IL-6 on admission was associated with an increased likelihood of mortality (Aziz *et al.*, 2020). A serum IL-6 cut-off of 55 pg/ml and 80 pg/ml has been proposed as predictors of severe disease and mortality in COVID-19, respectively (Aziz *et al.*, 2020; Chen *et al.*, 2020). Regarding C-reactive protein, a cut-off of 26.9 mg/l has been proposed as being predictive of aggravation of non-severe COVID-19 (Wang *et al.*, 2020).

As per as ferritin is concerned, Wu *et al.* found that higher serum levels of ferritin was associated with ARDS (hazard ratio 3.53); the association with survival however did not reach the level of significance (hazard ratio 5.28; *P* value=0.10) (Wu *et al.*, 2020a). At their univariate analysis, Zhou *et al.* pointed out at an association between higher serum ferritin levels and mortality, but subsequently, multivariate analysis was not presented (Zhou *et al.*, 2020). Similarly, non-survivors, as compared to survivors, presented more often with high LDH and high procalcitonin. Increased LDH has also been shown to be associated with a higher risk of ARDS (Wu *et al.*, 2020a), ICU support (Fan *et al.*, 2020) and death (Martins-Filho *et al.*, 2020; Wu *et al.*, 2020a) across multiple published studies. A meta-analysis of four published studies showed that increased procalcitonin values were associated with a nearly 5-fold higher risk of severe infection in COVID-19 (Lippi and Plebani, 2020).

Between 7% and 27.8% of COVID-19 patients may have elevated troponin levels (Guo *et al.*, 2020; Shi *et al.*, 2020; Wang *et al.*, 2020; Yang *et al.*, 2020). The plausible reasons for troponin elevation in patients with COVID-19 are multiple. First, SARS-CoV-2 induced cytokine storm can lead to myocardial inflammatory damage (Yang *et al.*, 2020). Second, SARS-CoV-2 can cause cardiac damage through direct viral invasion. Third, it is also possible that the elevated troponin levels are due to coronary microvascular ischemia mediated by direct binding of SARS-CoV-2 to the endothelial ACE2 receptor (Gupta *et al.*, 2020). Lastly, the hypercoagulable state seen in patients with COVID-19 can lead to microvascular thrombi and secondary myocardial infarction with subsequent elevation in serum troponins (Tang *et al.*, 2020). Several studies have shown that those with elevated troponin levels at baseline are predictive of severe disease, increased intensive care unit admissions and higher mortality (Guo *et al.*, 2020; Martins-Filho *et al.*, 2020; Shi *et al.*, 2020; Tang *et al.*, 2020; Tian *et al.*, 2020). In a cohort study, the presence of elevated troponin levels was associated with mortality with a hazard ratio of 4.26 (Shi *et al.*, 2020). In another single-center retrospective analysis of 187 COVID-19 patients, Guo *et al.* studied the relationship of baseline troponin levels and other comorbidities with mortality. They reported that the risk of death could be stratified according to the presence of elevated troponin and/or previous history of cardiovascular disease. Notably, elevated troponin levels carried a strong prognostic value even in the absence of cardiovascular disease history. In addition, the authors reported that in survivors, during the hospitalization period, the troponin levels remained stable and within normal limits. On the other hand, non-survivors showed a trend of gradual and progressive increase in troponin levels (Guo *et al.*, 2020). Du *et al.* reported that cardiac troponin I ≥ 0.05 ng/mL (odds ratio 4.077) was associated with an increased risk of mortality in COVID-19 independent of age, sex or presence of comorbid illness (Du *et al.*, 2020).

Amongst hematological parameters, elevated D-dimer has consistently been found to be associated with severe disease and mortality in COVID-19 (Martins-Filho *et al.*, 2020; Tang *et al.*, 2020; Tian *et al.*, 2020; Wu *et al.*, 2020a; Zhou *et al.*, 2020). Among 201 patients with COVID-19, increased levels of D-dimer were significantly associated with increased risk of both ARDS and death (Wu *et al.*, 2020a). In a multicenter retrospective cohort study from China, increased D-dimer levels (> 1µg/mL) were significantly associated with in-hospital death in the multivariable analysis. D-dimer levels also showed a sequential increase with time among non-survivors as against those who survived (Zhou *et al.*, 2020). In another retrospective study by Tang *et al.*, encompassing data from 183 consecutive patients with COVID-19, non-survivors had significantly higher D-dimer levels compared with survivors at initial evaluation (Tang *et al.*, 2020). Elevated D-dimer points towards the possibility of hyper-activation of the fibrinolytic system as an adaptive measure to counteract the hypercoagulable state induced by COVID-19. It could also imply an underlying state of compensated DIC (Terpos *et al.*, 2020).

Lastly, circulating blood cell counts can also help predict mortality. Significant lymphopenia in patients with COVID-19 often coincides with cytokine storm (Terpos *et al.*, 2020). Several factors may contribute to COVID-19 associated lymphopenia. Lymphocytes express ACE2 receptor on their membrane (Xu *et al.*, 2020); SARS-CoV-2 may directly infect them and lead to their lysis. Besides, the cytokine storm is characterized by markedly increased levels of interleukins and TNFα that may promote lymphocyte apoptosis (Terpos *et al.*, 2020). Cytokines may also lead to atrophy of lymphoid organs, like the spleen, and further impair lymphocyte turnover (Chan *et al.*, 2020). In addition, coexisting lactic acid acidosis may also impair lymphocyte proliferation (Fischer *et al.*, 2007). Whatever may be the underlying cause, lymphopenia is associated with severe disease (Guan *et al.*, 2020b; Huang *et al.*, 2020; Wang *et al.*, 2020), ARDS (Wu *et al.*, 2020b) and mortality in COVID-19 (Martins-Filho *et al.*, 2020; Ruan *et al.*, 2020). In addition, lymphocyte subtyping has shown that CD3+ CD8+ T-cell count ≤ 75 cell/µl is an independent predictor of mortality in COVID-19 (Du *et al.*, 2020). Apart from lymphocyte count, total leukocyte count and absolute neutrophil count have also been shown to predict mortality. Leukocytosis and neutrophilia have been reported to be associated with mortality in a few studies (Martins-Filho *et al.*, 2020; Ruan *et al.*, 2020; Wu *et al.*, 2020b).

CONCLUSION

The novel coronavirus disease (COVID-19) tends to be asymptomatic or mild in most of the patients. However, around 5% of the patients tend to have critical disease complicated by ARDS, shock and multiple organ failure. Mortality in COVID-19, as represented by the case-fatality rate, is around 6% (as of June 4, 2020) with maximum mortality being reported from the European nations. Respiratory failure ensuing from ARDS and pulmonary thromboembolism seem to be the most common cause of death in COVID-19. Advancing age and presence of comorbid illness are consistently associated with an increased risk of death, while certain biochemical and hematological parameters, notably C-reactive protein, IL-6, cardiac troponin, D-dimer and absolute count can also help predict mortality in patients with COVID-19.

ABBREVIATIONS

ACE2	Angiotensin converting enzyme 2
ARDS	Acute respiratory distress syndrome
CFR	Case-fatality rate
COVID-19	Novel coronavirus disease 2019
CRP	C-reactive protein
DM	Diabetes mellitus
DIC	Disseminated intravascular coagulation
DVT	Deep vein thrombosis
ICU	Intensive care unit

IL-6	Interleukin-6
MERS	Middle East Respiratory Syndrome
SARS	Sever Acute Respiratory Syndrome
WHO	World Health Organization

CONSENT FOR PUBLICATION

Not applicable.

CONFLICT OF INTEREST

The author declares no conflict of interest, financial or otherwise.

ACKNOWLEDGEMENTS

Declared none.

REFERENCES

Age, Sex, Existing Conditions of COVID-19 Cases and Deaths. https://www.worldometers.info/coronavirus/coronavirus-age-sex-demographics

Aziz, M, Fatima, R & Assaly, R (2020) Elevated interleukin-6 and severe COVID-19: A meta-analysis. *J Med Virol*, 92, 2283-5.
[http://dx.doi.org/10.1002/jmv.25948] [PMID: 32343429]

Batlle, D, Soler, MJ, Sparks, MA, Hiremath, S, South, AM, Welling, PA & Swaminathan, S COVID-19 and ACE2 in Cardiovascular, Lung, and Kidney Working Group (2020) Acute Kidney Injury in COVID-19: Emerging Evidence of a Distinct Pathophysiology. *J Am Soc Nephrol*, 31, 1380-3.
[http://dx.doi.org/10.1681/ASN.2020040419] [PMID: 32366514]

Becker, RC (2020) COVID-19 update: Covid-19-associated coagulopathy. *J Thromb Thrombolysis*, 50, 54-67.
[http://dx.doi.org/10.1007/s11239-020-02134-3] [PMID: 32415579]

Brake, SJ, Barnsley, K, Lu, W, McAlinden, KD, Eapen, MS & Sohal, SS (2020) Smoking Upregulates Angiotensin-Converting Enzyme-2 Receptor: A Potential Adhesion Site for Novel Coronavirus SARS-CoV-2 (Covid-19). *J Clin Med*, 9, 841.
[http://dx.doi.org/10.3390/jcm9030841] [PMID: 32244852]

Cariou, B, Hadjadj, S, Wargny, M, Pichelin, M, Al-Salameh, A, Allix, I, Amadou, C, Arnault, G, Baudoux, F, Bauduceau, B, Borot, S, Bourgeon-Ghittori, M, Bourron, O, Boutoille, D, Cazenave-Roblot, F, Chaumeil, C, Cosson, E, Coudol, S, Darmon, P, Disse, E, Ducet-Boiffard, A, Gaborit, B, Joubert, M, Kerlan, V, Laviolle, B, Marchand, L, Meyer, L, Potier, L, Prevost, G, Riveline, J-P, Robert, R, Saulnier, P-J, Sultan, A, Thébaut, J-F, Thivolet, C, Tramunt, B, Vatier, C, Roussel, R, Gautier, J-F & Gourdy, P CORONADO investigators (2020) Phenotypic characteristics and prognosis of inpatients with COVID-19 and diabetes: the CORONADO study. *Diabetologia*, 63, 1500-15.
[http://dx.doi.org/10.1007/s00125-020-05180-x] [PMID: 32472191]

Chan, JF-W, Zhang, AJ, Yuan, S, Poon, VK-M, Chan, CC-S, Lee, AC-Y, Chan, W-M, Fan, Z, Tsoi, H-W, Wen, L, Liang, R, Cao, J, Chen, Y, Tang, K, Luo, C, Cai, J-P, Kok, K-H, Chu, H, Chan, K-H, Sridhar, S, Chen, Z, Chen, H, To, KK-W & Yuen, K-Y (2020) Simulation of the clinical and pathological manifestations of Coronavirus Disease 2019 (COVID-19) in golden Syrian hamster model: implications for disease pathogenesis and transmissibility. *Clin Infect Dis*, 71, 2428-46.

[http://dx.doi.org/10.1093/cid/ciaa325] [PMID: 32215622]

Channappanavar, R & Perlman, S (2017) Pathogenic human coronavirus infections: causes and consequences of cytokine storm and immunopathology. *Semin Immunopathol,* 39, 529-39.
[http://dx.doi.org/10.1007/s00281-017-0629-x] [PMID: 28466096]

Chen, N, Zhou, M, Dong, X, Qu, J, Gong, F, Han, Y, Qiu, Y, Wang, J, Liu, Y, Wei, Y, Xia, J, Yu, T, Zhang, X & Zhang, L (2020) Epidemiological and clinical characteristics of 99 cases of 2019 novel coronavirus pneumonia in Wuhan, China: a descriptive study. *Lancet,* 395, 507-13.
[http://dx.doi.org/10.1016/S0140-6736(20)30211-7] [PMID: 32007143]

Chen, T, Wu, D, Chen, H, Yan, W, Yang, D, Chen, G, Ma, K, Xu, D, Yu, H, Wang, H, Wang, T, Guo, W, Chen, J, Ding, C, Zhang, X, Huang, J, Han, M, Li, S, Luo, X, Zhao, J & Ning, Q (2020) Clinical characteristics of 113 deceased patients with coronavirus disease 2019: retrospective study. *BMJ,* 368, m1091.
[http://dx.doi.org/10.1136/bmj.m1091] [PMID: 32217556]

Chertow, DS & Memoli, MJ (2013) Bacterial coinfection in influenza: a grand rounds review. *JAMA,* 309, 275-82.
[http://dx.doi.org/10.1001/jama.2012.194139] [PMID: 23321766]

Coperchini, F, Chiovato, L, Croce, L, Magri, F & Rotondi, M (2020) The cytokine storm in COVID-19: An overview of the involvement of the chemokine/chemokine-receptor system. *Cytokine Growth Factor Rev,* 53, 25-32.
[http://dx.doi.org/10.1016/j.cytogfr.2020.05.003] [PMID: 32446778]

Coronavirus (COVID-19) Available at: https://news.google.com/covid19/map?hl=en-IN&gl=IN&ceid=IN%3Aen

Coronavirus disease (2019) (COVID-19) Situation Report – 24. Available at: https://www.who.int/docs/default-source/coronaviruse/situation-reports/ 20200213-sitrep-24-covid-19.pdf?sfvrsn=9a7406a4_4

Coronavirus disease (2019) (COVID-19) Situation Report – 24. Available at: https://www.who.int/docs/default-source/coronaviruse/situation-reports/20200225-sitrep-36-covid-19.pdf?sfvrsn=2791b4e0_2

Coronavirus disease (COVID-19) Situation Report – 135. Available from: https://www.who.int/docs/default-source/coronaviruse/situation-reports/ 20200603-covid-19-sitrep-135.pdf?sfvrsn=39972feb_2

Coronavirus: Europe "wary of confronting China over deaths". Available from: https://www.bbc.com/news/world-asia-china-52404612

Danzi, GB, Loffi, M, Galeazzi, G & Gherbesi, E (2020) Acute pulmonary embolism and COVID-19 pneumonia: a random association? *Eur Heart J,* 41, 1858-8.
[http://dx.doi.org/10.1093/eurheartj/ehaa254] [PMID: 32227120]

Dietz, W & Santos-Burgoa, C (2020) Obesity and its Implications for COVID-19 Mortality. *Obesity (Silver Spring),* 28, 1005-5.
[http://dx.doi.org/10.1002/oby.22818] [PMID: 32237206]

Disease Burden of Influenza Available from: https://www.cdc.gov/flu/about/burden/index.html

Du, R-H, Liang, L-R, Yang, C-Q, Wang, W, Cao, T-Z, Li, M, Guo, G-Y, Du, J, Zheng, C-L, Zhu, Q, Hu, M, Li, X-Y, Peng, P & Shi, H-Z (2020) Predictors of mortality for patients with COVID-19 pneumonia caused by SARS-CoV-2: a prospective cohort study. *Eur Respir J,* 55, 2000524.
[http://dx.doi.org/10.1183/13993003.00524-2020] [PMID: 32269088]

Ebrahim, SH & Memish, ZA (2020) COVID-19: preparing for superspreader potential among Umrah pilgrims to Saudi Arabia. *Lancet,* 395, e48.
[http://dx.doi.org/10.1016/S0140-6736(20)30466-9] [PMID: 32113506]

Fan, BE, Chong, VCL, Chan, SSW, Lim, GH, Lim, KGE, Tan, GB, Mucheli, SS, Kuperan, P & Ong, KH (2020) Hematologic parameters in patients with COVID-19 infection. *Am J Hematol,* 95, E131-4.

[http://dx.doi.org/10.1002/ajh.25774] [PMID: 32129508]

Faust, JS & Del Rio, C (2020) Assessment of deaths from COVID-19 and from seasonal influenza. *JAMA Intern Med,* 180, 1045-6.
[http://dx.doi.org/10.1001/jamainternmed.2020.2306] [PMID: 32407441]

Ferrara, JL, Abhyankar, S & Gilliland, DG (1993) Cytokine Storm of graft-*versus*-host disease: a critical effector role for interleukin-1. *Transplantion Proceedings,* 25, 1216-7.

Fischer, K, Hoffmann, P, Voelkl, S, Meidenbauer, N, Ammer, J, Edinger, M, Gottfried, E, Schwarz, S, Rothe, G, Hoves, S, Renner, K, Timischl, B, Mackensen, A, Kunz-Schughart, L, Andreesen, R, Krause, SW & Kreutz, M (2007) Inhibitory effect of tumor cell-derived lactic acid on human T cells. *Blood,* 109, 3812-9.
[http://dx.doi.org/10.1182/blood-2006-07-035972] [PMID: 17255361]

García-Valero, J, Olloquequi, J, Montes, JF, Rodríguez, E, Martín-Satué, M, Texidó, L & Ferrer Sancho, J (2019) Deficient pulmonary IFN-β expression in COPD patients. *PLoS One,* 14, e0217803.
[http://dx.doi.org/10.1371/journal.pone.0217803] [PMID: 31170225]

Geerlings, SE & Hoepelman, AIM (1999) Immune dysfunction in patients with diabetes mellitus (DM). *FEMS Immunol Med Microbiol,* 26, 259-65.
[http://dx.doi.org/10.1111/j.1574-695X.1999.tb01397.x] [PMID: 10575137]

Guan, W., Liang, W., Zhao, Y., Liang, H., Chen, Zi-sheng, Li, Y., Liu, X., Chen, R., Tang, C., Wang, T., Ou, C., Li, L., Chen, P., Sang, L., Wang, W., Li, J., Li, C., Ou, L., Cheng, B., Xiong, S., Ni, Z., Xiang, J., Hu, Yu, Liu, L., Shan, H., Lei, C., Peng, Y., Wei, L., Liu, Y., Hu, Ya-hua, Peng, P., Wang, J., Liu, J., Chen, Zhong, Li, G., Zheng, Z., Qiu, S., Luo, J., Ye, C., Zhu, S., Cheng, L., Ye, F., Li, S., Zheng, J., Zhang, N., Zhong, N., He, J. (2020) Comorbidity and its impact on 1590 patients with Covid-19 in China: a nationwide analysis. *Eur Res J,* 2000547.

Guan, W., Ni, Z., Hu, Yu, Liang, W., Ou, C., He, J., Liu, L., Shan, H., Lei, C., Hui, D.S.C., Du, B., Li, L., Zeng, G., Yuen, K.-Y., Chen, R., Tang, C., Wang, T., Chen, P., Xiang, J., Li, S., Wang, Jin-lin, Liang, Z., Peng, Y., Wei, L., Liu, Y., Hu, Ya-hua, Peng, P., Wang, Jian-ming, Liu, J., Chen, Z., Li, G., Zheng, Z., Qiu, S., Luo, J., Ye, C., Zhu, S., Zhong, N. (2020) Clinical characteristics of coronavirus disease 2019 in China. *New Engl J Med,* 382, 1708-20.
[http://dx.doi.org/10.1056/NEJMoa2002032] [PMID: 32109013]

Guidance for appropriate recording of COVID-19 related deaths in India. Available at: https://www.ncdirindia.org/ Downloads/CoD_COVID-19_Guidance.pdf

Guo, T, Fan, Y, Chen, M, Wu, X, Zhang, L, He, T, Wang, H, Wan, J, Wang, X & Lu, Z (2020) Cardiovascular implications of fatal outcomes of patients with coronavirus disease 2019 (COVID-19). *JAMA Cardiol,* 5, 811-8.
[http://dx.doi.org/10.1001/jamacardio.2020.1017] [PMID: 32219356]

Guo, W, Li, M, Dong, Y, Zhou, H, Zhang, Z, Tian, C, Qin, R, Wang, H, Shen, Y, Du, K, Zhao, L, Fan, H, Luo, S & Hu, D (2020) Diabetes is a risk factor for the progression and prognosis of COVID-19. *Diabetes Metab Res Rev,* e3319.
[http://dx.doi.org/10.1002/dmrr.3319] [PMID: 32233013]

Gupta, AK, Jneid, H, Addison, D, Ardehali, H, Boehme, AK, Borgaonkar, S, Boulestreau, R, Clerkin, K, Delarche, N, DeVon, HA, Grumbach, IM, Gutierrez, J, Jones, DA, Kapil, V, Maniero, C, Mentias, A, Miller, PS, May Ng, S, Parekh, JD, Sanchez, RH, Teodor Sawicki, K & te Riele, SJM (2020) Current perspectives on coronavirus 2019 (COVID-19) and cardiovascular disease: A white paper by the JAHA editors. *J Am Heart Assoc,* 9, e017013.
[http://dx.doi.org/10.1161/JAHA.120.017013]

Huang, C, Wang, Y, Li, X, Ren, L, Zhao, J, Hu, Y, Zhang, L, Fan, G, Xu, J, Gu, X, Cheng, Z, Yu, T, Xia, J, Wei, Y, Wu, W, Xie, X, Yin, W, Li, H, Liu, M, Xiao, Y, Gao, H, Guo, L, Xie, J, Wang, G, Jiang, R, Gao, Z, Jin, Q, Wang, J & Cao, B (2020) Clinical features of patients infected with 2019 novel coronavirus in Wuhan, China. *Lancet,* 395, 497-506.
[http://dx.doi.org/10.1016/S0140-6736(20)30183-5] [PMID: 31986264]

Inaccurate COVID-19 death reporting can lower international health assistance. Available at: https://tbsnews.net/thoughts/inaccurate-covid-19-death-reporting-can-lower-international-health-assistance-87601#main-content

Inciardi, RM, Lupi, L, Zaccone, G, Italia, L, Raffo, M, Tomasoni, D, Cani, DS, Cerini, M, Farina, D, Gavazzi, E, Maroldi, R, Adamo, M, Ammirati, E, Sinagra, G, Lombardi, CM & Metra, M (2020) Cardiac involvement in a patient with coronavirus disease 2019 (COVID-19). *JAMA Cardiol,* 5, 819-24.
[http://dx.doi.org/10.1001/jamacardio.2020.1096] [PMID: 32219357]

Iran uses arrests Censorship to silence critical COVID-19 coverage. Available from: https://www.voanews.com/extremism-watch/iran-uses-arrests-censorship-silence-critical-covid-19-coverage

Jafar, N, Edriss, H & Nugent, K (2016) The effect of short-term hyperglycemia on the innate immune system. *Am J Med Sci,* 351, 201-11.
[http://dx.doi.org/10.1016/j.amjms.2015.11.011] [PMID: 26897277]

Jin, J-M, Bai, P, He, W, Wu, F, Liu, X-F, Han, D-M, Liu, S & Yang, J-K (2020) Gender differences in patients With COVID-19: focus on severity and mortality. *Frontiers in Public Health,* no. 8.

Kassir, R (2020) Risk of COVID-19 for patients with obesity. *Obes Rev,* 21, e13034.
[http://dx.doi.org/10.1111/obr.13034] [PMID: 32281287]

Klok, FA, Kruip, MJHA, van der Meer, NJM, Arbous, MS, Gommers, DAMPJ, Kant, KM, Kaptein, FHJ, van Paassen, J, Stals, MAM, Huisman, MV & Endeman, H (2020) Incidence of thrombotic complications in critically ill ICU patients with COVID-19. *Thromb Res,* 191, 145-7.
[http://dx.doi.org/10.1016/j.thromres.2020.04.013] [PMID: 32291094]

Lax, SF, Skok, K, Zechner, P, Kessler, HH, Kaufmann, N, Koelblinger, C, Vander, K, Bargfrieder, U & Trauner, M (2020) Pulmonary arterial thrombosis in COVID-19 with fatal outcome: results from a prospective, single-center, clinicopathologic case series. *Ann Intern Med,* 173, 350-61.
[http://dx.doi.org/10.7326/M20-2566] [PMID: 32422076]

Lippi, G & Henry, BM (2020) Active smoking is not associated with severity of coronavirus disease 2019 (COVID-19). *Eur J Intern Med,* 75, 107-8.
[http://dx.doi.org/10.1016/j.ejim.2020.03.014] [PMID: 32192856]

Lippi, G & Plebani, M (2020) Laboratory abnormalities in patients with COVID-2019 infection. *Clin Chem Lab Med,* 58, 1131-4.
[http://dx.doi.org/10.1515/cclm-2020-0198] [PMID: 32119647]

Liu, K, Chen, Y, Lin, R & Han, K (2020) Clinical features of COVID-19 in elderly patients: A comparison with young and middle-aged patients. *J Infect,* 80, e14-8.
[http://dx.doi.org/10.1016/j.jinf.2020.03.005] [PMID: 32171866]

Liu, Y, Gayle, AA, Wilder-Smith, A & Rocklöv, J (2020) The reproductive number of COVID-19 is higher compared to SARS coronavirus. *J Travel Med,* 27.
[http://dx.doi.org/10.1093/jtm/taaa021]

MacIntyre, CR, Chughtai, AA, Barnes, M, Ridda, I, Seale, H, Toms, R & Heywood, A (2018) The role of pneumonia and secondary bacterial infection in fatal and serious outcomes of pandemic influenza a (H1N1). *BMC Infect Dis,* 18.
[http://dx.doi.org/10.1186/s12879-018-3548-0]

Maier, CL, Truong, AD, Auld, SC, Polly, DM, Tanksley, C-L & Duncan, A (2020) COVID-19-associated hyperviscosity: a link between inflammation and thrombophilia? *Lancet,* 395, 1758-9.
[http://dx.doi.org/10.1016/S0140-6736(20)31209-5] [PMID: 32464112]

Martins-Filho, PR, Tavares, CSS & Santos, VS (2020) Factors associated with mortality in patients with COVID-19. A quantitative evidence synthesis of clinical and laboratory data. *Eur J Intern Med,* 76, 97-9.
[http://dx.doi.org/10.1016/j.ejim.2020.04.043] [PMID: 32345526]

McGonagle, D, Sharif, K, O'Regan, A & Bridgewood, C (2020) The role of cytokines including interleukin-6 in COVID-19 induced pneumonia and macrophage activation syndrome-like disease. *Autoimmune Rev,* 19, 102537.
[http://dx.doi.org/10.1016/j.autrev.2020.102537]

Middle East respiratory syndrome coronavirus (MERS-CoV). Available from: https://www.who.int/emergencies/mers-cov/en

Mortality Risk of COVID-19 Available at: https://ourworldindata.org/mortality-risk-covid#the-current--ase-fatality-rate-of-covid-19

Onder, G, Rezza, G & Brusaferro, S (2020) Case-fatality rate and characteristics of patients dying in relation to COVID-19 in Italy. *JAMA,* 323, 1775-6.
[http://dx.doi.org/10.1001/jama.2020.4683] [PMID: 32203977]

Pal, R (2020) COVID-19, hypothalamo-pituitary-adrenal axis and clinical implications. *Endocrine,* 68, 251-2.
[http://dx.doi.org/10.1007/s12020-020-02325-1] [PMID: 32346813]

Pal, R & Banerjee, M (2020) COVID-19 and the endocrine system: exploring the unexplored. *J Endocrinol Invest,* 43, 1027-31.
[http://dx.doi.org/10.1007/s40618-020-01276-8] [PMID: 32361826]

Pal, R & Bhadada, SK (2020) COVID-19 and non-communicable diseases. *Postgrad Med J,* postgradmedj-2020-137742 .
[http://dx.doi.org/10.1136/postgradmedj-2020-137742]

Pal, R & Bhadada, SK (2020) COVID-19 and diabetes mellitus: An unholy interaction of two pandemics. *Diabetes Metab Syndr,* 14, 513-7.
[http://dx.doi.org/10.1016/j.dsx.2020.04.049] [PMID: 32388331]

Pal, R & Bhadada, SK (2020) Should anti-diabetic medications be reconsidered amid COVID-19 pandemic? *Diab Res Clin Pract,* 108146.
[http://dx.doi.org/10.1016/j.diabres.2020.108146]

Pal, R & Bhansali, A (2020) COVID-19, diabetes mellitus and ACE2: the conundrum. *Diab Res Clin Pract,* 108132.
[http://dx.doi.org/10.1016/j.diabres.2020.108132]

Pneumonia of unknown cause – China. Available from: https://www.who.int/csr/don/05-january-20-0-pneumonia-of-unkown-cause-china/en (2020)

Richard, C, Wadowski, M, Goruk, S, Cameron, L, Sharma, AM & Field, CJ (2017) Individuals with obesity and type 2 diabetes have additional immune dysfunction compared with obese individuals who are metabolically healthy. *BMJ Open Diabetes Res Care,* 5, e000379.
[http://dx.doi.org/10.1136/bmjdrc-2016-000379] [PMID: 28761653]

Ruan, Q, Yang, K, Wang, W, Jiang, L & Song, J (2020) Clinical predictors of mortality due to COVID-19 based on an analysis of data of 150 patients from Wuhan, China. *Intensive Care Med,* 46, 846-8.
[http://dx.doi.org/10.1007/s00134-020-05991-x] [PMID: 32125452]

Schiffrin, EL, Flack, JM, Ito, S, Muntner, P & Webb, RC (2020) Hypertension and COVID-19. *Am J Hypertens,* 33, 373-4.
[http://dx.doi.org/10.1093/ajh/hpaa057] [PMID: 32251498]

Scialpi, M, Scialpi, S, Piscioli, I, Battista Scalera, G & Longo, F (2020) Pulmonary thromboembolism in critical ill COVID-19 patients. *Int J Infect Dis,* 95, 361-2.
[http://dx.doi.org/10.1016/j.ijid.2020.04.056] [PMID: 32339717]

Shi, S, Qin, M, Shen, B, Cai, Y, Liu, T, Yang, F, Gong, W, Liu, X, Liang, J, Zhao, Q, Huang, H, Yang, B & Huang, C (2020) Association of cardiac injury with mortality in hospitalized patients with COVID-19 in Wuhan, China. *JAMA Cardiol,* 5, 802-10.
[http://dx.doi.org/10.1001/jamacardio.2020.0950] [PMID: 32211816]

Siripanthong, B, Nazarian, S, Muser, D, Deo, R, Santangeli, P, Khanji, MY, Cooper, LT, Jr & Chahal, CAA (2020) Recognizing COVID-19-related myocarditis: The possible pathophysiology and proposed guideline for diagnosis and management. *Heart Rhythm,* 17, 1463-71.
[http://dx.doi.org/10.1016/j.hrthm.2020.05.001] [PMID: 32387246]

Spychalski, P, Błażyńska-Spychalska, A & Kobiela, J (2020) Estimating case fatality rates of COVID-19. *Lancet Infect Dis,* 20, 774-5.
[http://dx.doi.org/10.1016/S1473-3099(20)30246-2] [PMID: 32243815]

Summary of probable SARS cases with onset of illness from 1 November 2002 to 31 July 2003. Available from: https://www.who.int/csr/sars/country/table2004_04_21/en

Tang, N, Li, D, Wang, X & Sun, Z (2020) Abnormal coagulation parameters are associated with poor prognosis in patients with novel coronavirus pneumonia. *J Thromb Haemost,* 18, 844-7.
[http://dx.doi.org/10.1111/jth.14768] [PMID: 32073213]

Terpos, E, Ntanasis-Stathopoulos, I, Elalamy, I, Kastritis, E, Sergentanis, TN, Politou, M, Psaltopoulou, T, Gerotziafas, G & Dimopoulos, MA (2020) Hematological findings and complications of COVID-19. *Am J Hematol,* 95, 834-47.
[http://dx.doi.org/10.1002/ajh.25829] [PMID: 32282949]

Tian, W, Jiang, W, Yao, J, Nicholson, CJ, Li, RH, Sigurslid, HH, Wooster, L, Rotter, JI, Guo, X & Malhotra, R (2020) Predictors of mortality in hospitalized COVID-19 patients: A systematic review and meta-analysis. *J Med Virol,* 92, 1875-83.
[http://dx.doi.org/10.1002/jmv.26050] [PMID: 32441789]

Tikellis, C & Thomas, MC (2012) Angiotensin-converting enzyme 2 (ACE2) is a key modulator of the renin angiotensin system in health and disease. *Internal J Peptide Res Therapeut,* 1–8.
[http://dx.doi.org/10.1155/2012/256294]

Tisoncik, JR, Korth, MJ, Simmons, CP, Farrar, J, Martin, TR & Katze, MG (2012) Into the eye of the cytokine storm. *Microbiol Mol Biol Rev,* 76, 16-32.
[http://dx.doi.org/10.1128/MMBR.05015-11] [PMID: 22390970]

Vardavas, C & Nikitara, K (2020) COVID-19 and smoking: A systematic review of the evidence. *Tobacco Ind Dis,* 18.
[http://dx.doi.org/10.18332/tid/119324]

Vincent, J-L & Taccone, FS (2020) Understanding pathways to death in patients with COVID-19. *Lancet Respir Med,* 8, 430-2.
[http://dx.doi.org/10.1016/S2213-2600(20)30165-X] [PMID: 32272081]

Wang, D, Hu, B, Hu, C, Zhu, F, Liu, X, Zhang, J, Wang, B, Xiang, H, Cheng, Z, Xiong, Y, Zhao, Y, Li, Y, Wang, X & Peng, Z (2020) Clinical characteristics of 138 hospitalized patients with 2019 novel coronavirus-infected pneumonia in Wuhan, China. *JAMA,* 323, 1061-9.
[http://dx.doi.org/10.1001/jama.2020.1585] [PMID: 32031570]

Wang, F Wang, Haizhou, Fan, J., Zhang, Y., Wang, Hongling, Zhao, Q., (2020), Pancreatic injury patterns in patients with COVID-19 pneumonia. *Gastroenterology,* 159, 367-70.
[http://dx.doi.org/10.1053/j.gastro.2020.03.055] [PMID: 32247022]

Wang, G, Wu, Chenfang, Zhang, Q, Zhang, Q, Wu, F, Yu, B, Lv, J & Li, Y (2020) Li T, Zhang S, Wu C, Wu G, Zhong Y. C-reactive protein level may predict the risk of COVID-19 aggravation. *Open Forum Infect Dis,* ofaa153.
[http://dx.doi.org/10.1093/ofid/ofaa153] [PMID: 32455147]

WHO Director-General's opening remarks at the media briefing on COVID-19 (2020) Available from: https://www.who.int/dg/speeches/detail/who-director-general-s-opening-remarks-at-the-media-briefing-on-covid-19-3-march-2020

Wichmann, D, Sperhake, J-P, Lütgehetmann, M, Steurer, S, Edler, C, Heinemann, A, Heinrich, F, Mushumba, H, Kniep, I, Schröder, AS, Burdelski, C, de Heer, G, Nierhaus, A, Frings, D, Pfefferle, S, Becker,

H, Bredereke-Wiedling, H, de Weerth, A, Paschen, H-R, Sheikhzadeh-Eggers, S, Stang, A, Schmiedel, S, Bokemeyer, C, Addo, MM, Aepfelbacher, M, Püschel, K & Kluge, S (2020) Autopsy findings and venous thromboembolism in patients with COVID-19: A prospective cohort study. *Ann Intern Med,* 173, 268-77.
[http://dx.doi.org/10.7326/M20-2003] [PMID: 32374815]

Wu, C, Chen, X, Cai, Y, Xia, J, Zhou, X, Xu, S, Huang, H, Zhang, L, Zhou, X, Du, C, Zhang, Y, Song, J, Wang, S, Chao, Y, Yang, Z, Xu, J, Zhou, X, Chen, D, Xiong, W, Xu, L, Zhou, F, Jiang, J, Bai, C, Zheng, J & Song, Y (2020) Risk factors associated with acute respiratory distress syndrome and death in patients with coronavirus disease 2019 pneumonia in Wuhan, China. *JAMA Intern Med,* 180, 934-43.
[http://dx.doi.org/10.1001/jamainternmed.2020.0994] [PMID: 32167524]

Wu, Z & McGoogan, JM (2020) Characteristics of and important lessons from the coronavirus disease 2019 (COVID-19) outbreak in China: summary of a report of 72 314 cases from the chinese center for disease control and prevention. *JAMA,* 323, 1239-42.
[http://dx.doi.org/10.1001/jama.2020.2648] [PMID: 32091533]

Xie, J, Covassin, N, Fan, Z, Singh, P, Gao, W, Li, G, Kara, T & Somers, VK (2020) Association between hypoxemia and mortality in patients with COVID-19. *Mayo Clin Proc,* 95, 1138-47.
[http://dx.doi.org/10.1016/j.mayocp.2020.04.006] [PMID: 32376101]

Xie, Y, Wang, X, Yang, P & Zhang, S (2020) COVID-19 complicated by acute pulmonary embolism. *Radiol Cardiothorac Imag,* 2, e200067.
[http://dx.doi.org/10.1148/ryct.2020200067]

Xu, H, Zhong, L, Deng, J, Peng, J, Dan, H, Zeng, X, Li, T & Chen, Q (2020) High expression of ACE2 receptor of 2019-nCoV on the epithelial cells of oral mucosa. *Int J Oral Sci,* 12, 8.
[http://dx.doi.org/10.1038/s41368-020-0074-x] [PMID: 32094336]

Xu, Z, Shi, L, Wang, Y, Zhang, J, Huang, L, Zhang, C, Liu, S, Zhao, P, Liu, H, Zhu, L, Tai, Y, Bai, C, Gao, T, Song, J, Xia, P, Dong, J, Zhao, J & Wang, F-S (2020) Pathological findings of COVID-19 associated with acute respiratory distress syndrome. *Lancet Respir Med,* 8, 420-2.
[http://dx.doi.org/10.1016/S2213-2600(20)30076-X] [PMID: 32085846]

Yang, X, Yu, Y, Xu, J, Shu, H, Xia, J, Liu, H, Wu, Y, Zhang, L, Yu, Z, Fang, M, Yu, T, Wang, Y, Pan, S, Zou, X, Yuan, S & Shang, Y (2020) Clinical course and outcomes of critically ill patients with SARS-CoV-2 pneumonia in Wuhan, China: a single-centered, retrospective, observational study. *Lancet Respir Med,* 8, 475-81.
[http://dx.doi.org/10.1016/S2213-2600(20)30079-5] [PMID: 32105632]

Zhang, C, Wu, Z, Li, J-W, Zhao, H & Wang, G-Q (2020) Cytokine release syndrome in severe COVID-19: interleukin-6 receptor antagonist tocilizumab may be the key to reduce mortality. *Int J Antimicrob Agents,* 55, 105954.
[http://dx.doi.org/10.1016/j.ijantimicag.2020.105954] [PMID: 32234467]

Zhang, W, Zhao, Y, Zhang, F, Wang, Q, Li, T, Liu, Z, Wang, J, Qin, Y, Zhang, X, Yan, X, Zeng, X & Zhang, S (2020) The use of anti-inflammatory drugs in the treatment of people with severe coronavirus disease 2019 (COVID-19): The Perspectives of clinical immunologists from China. *Clin Immunol,* 214, 108393.
[http://dx.doi.org/10.1016/j.clim.2020.108393]

Zhao, Q, Meng, M, Kumar, R, Wu, Y, Huang, J, Lian, N, Deng, Y & Lin, S (2020) The impact of COPD and smoking history on the severity of COVID-19: A systemic review and meta-analysis. *J Med Virol,* 92, 1915-21.
[http://dx.doi.org/10.1002/jmv.25889] [PMID: 32293753]

Zhou, F, Yu, T, Du, R, Fan, G, Liu, Y, Liu, Z, Xiang, J, Wang, Y, Song, B, Gu, X, Guan, L, Wei, Y, Li, H, Wu, X, Xu, J, Tu, S, Zhang, Y, Chen, H & Cao, B (2020) Clinical course and risk factors for mortality of adult inpatients with COVID-19 in Wuhan, China: a retrospective cohort study. *Lancet,* 395, 1054-62.
[http://dx.doi.org/10.1016/S0140-6736(20)30566-3] [PMID: 32171076]

Zhou, P, Liu, Z, Chen, Y, Xiao, Y, Huang, X & Fan, X-G (2020) Bacterial and fungal infections in COVID-19 patients: A matter of concern. *Infect Control Hosp Epidemiol,* 1–2.

CHAPTER 4

Long Term Complications of COVID-19

Ankita Sood[1], Bimlesh Kumar[1,*], Indu Melkani[1], Archit Sood[2], Pankaj Prashar[1], Anamika Gautam[1], Kardam Joshi[3] and Dhara Patel[3]

[1] *School of Pharmaceutical Sciences, Lovely Professional University, Phagwara, Punjab, India*

[2] *Punjab University, Chandigarh, Punjab, India*

[3] *Topicals Research and Development, Amneal Pharmaceuticals, Piscataway, New Jersey, USA*

Abstract: Coronavirus disease 2019 (COVID-19) is an acute respiratory illness. It is caused by a novel coronavirus (SARS-CoV-2). It has gained widespread recognition after it originated from China. The World Health Organisation (WHO) declared the outbreak of COVID-19 as an international public health emergency. Patients of COVID-19 develop long-time complications along with severe health problems as it majorly affects the respiratory system, utilizing angiotensin-converting enzyme 2. Characteristic symptoms include fever, cough, and dyspnea, although some patients may be asymptomatic. People need extensive care to be protected from anxiety and depression. This outbreak harmed various organ systems and led to the development of long-term complications such as respiratory failure, pneumonia, pancreatic complications, cardiac injury, secondary infections, renal disorders, disseminated intravascular coagulation, and rhabdomyolysis. Individuals with comorbidities are at higher risk of illness and mortality. The risk is also increasing in older people, especially people the age of 60-80 years or more. The most prevalent comorbidities are asthma, neurologic disorders, diabetes, obesity, cardiovascular disease, and malignancy/hematologic conditions. As there is no specific treatment available so far, therefore complications of this disease are also increased by the use of non-specific drugs. The recovery of these patients is another major challenge for health care professionals. So in this chapter, we will discuss long-term complications associated with COVID-19.

Keywords: Cardiovascular diseases, Coronavirus, COVID-19, Diabetes, Mortality, Neurological effect, Pandemic, Renal effect, Respiratory effect, Rheumatoid arthritis.

INTRODUCTION

The latest coronavirus 2019 (2019-nCoV) or SARS-COV-2, a respiratory synd-

---

* **Corresponding author Bimlesh Kumar:** School of Pharmaceutical Sciences, Lovely Professional University, Jalandhar, Punjab, India; Fax: +91-1824-240830; Tel: +919872260354;
E-mails: bimlesh1Pharm@gmail.com and bimlesh.12474@lpu.co.in

Neeraj Mittal, Sanjay Kumar Bhadada, O. P. Katare and Varun Garg (Eds.)

rome, has rapidly spread from the Wuhan Town of Hubei, China, to the rest of the world. Coronavirus 2019 (COVID-19) is a consequence of severe acute respiratory syndrome that is now a significant concern for global public safety and local communities (Li *et al.*, 2020b). More importantly, following considerable initiatives and a rising number of remedies in China, the disease has now started to spread from China to Europe, North America, and other Asian countries (Wu and McGoogan, 2020). Coronavirus is a positive-sense RNA virus with spike-like projections having a diameter of about 60-140 nm. Under the electron microscope, it shows its crown-like appearance; thus, the term coronavirus has been used for it. There are four different types of coronaviruses (HKU1, NL63, 229E, and OC43). They are responsible for causing mild respiratory diseases in humans (Singhal, 2020). If an individual is suffering from COVID-19, their clinical symptoms range from asymptomatic disease to respiratory failure and finally leading to multiple organ dysfunction. Such kind of developed complication leads to the death of patients. The commonest health symptoms in COVID-19 include fever, cough, headache, sore throat, myalgia, fatigue, and respiratory illness. Conjunctivitis is also reported in some of the patients of COVID-19. Therefore it is difficult to distinguish this from other respiratory infections (Lima, 2020).

By the completion of the first week after the reports of the spread of COVID-19, cases of pneumonia, respiratory failure, and death were reported. This breakthrough is related to the significant increase in inflammatory cytokines like IL2, IL7, IL10, and TNFα. A person of any age group is susceptible to this disease. Symptomatic patients of COVID-19 release their large droplets through cough and sneezing. These incidences cause the spreading of infection of COVID-19. This spread of infection may also arise from asymptomatic individuals even before the occurrence of symptoms. In contrast with the mouth, higher viral loads have been observed in the nasal cavity. Moreover, patients can remain contagious as long as the virus survives in them, and also after they are fully recovered (Wu *et al.*, 2020a, Singhal, 2020). The development of such a condition of infection is due to the passing of the virus through the mucous membranes. It enters the human body through nasal and larynx mucosa. After that, it enters into the lungs through the respiratory tract. As a result of this, fever and cough are the most common symptoms of infection to appear. Further, it causes viremia when it invades into peripheral blood through the lungs. Then the virus attacks the targeting organs that express Angiotensin-converting enzyme 2 (ACE2), such as the lungs, heart, renal, gastrointestinal tract. The fecal samples have also been found to have evidence of SARS-CoV-2. The reason behind this detection is due to the entry of this virus takes place through the lung to blood and then it propagates from the blood to the intestines. During the process of infection, the count of white blood cells is normally or slightly less in peripheral blood at an early stage only. But as time progresses the lymphopenia is observed in patients (Cheng *et al.,* 2020a). The critical stage is appearing in this disease as a reduction of B lymphocyte occurs in the early stage of this disease only, which may affect the production of antibodies. It is also noticed that the patients having a severe stage of the COVID-19 reduction of lymphocytes significantly takes place (Cheng *et al.,* 2020a). The increased level of neutrophils, D-Dimer, blood urea nitrogen, and creatinine was reported in non-survivors than the survivors. Based on these recently reported facts and assumptions, the clinical stages can be divided as follows:

a. The viremia stage.
b. The acute stage (pneumonia phase) and
c. The recovery stage (Guan *et al.*, 2020, Wang *et al.*, 2020a, Letko *et al.*, 2020).

The coronavirus disease pandemic is causing significant morbidity and mortality in patients having a long history of any diseases associated with primary disease. Older age, diabetes mellitus, cancer, chronic kidney disease, rheumatoid arthritis, hypertension, and obesity greatly raise the likelihood of hospitalization and mortality in patients with COVID-19 (Guo *et al.*, 2020a). In this context, we explore the long-term complications of COVID-19 in patients suffering from various diseases.

LONG TERM COMPLICATIONS OF COVID-19

The meaning of the long history of diseases is chronic complications and it can be defined as the clinical state of suffering that tends to arise over the years and persists for decades. In this, patients used to suffer from not only the various complications of primary diseases but also secondary or multiple diseased states. Even though a large number of people are impacted by the COVID-19 pandemic, the most vulnerable are the aged, under-represented minorities, and underlying diseases. The increasing consumption of an unhealthy diet with excessive amounts of saturated fats, carbohydrates, and sugar persuade the pervasiveness of obesity and type 2 kind of diabetes and may raise the likelihood of seriousness of COVID-19 disease and its mortality (Butler and Barrientos, 2020). A healthy diet is very important for the development of immunity. Immunity and lifestyle (daily habit of food intake) are related to each other. So if the person taking an unhealthy diet or careless about the daily nutritious diet intake invites stimulation of the innate immune response and impairment of adaptive immunity which is inducing persistent inflammation, and finally brings disruption of the host defense system. Besides, the long-standing impact of peripheral inflammation induced by COVID-19 contributes to chronic medical disorders such as neurodegenerative disorder and dementia. These conditions are developed possibly through

Long Term Complications   *COVID-19: Diagnosis and Management-Part II* **99**

neuroinflammatory pathways, which can be accelerated by an unhealthy diet (Connaughton *et al.*, 2016).

All these diseases are responsible for long-term complications of COVID-19 (Table **1**). Moreover, there is no specific treatment of COVID-19 available so far therefore various nonspecific drugs that are used nowadays also lead to serious complications. Pre-exposure prophylaxis or post-exposure vaccination is not yet authorized. At this moment, there is no approved specific antiviral therapy for is available for COVID-19. The medication is given to the patients is primarily symptomatic and in special circumstances respiratory medication and ventilator assistance being the primary recovery methods for severely infected patients. Supported mechanical ventilation is essential for the prevention of respiratory collapse in serious patients. Hemodynamic assistance is provided to treat circulatory dysfunction and a septic diseased state (Wu and McGoogan, 2020). In the absence of any FDA-approved COVID-19 therapies, several physicians and scientists are shifting to established medicines for the prevention or treatment of the disease (Harrison, 2020). Many medicines that have been studied based on hypothesis or insufficient data include antiviral (Lopinavir, Ritonavir, and Remdesivir), monoclonal antibodies (Tocilizumab), chloroquine/Hydroxychloro-quine, arbidol, and azithromycin, *etc.*, which have multiple side effects and toxicities even they are failed to provide relief to the patients. Hence, other studies have pointed out that repurposing of some drugs, rationalized identification and strict clinical testing may provide a step forward for the treatment of COVID-19. These drugs could be chloroquine, hydroxychloroquine, and Azithromycin, as well as anti-diabetics such as metformin, angiotensin receptor inhibitors such as sartans, or statins such as simvastatin (Nabirotchkin *et al.*, 2020), Human immunoglobulin, Darunavir-cobicistat combination, Recombinant human interferon α2β, Carrimycin or lopinavir-ritonavir or arbidol or chloroquine phosphate, Danoprevir-ritonavir and interferon inhalation or lopinavir-ritonavir or TCM plus interferon inhalation, Xiyanping or lopinavir-ritonavir-interferon inhalation, Thalidomide, Vitamin C, Pirfenidone and Methylprednisolone, *etc.* (Rosa and Santos, 2020, Mercorelli *et al.*, 2018).

Table 1. Complications in patients with COVID-19.

No. of Patients	Diabetes (%)	HTN (%)	CVD (%)	COPD (%)	CKD (%)	Reference
1099	7.4	15.0	3.8	1.1	0.7	(Guan *et al.*, 2019)
7162	10.9	-	9.0	9.2	3	(Gangopadhyay, 2020)
138	10.1	31.2	19.6	2.9	2.9	(Wang *et al.*, 2020a)
191	19.0	30	8.0[+]	3.0	1.0	(Zhou *et al.*, 2020a)

(Table 1) cont.....

No. of Patients	Diabetes (%)	HTN (%)	CVD (%)	COPD (%)	CKD (%)	Reference
201	10.9	19.4	4.0	2.5	1.0	(Wu *et al.*, 2020a)
140	12.1	30	8.6	1.4	1.4	(Zhang *et al.*, 2020a)

[a] Dead COVID-19 Patients, [+] coronary heart disease only, CVD-cardiovascular disease, HTN-Hypertension, CKD-chronic kidney disease, COPD-chronic obstructive pulmonary disease.

COMPLICATIONS OF COVID-19 IN VARIOUS DISEASES

Diabetes Mellitus (DM)

Older age groups and the presence of diabetes mellitus (DM), extreme obesity, and hypertension (HTN) have now been well-known to raise morbidity and mortality in COVID-19 patients. Despite the increased incidence of cardiovascular diseases (CVD), HTN, and obesity, in DM patients, it is unclear whether DM individually leads to an elevated risk. However, plasma glucose and DM are acting as a predictor for mortality and morbidity separately for Severe Acute Respiratory Syndrome (SARS) patients. Potential pathways are represented in Fig. (**1**). May cause elevation of COVID-19 responsiveness in DM patients. It involves viruses that have:

a. High cellular entry (in terms of its affinity and efficiency)
b. Reduction of its clearance and reduction in the function of T cells
c. Increased sensitivity to hyper-inflammation as well as cytokine storm syndrome; and
d. Presence of CVD (Muniyappa and Gubbi, 2020).

The binding of SARS-CoV-2 at a cellular level is supported by an increase in expression of ACE2 in alveolary AT2 cells, kidney, myocardium, and pancreas. Its excessive expression was investigated and reported in the liver, intestine, heart, and pancreas when the preclinical evaluation was conducted in diabetic animals. Further, it was also reported that insulin therapy causes suppression inactivation of ACE2. On the other hand, glucagon-like peptide 1 (GLP-1) agonists, ACE inhibitors, and statins are known to use as hypoglycemic medication increase the expression of ACE2 (Guo *et al.*, 2020b). Till now, it was not clear that DM was causally related to ACE2 expression in humans in the lung. But recently Rao *et al.* studied that diseases or their characteristics could induce a rise in ACE2 expression in the lungs and found that DM. It was also indicated that it is correlated with increased expression of ACE2 in the lungs. It is also found that Furin, a cell protease promotes viral entry through the breakdown of the S1 and S2 spike protein and the level of this is also increased in the patient of DM (Rao *et al.*, 2020). ACE is responsible for the conversion of angiotensin (Ang) I to octapeptide, Ang II. ACE2 causes the transformation of Ang II to Ang1–7. Ang II causes Vasoconstriction and proliferation kind of activity performed by Ang II *via* stimulation of Ang II type 1a. On the other hand, it is very important to note that Ang1–7causes vasodilation with the reduction of proliferation of cells. The increased pulmonary ratio of ACE/ACE2, favors the development of Ang II in patients of respiratory distress syndrome (ARDS) (Wösten-van Asperen *et al.*, 2013, Kuba *et al.*, 2005). SARS-CoV causes decreases in the expression of ACE2 but the non-opposed activity of Ang II leads to lung damage. The ACE2 attachment alone will not do significant harm to the heart, as can be seen with other CoVs (NL63) (Case *et al.*, 2010). The evidence about SARS-CoV-2 triggers the pulmonary downregulation of ACE2 is still uncertain and imprecise. In the absence of more risk or benefit data, the United States Heart Association as well as the American Society of Hypertension advised the patients to start their regular antihypertensive treatment (Danser *et al.*, 2020).

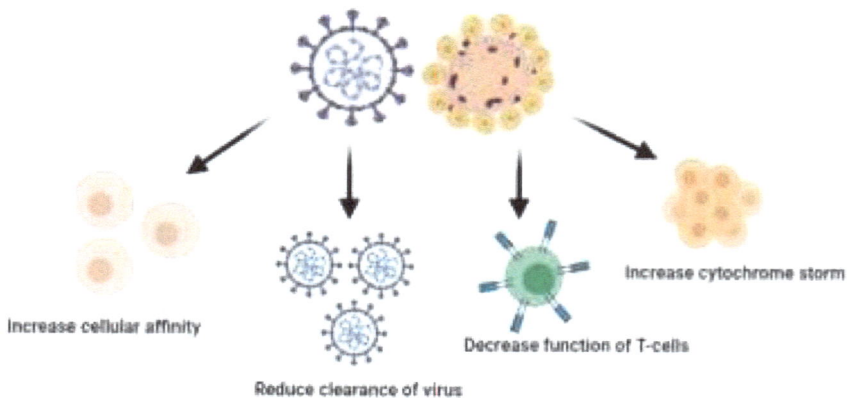

Fig. (1). Influence of COVID-19 in patients of diabetes.

Moreover, diabetes is a metabolic disorder and its complications are so vast that it can not only cause vascular diseases but also responsible to develop the chronic inflammatory disease. In case of infection with DM can impair pathogenic responses of individuals. The chronic inflammatory responses in the case of DM are because of the appearance of glycosylation (AGE), pro-inflammatory cytokines lead to evoke oxidative stress, as well as activation of adhesive molecules. This condition can be more aggravated with an increase in hyperglycemia and insulin resistance (Knapp, 2013). The inflammatory cycle contributing to higher infection susceptibility, this is worse in diabetes patients.

Several immune deficiencies have been attributed to hyperglycemia, but the therapeutic significance of these *in vitro* abnormalities remains uncertain (Petrie *et al.*, 2018). Poorly regulated diabetes has been associated with the suppressed proliferative lymphocyte response to various forms of stimuli, as well as the disrupted activities of macrophages and neutrophils. In patients having diabetes, irregular hypersensitivity reaction, and disruption in complement activation were also identified (Geerlings and Hoepelman, 1999). An increase in influenza virus infection, as well as its replication, was observed in *in vitro* experiments in which lung epithelial cells have also shown access to elevated glucose cells. This experiment suggesting that hyperglycemia can increase *in vivo* viral replication(Kohio and Adamson, 2013). Structural pulmonary modifications in animal models have been connected to diabetes, such as increased permeability of the vasculature and also the disintegrated alveolar epithelium. Forced vital capacity and forced expiratory volumes are related to the increased glucose level in the blood. Patients with DM typically have a significant decrease in their forced vital capacity and forced expiratory volumes (Popov and Simionescu, 1997, Lange *et al.*, 1989). There are no data available so far for the effective management of SARS-CoV-2 in diabetes patients and no treatment approach also available for COVID-19 patients who develop glycaemic decompensation. Rigorous control of glucose and careful consideration of drug reactions may reduce the severity of symptoms and adverse effects. While hyperglycemia is typically the major concern, in this case, the risk for hypoglycemic episodes should not be ignored due to the relationship between medication usage, viral pathogenesis, and normal diabetes metabolic disturbances. Patient treatment approaches and optimal control thresholds of glucose should be developed based on disease seriousness, co-existence and risks, age, and other aspects correlated with diabetes (Zhang *et al.*, 2020a). In Wuhan, China, 258 confirmed COVID-19 patients who suffered from diabetes had a significant increase level of leukocyte, neutrophil with higher levels of fasting blood glucose, serum creatinine, urea nitrogen, and creatine kinase isoenzyme MB in comparison with non-diabetic patients (Zhang *et al.*, 2020b). In Hong Kong also patients who suffered from diabetes had an increased mortality rate from pneumonia. The age of these patients was observed as ≥ 75 and reported to have CVD and cancer causes increases in the risk of mortality (Bloomgarden, 2020). Hence, during the prolonged hospitalization and recovery periods, a collaborative team strategy, involving infectologists, endocrinologists, lung biologists, psychiatrists, nutritionists, and fitness therapy specialists, can be essential. Special attention should be paid to diabetes nephropathic patients or heart disorders related to diabetes (Hussain *et al.*, 2020) as it can be fatal.

Hematological Complications

In the case of viremia, SARS-CoV-2 prominently damages the tissues responsible to express elevated ACE2. It generally takes place in the lungs, heart, and gastrointestinal tract. As the day progresses initial symptoms become worst and it is observed from day 7 to 14. Further, an unexpected rise in other clinical manifestations also occurs. It is characterized by the systemic surge of inflammatory mediators and cytokines storm. This is the time when significant lymphopenia becomes evident in patients. Here the meaning of cytokine storm can be stated as an abnormal increase in the levels of interleukins. The components that take part in this storm are helpful to promote the apoptosis of lymphocytes. It includes IL-2, 6, and 7, granulocyte colony-stimulating factor, interferon-γ inducible protein 10, MCP-1, MIP1-a, and TNF-α. (Li *et al.*, 2020d, Xu *et al.*, 2020a, Singh *et al.*, 2014, Liao *et al.*, 2002). COVID-19 is a systemic infection that affects the hematopoietic and hemostasis systems significantly. Lymphopenia is considered as a cardinal laboratory observation having prognostic value. The ratio and amount of neutrophil/lymphocytes can also be used to determine severe cases (Table **2**). Coagulation disorders are fairly common among patients with COVID-19, especially those with severe disease. During the first 2 months of an outbreak in China, the longitudinal multi-center analysis showed that 260 out of 560 patients having COVID-19 was confirmed with an increased level of D-dimer and the elevation was more prominent in severe patients (Guan *et al.*, 2020). Sepsis is another factor to be considered in patients with a severe case of COVID-19.

Table 2. Impact of COVID-19 on lymphocyte count.

Location	Duration of Study	No. of Patients	Identifying Features	Remarks	References
General Hospital of Central Theater Command, Wuhan, China	-	90	Lymphocytes at time point 1. day 10-12 from symptom onset (>20% or < 20%) and on day 17-19 (>20%, 5-20%, and < 5%).	Pre-severe disease state was observed at time point 1 while on time point 2 it turns to critical illness.	(Tan *et al.*, 2020)

(Table 2) cont.....

Location	Duration of Study	No. of Patients	Identifying Features	Remarks	References
Tongji Hospital, Hankou branch of Central Hospital Wuhan, China	1 Jan 2020 to 21 February 2020	-	Lower lymphocyte count (median: 0.63) at admission . Non-survivors have a lower lymphocyte/WBC ratio (median: 7.10)	A significantly lower level of lymphocytes was observed in the non-survivor group of patients The lymphocyte/WBC ratio decreased continuously from the time of admission to death during hospitalization.	(Deng *et al.*, 2020)
Seattle region, Washington State, USA	24 February 2020, to 9 March 2020	24 ICU patients	Lymphocyte counts were a continuous variable	The exact causes of lymphocytopenia were not provided.	(Bhatraju *et al.*, 2020)
Evergreen Hospital, Washington State, USA	20 February 2020, to 5 March 2020	21 ICU patients	Less than 1000 cells/µL	Low lymphocyte count was observed in 67% of critically ill patients.	(Arentz *et al.*, 2020)
Jinyintan Hospital and Wuhan Pulmonary Hospital, Wuhan, China	25 December 2019, to 31 January 2020	191	Lymphocyte counts treated as a continuous variable ($\times 10^9$/L)	Lower lymphocyte count was associated with higher odds of death at the univariate analysis.	(Zhou *et al.*, 2020a)
Jinyintan Hospital, Wuhan, China	24 December 2019, to 9 February 2020	52 critically ill patients		85% of lymphocytopenia in critically ill patients	(Yang *et al.*, 2020)
National Centre for Infectious Diseases, Singapore	23 January to 28 February 2020	69	Lymphocyte count =<0.5×10^9/L.	Lymphopenia at admission (4/9 of ICU patients vs 1/58 non-ICU patients, $P < .001$) and nadir lymphopenia during hospital stay (7/9 of ICU patients vs 1/58 non-ICU patients, $P < .001$) were associated with the need for ICU.	(Fan *et al.*, 2020)

It leads to increased activation of neutrophils, delaying of apoptosis, depletion with the exhaustion of CD4 and CD8 T cells in patients having the severe condition of COVID-19(van der Poll *et al.*, 2017, Zhou *et al.*, 2020c). The level of disseminated intravascular coagulation (DIC) can be measured to check the condition of sepsis in patients. It was observed that the DIC level increases in nonsurvivors of COVID-19. Similarly, sepsis-induced coagulopathy (SIC) is a newly proposed category of global coagulation tests, which has been established as an early warning signal of DIC. Hence, hematological parameters might provide a method for classifying the severity of COVID-19 and the SIC scoring system might be a useful tool to manage critically ill patients (Iba *et al.*, 2020, Liao *et al.*, 2020).

The dynamics of the D-dimer can represent severity and are associated with increased rates of adverse effects for community-acquired patients. Hypercoagulation of the blood is normal in COVID-19 patients. High rates of D-Dimers and its gradual rise during disease are regularly recorded particularly linked with the worsening of disease (Snijders *et al.*, 2012). SARS-CoV-2 is likely to boost a massive increase in fibrin formation and its deposition. It causes a very high level of D-dimer in these patients. Hence, deposition of fibrin in the alveolar sac and interstitial lung spaces may contribute to worsening of respiratory condition which turns to its failure and advocates prolonged mechanical ventilation, poor prognosis, and death (Tang *et al.*, 2020, Spiezia *et al.*, 2020). Some abnormalities of coagulation contribute to life-threatening conditions. It includes an increase in fibrin degradation products with severe intravascular thrombocytopenia which disseminated intravascular coagulation. This shows that hospital-based and ambulatory COVID-19 infected patients are at elevated risk for venous thromboembolism. Apart from this, venous thromboembolism was also recorded in 20% to 69% of patients with extreme COVID-19 and may be linked to poor prognosis. Warm or cold autoimmune hemolytic anemia has been documented after the beginning of COVID-19 symptoms that may be due to cytokine release syndrome (Fig. **2**). It is still not clear whether hemolytic anemia is correlated with COVID-19 infection or not (Lazarian *et al.*, 2020). On the other hand, venous thromboembolism was recorded in 20% to 69% of patients with extreme COVID-19 and may be linked to poor prognosis. Pulmonary embolism in 23% of patients at one US center and 20% to 30% of patients in France were also recorded (Llitjos *et al.*, 2020). Such patients were more likely to require intensive treatment and artificial ventilation than those having no pulmonary embolism (Fig. **3**). The level of D-dimer changes from mild to a significant level as per the occurrence and development of dyspnoea as well as chest imaging changes from mild to severe. It is also very important to note that these fluctuations also affect the prolongation of prothrombin time and a gradual decrease of fibrinogen with platelet.

The identification of patients at high risk with the COVID-19 is essential for the implementation of venous thromboembolism prophylaxis measures (van Nieuwkoop, 2020). Ischemic changes comprise ecchymosis of the fingers and toes. In many non-survivors of ischemic changes, it has been clinically observed that they were also suffered from the worse condition of kidney and heart function. Hence, it is indicated that early anticoagulation may be the reason for the blocking of clot formation and causes the reduction of microthrombus. It causes a decrease in the risk of major organ damages (Li, 2020, Lin *et al.*, 2020).

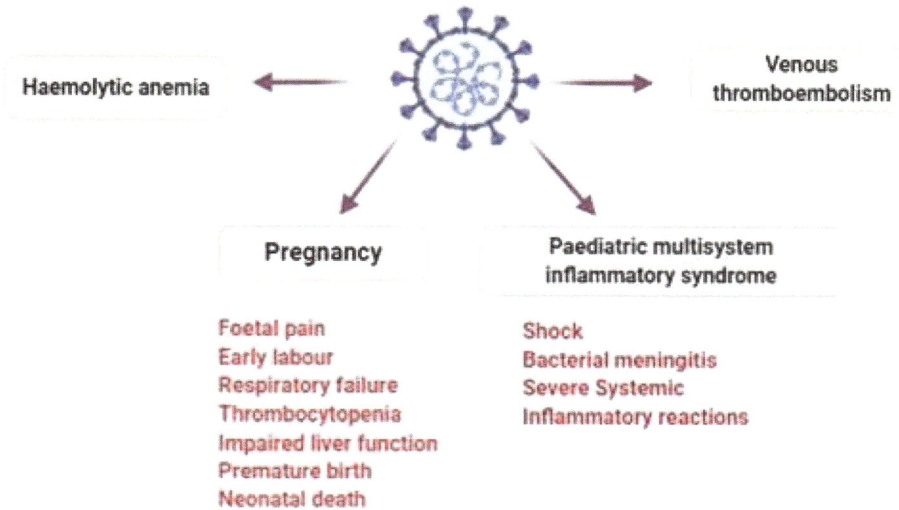

Fig. (2). Effects of COVID-19 in hemolytic anemia and venous thromboembolism.

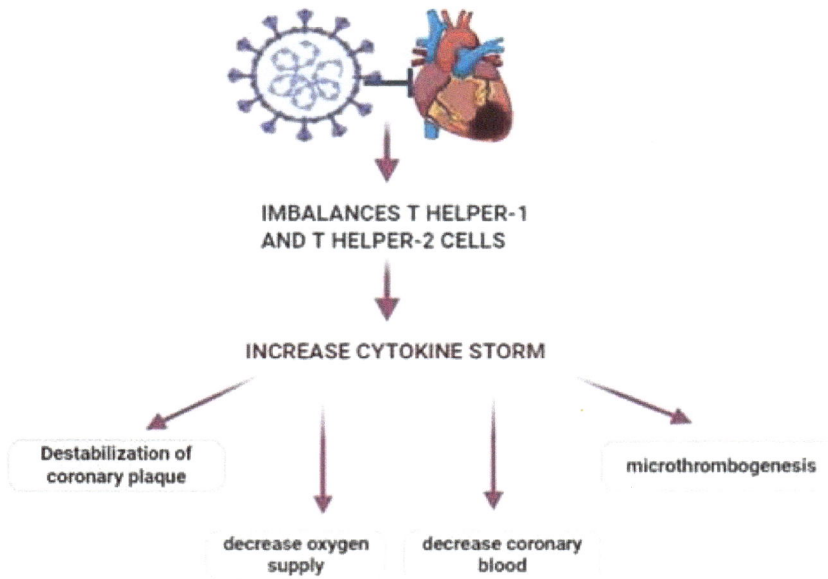

Fig. (3). Impact of COVID-19 in cardiovascular diseases.

Cardiovascular Diseases

A meta-analysis found that patients having CVD were more prone to MERS-CoV. 50% of MERS-CoV disease patients were suffering from hypertension and diabetes and up to 30% of people were suffering from other heart diseases. Likewise, for the Latest Coronavirus Infection, the people with comorbidities are more susceptible to infection caused by SARS-CoV-2, especially to the individual having a history of hypertension, cardiac disease, or diabetes. Besides, these infections a patient having CVD are liable for the development of complications of COVID-19. Moreover, such patients account for a significant proportion of deaths due to COVID-19. This can be understood properly by one of the case studies in which, 58%, 25%, and 44% cases have hypertension, heart disease, and have arrhythmias respectively among patients with severe COVID-19 conditions. As per the report released by NHC, mortality occurs in SARS-CoV-2 patients who had a history of high blood pressure (35% cases) and had a background of cardiac disease (17% cases). Moreover, these results suggested that more chronic and serious pneumonia occurred in patients having on or above 60 years of age diagnosed with SARS-CoV-2 as compare to the patients aged lesser than 60 years (Chan *et al.*, 2020). Therefore, it suggests that if the individual suffering from an infection of SARS-CoV-2 associated with clinical evidence of CVD will be also suffered from pneumonia, and such condition may raise the severity state to the patients.

Moreover, patients infected with SARS-CoV-2 with the coronary syndrome (CS) often have a poor prognosis. Heart disease is more likely to appear in a patient infected with SARS-CoV-2 and the situation of these patients suddenly deteriorates. In Wuhan, it was also observed that the patient of COVID-19 had prior ACS resulted in serious illness and a high mortality rate. The infection of SARS-CoV-2 may act as an exacerbating indicator in patients having cardiac insufficiency that leads to death. The present research indicates that patients with existing CVD and other co-morbid disorders are more likely to develop myocardial damage during COVID-19. The viral disease may destroy more myocardial cells *via* a variety of pathways, including direct exposure to the virus, systemic inflammation reaction, destabilized coronary plaque, as well as exacerbated hypoxia, in patients having CVD, including coronary heart disease, hypertension (HTN), and cardiomyopathy (Fig. **3**). Therefore in CVD patients, there is a greater risk of myocardial injury after COVID-19 and a higher risk of mortality (Zheng *et al.*, 2020). While the actual pathophysiological process of myocardial damage triggered by COVID-19 is not well known, an earlier study has revealed that 35% of patients with severe acute corona viral syndrome (SARS-CoV) infection had severe cardiovascular disease and virus genome was identified in the heart of patients. This increases the possibility of direct cardiomyocyte disruption by the virus. SARS-CoV-2 could have the same mechanism as SARS-COV because the genome of the two viruses is highly homologous (Li *et al.*, 2020b).

Current scientific reports providing a shred of evidence for the progression of the disease, myocardial damage could directly join the inflammatory pathogenesis. Invading of viral particles takes place through respiratory mucosa and as time progresses it simultaneously infects other cells. Such kind events further lead to cause a cytokine storm, as well as a series of immune reactions, occur. Huang *et al.*, also illustrated that in the patient of COVID-19 inequality of T-Helper 1 and 2 develops, which leads to an increase in cytokine storms and acts as a contributing factor to cause myocardial injury (Li *et al.*, 2020b). The inflammatory cytokines release following infection can lead to a reduction in coronary blood flow, reduced oxygen supply, microthrombogenesis, and destabilization of coronary plaque (Guo *et al.*, 2020a).

Central Nervous System Complications

Viral Encephalitis

Encephalitis leads to inflammatory disorders, including neural disruption and inflammation, in the brain's parenchyma triggered by pathogens. It leads to fatigue, fever (primarily elevated temperature), diarrhea, convulsions, and disruption of awareness (Ellul and Solomon, 2018). The Beijing Ditan Hospital research team reported that SARS-CoV-2 was present in the cerebrospinal fluid of patients having COVID-19, which culminated that is responsible for viral encephalitis(Xiang *et al.*, 2020). It gives strong evidence that encephalitis is induced by CoV (Fig. **4**). Viral infections such as Herpes simplex virus (HSV), Varicella zoster (VZV), cytomegalovirus (CMV), influenza virus, and various other respiratory-influenza viruses, such as Severe SARS-CoV and Middle East Airborne Virus (MERS-CoV) are part of a more severe underlying etiology of encephalitis or inflammation. SARS-CoV-2 may also have neurotrophic effects as well as typical respiratory symptoms. Poyiadji *et al.*, recorded another case of a female who had 3 days of experience of fever, coughing, and impaired mental state during their fifties, and diagnosed with COVID-19 through the identification of SARS-Cov-2 nucleic acid. Her CSF analysis was negative for bacteria, type 1 and 2 HSV, and varicella-zoster virus. Throughout, the longitudinal thalami, medial temporal lobes, and subinsular areas, hemorrhagic ring enhanced lesions associated with necrotizing encephalitis are seen. The above case report could support the possible idea of encephalitis by SARS-CoV-2. Poyiadji *et al.,* reported that the SARS COV-2 virus will not penetrate the blood-brain barrier explicitly, and cause necrosis encephalitis (Ahmed *et al.*, 2020).

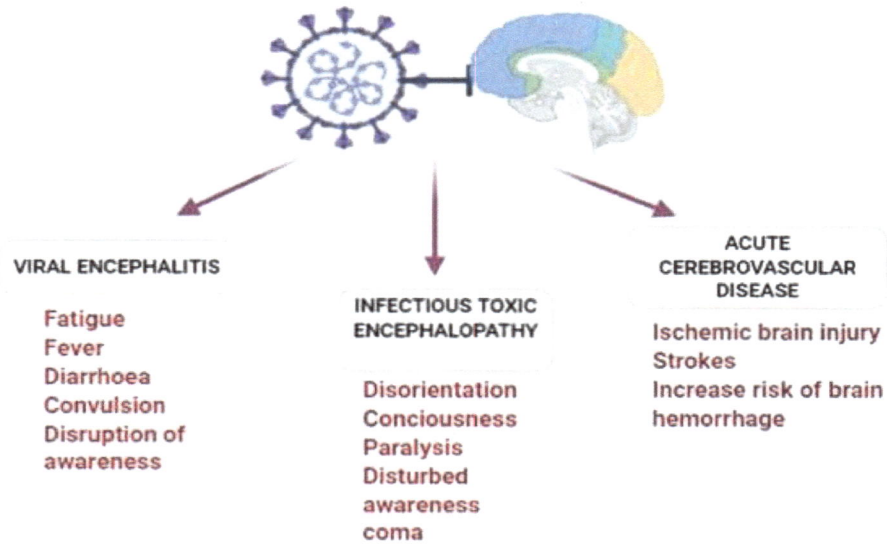

Fig. (4). Impact of COVID-19 in CNS.

Infectious Toxic Encephalopathy and Cerebrovascular Disease

A type of brain impairment syndrome is induced by various reasons which include systemic toxemia, abnormalities linked with metabolism, and hypoxia. At the time of the development of infection, it is referred to as infectious toxic encephalopathy. Cerebral edema with little proof of inflammation on the cerebrospinal fluid analysis is the fundamental pathological change to this disease. It has diverse and varied health manifestations (Tauber *et al.*, 2017). Headache, mental disorder, delirium, and dysphoria may develop in patients with a minor course of the disease. Patients who are seriously impaired will suffer from disorientation, consciousness loss, paralysis, and coma. Acute virus infection is also a significant source of the illness, as in the case of COVID-19 infection. COVID-19 patients also suffer extreme hypoxia and viremia possibly contributing to toxic encephalopathy (Guo *et al.*, 2020c). Additionally, about 40 percent of COVID-19 patients experience pain, disturbed awareness, and other signs of brain impairment, and an autopsy analysis recorded edema in brain tissue (Mao *et al.*, 2020, Xu *et al.*, 2020b). It collectively explored that COVID-19 can induce infectious toxic encephalopathy, although comprehensive studies are still required. Substantial data suggest that a respiratory infection, in particular, is a distinct risk factor for severe cerebrovascular disorders. Data obtained from experimental animal models indicate that influenza will exacerbate ischemia brain injury by causing a cytokine cascade as well as increasing the risk of brain hemorrhage COVID virus infection (Fig. **4**).

Specifically, SARS-CoV-2 is widely reported for cytokine storm syndrome, which may cause CBD (Cerebrovascular disease) (Warren-Gash *et al.*, 2018). Seriously ill patients with serious SARS-CoV-2 infections also generally have high concentrations of D-dimer and drastic platelet reduction, which can make them more likely to develop strokes. Thereby, people at risk of developing cerebrovascular disease during CoV infections (Wang *et al.*, 2020b, Wu *et al.*, 2020b).

Chronic Kidney Disease (CKD)

The elevated incidence of inpatient, as well as outpatient pneumonia, is correlated with chronic kidney disease (CKD). The death rate associated with pneumonia further appears to be 14–16 times greater in CKD patients than in the general population (Henry and Lippi, 2020). The pathogenesis of the occurrence of kidney failure in COVID-19 patients is probably more common. First, the current coronavirus may have immediate kidney tissue cytotoxic consequences. Current coronavirus using ACE 2 receptor is the same as SARS-CoV which was recorded in 2003. Also, it is confirmed by a polymerase chain reaction. In this reaction, it was observed that the chain reaction fragments of coronavirus are available in both the blood and the urine (Peiris *et al.*, 2003, Zhou *et al.*, 2020b). Second, the accumulation of immune complex of the viral antigen or unique immunological effector processes triggered by the virus (primary T cell lymphocyte) may be devasting for the renal system which severely affects the kidney.

However, kidney microscopy samples also provided evidence of normal architecture of glomerular components as well as lack of electron-dense deposits in patients who already had SARS (Chu *et al.*, 2005). Potential pathological shifts in the kidney of COVID-19 patients need further analysis. Thirdly, cytokines induced by viruses or mediators can have indirect consequences, like hypoxia, shock, and even rhabdomyolysis (Fig. **5**). In some patients with the 2009 H1N1 virus relatively had an elevated level of serum creatinine (Kumar *et al.*, 2009). According to a recent report, patients admitted to an intensive care facility having COVID-19 appeared to have elevated levels of creatinine and the patients with renal involvement may even have increased levels of creatine kinase (Wang *et al.*, 2020a, Cheng *et al.*, 2020b). The increased incidence of serious COVID-19 infection tends to be correlated with CKD. Therefore, extra care should be taken to reduce the risk of the virus in patients with CKD. Doctors should also be closely scrutinized the potential COVID-19 CKD cases, to detect the signals of disease development. Finally, in forthcoming COVID-19 risk stratification models the existence of CKD is deemed to be a significant factor (Henry and Lippi, 2020). Cheng and his colleagues examined a large cohort of 710 patients (more than 18 years of age) having COVID-19 infection for kidney disease. Those with a history of renal transplantation and maintenance dialysis were omitted from the study. In 110 hospitalized cases, base-line serum creatinine was increased. In the elevated serum creatinine community, most of the cases were older with a greater proportion of males and shorter days from the initiation of the illness to hospital entry. Those individuals were also seriously sick and having co-morbidities contrary to those having normal baseline creatinine levels. Also in these patients, the kidney injury was more severe, rates of mechanical ventilation and mortality were also high (Adapa *et al.*, 2020).

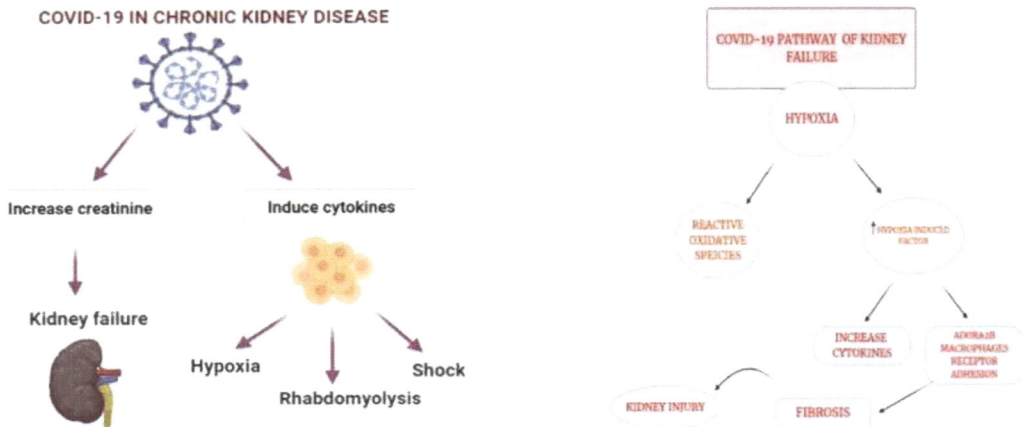

Fig. (5). Effect of COVID-19 in CKD.

Asthma and Respiratory Disorders

There is already considerable evidence that asthma patients are highly represented among the adult patients admitted to Hospital having (COVID-19). This overrepresentation could be triggered by asthma exacerbations, like other infections, which render asthma a contributing factor for the morbidity of COVID-19. The most severe symptoms of COVID-19 are dry cough and air scarcity. Fever is correlated most frequently with COVID-19 but can express any infection-induced asthma exacerbation. COVID-19 screening protocols will apply to someone who has intensified respiratory signs, like asthma. The incidence of asthma did not seem to raise previous novel coronaviruses, SARS-CoV, and MERS-CoV, unlike COVID-19 that increases the risk of asthma (Zheng *et al.*, 2018). The most severe symptoms related to COVID-19 cover fever, exhaustion, dry cough, myalgia anorexia, and dyspnea. Most complications of asthma do not escalate to fever, exhaustion, and anorexia. Typical asthma patients can exacerbate even the signs of COVID-19, indicative should be viewed with good treatment.

Oral steroids would be confined to the lowest dosage possible for the shortest duration. Patients with COVID-19 infection also have asthma should keep on their current regime of asthma (Fig. **6**). Oral corticosteroids should only be used when COVID-19 causes exacerbation of asthma, again restricting treatment dosage and duration as much as practicable (Pennington, 2020). The risk factors and worsening of Acute Respiratory distress syndrome (ARDS) to death were older age, neutrophilia, and dysfunction of an organ as well as coagulation. It has been found that some ARDS growth factors (*e.g.* comorbidity, CD3 and CD4 numbers, T-cell numbers, AST, pre-albumins, creatinine, low-density lipoprotein, serum ferritin, *etc.*) have not been linked with death. The gap between mortality and recovery classes in median D-dimer was greater than the one between ARDS and non-ARDS, suggesting that certain patients were on their path to mortality with disseminated intravascular coagulation. Also, the production of ARDS was positively linked to high fever and was negative to death which indicates the findings of a Schell-Chaple *et al.*, 2015.

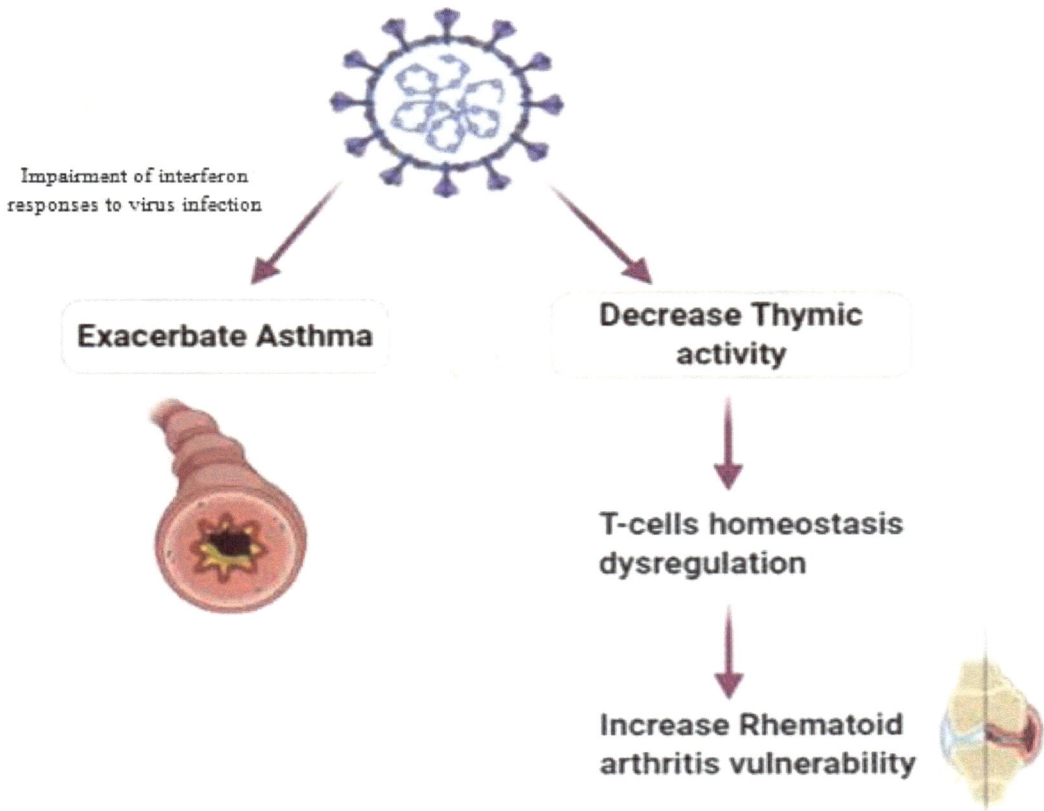

Impairment of interferon responses to virus infection

Exacerbate Asthma

Decrease Thymic activity

T-cells homeostasis dysregulation

Increase Rhematoid arthritis vulnerability

Fig. (6). Role of COVID-19 in asthma and rheumatoid arthritis.

The variations in patient temperature among groups were quite low and self-reported before hospital admission, so evidence on high fever should be viewed cautiously. Extremely pathogenic human coronavirus exact pathophysiology is still not completely known. Cytokine storms, as well as cellular immune responses, are believed to play a significant role in the seriousness of the disease (Fig. **7**). Neutrophilia has been recognized in patients suffering from both peripheral as well as lungs infected with SARS-CoV. In MERS patients, lung infections were linked with the substantial pulmonary accumulation of neutrophils and macrophages and higher levels of these cells in their peripheral blood. The primary causes of chemokines and cytokines storm are neutrophils that are responsible for the extreme acute respiratory syndrome that is a major cause of death (Cui *et al.*, 2003). In recent research, it has been found that patients with pneumonia COVID-19 who developed ARDS had slightly greater numbers of neutrophils than those without ARDS, which could contribute to the stimulation of neutrophils to carry out an immune response against the virus but also cause cytokine storm. This clarifies the favorable correlation between high fever and ARDS observed at the early stages of COVID-19. However, the findings of recent research revealed that older age is linked with a reduced immune capacity which's why they are more prone to ARDS and mortality. Older age correlated with mortality may also be related to less effective immune responses. From studies, it is also revealed that higher T-cell counts of CD3 and CD4 could protect patients against ARDS. CD8 numbers in those who were alive were slightly higher. These findings show the important functions of CD4 and CD8 T cells in the pneumonia of COVID-19. Previous studies have shown that SARS-CoV which has the same receptor as SARS-CoV-2, could invade immune cells, including T lymphocytes, monocytes, and macrophages. T-cell counts for CD3, CD4, and CD8 were reduced at the start of illness; this decline lasted until SARS-CoV pneumonia was restored. CD4 and CD8 numbers of T cells have reduced in the peripheral blood serum of patients with lethal SARS-CoV pneumonia. Studies have shown that T-cell reactions can prevent the over-activation of innate immunity. T-cells were recorded to help remove SARS-CoV, and a suboptimal T-cell response was observed in the mice with SARS-CoV to induce pathological changes (Li *et al.*, 2004, Wu *et al.*, 2020a). We presumed the need for persistent and gradual changes in lymphocyte response for successful immunity to SARS-CoV-2 infection.

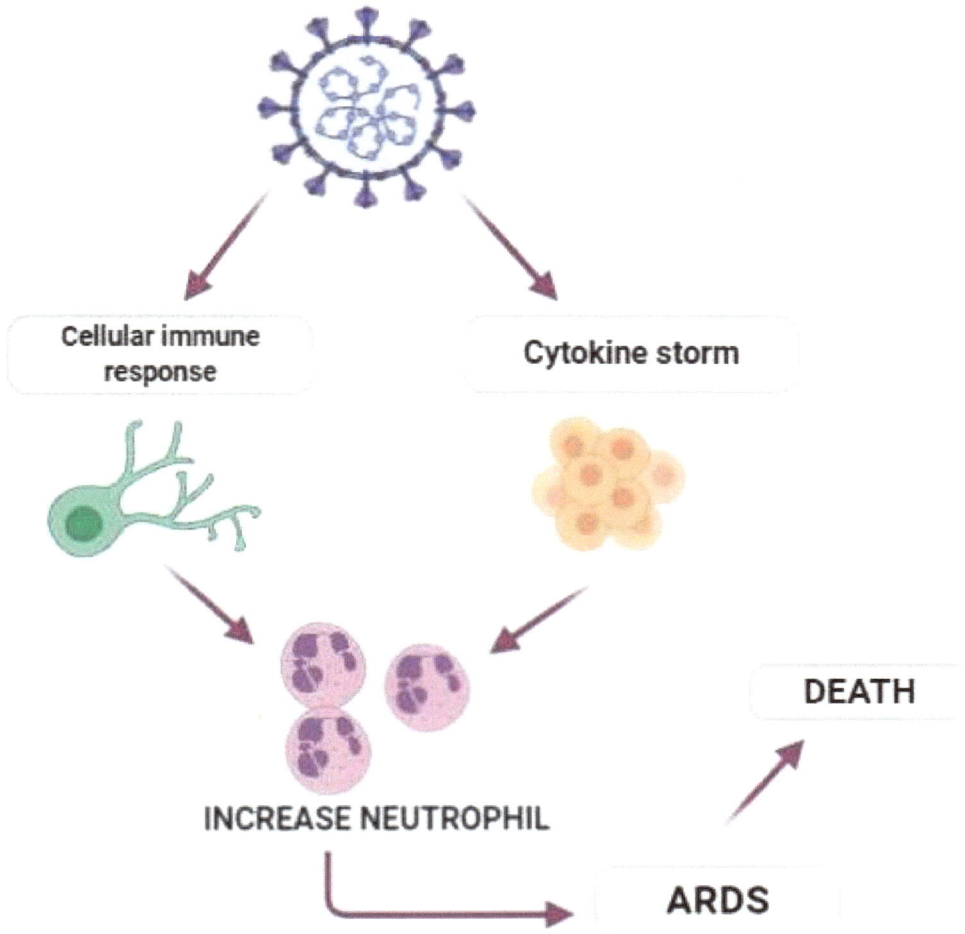

Fig. (7). Impact of COVID-19 in acute respiratory syndrome.

Apart from that Pulmonary fibrosis is also an important factor to consider as a challenging issue in the patients of COVID-19. It was reported in about 62% of the survivors. Its manifestation includes fibrous stripes, subpleural lines, and traction bronchiectasis. It may develop in the early stage in patients with SARS and diagnostic reports after recovery also suggest it as long-term complications (Antonio *et al.*, 2003) (Chan *et al.*, 2003). The reason behind the clinical state is deregulated release of metalloproteinases during the inflammatory phase of ARDS. It causes injury of epithelial as well as endothelial cells with unchecked fibroproliferation (Davey *et al.*, 2011, Zemans *et al.*, 2009).

The most fundamental aspect of all respiratory conditions is increased ACE2 expression after infection. 48h after all the pathogenesis of COVID-19 begins to start along with its transcription. Inflammatory responses associated with the ACE2 expression indicated by the availability of RPS3, RPS8, and PRS9 kind of ribosomal proteins. Along with this VCP, LARP1, UBA52, PRKN, EIF3A, and EIF3L are also important for protein-protein interaction. Finally, SRC, CASP1, and RIPK were Hub proteins responsible for cytokine secretion. Hence, patients with such conditions are at higher risk of death (Li *et al.*, 2020a).

Rheumatoid Arthritis (RA)

Previous reports provided evidence that rheumatoid arthritis (RA) is associated with an increased incidence and complications of respiratory infections (Vinogradova *et al.*, 2009, Blumentals *et al.*, 2012). These findings may be attributed to the immunological impairment of circulating T cells in patients suffering from RA (Fig. **6**). Consequently, it stops patients from responding to the infections caused by an infectious agent. The decreased thymic activity and enhanced peripheral T-cell turnover, which may lead to peripheral T-cell homeostasis dysregulation, may also increase the RA vulnerability to infection (Koetz *et al.*, 2000). Such fundamental aspects of scientific knowledge suggested a complex relationship between RA and infection as external microorganism can develop the chronic state of RA either by:

a. Direct colonization by the pathogen at joints or
b. It may be due to an aberrant autoimmune response

Several scientific works of literature are also available indicated the severity of RA due to respiratory viral infections (Arleevskaya *et al.*, 2017, Mathew and Ravindran, 2014, Bogdanos *et al.*, 2013). Besides, RA patients are often diagnosed with drugs including steroids or DMARDs, which are immunosuppressive. Giving these immunosuppressive agents further enhances the prevalence of infections in RA patients (Bernatsky *et al.*, 2007). COVID-19 therapy in RA patients is scientifically problematic as COVID-19 infection could worsen by immunosuppressive agents. Temporary cessation of most DMARDs is advised for patients hospitalized with severe infections to facilitate RA patients to acquire defensive immunity and remove pathogens. Besides, stopping the administration of DMARDs may lead to an increased incidence of RA, which is normally controlled by increased doses of immunosuppressives (Ledingham *et al.*, 2017). The impact of steroids on COVID-19 infection is still uncertain. Steroids may exacerbate infections by decreasing the immune response, but systemic steroid treatment will prevent the inflammatory cascade of pneumonia (Ni *et al.*, 2019). Earlier studies have indicated that steroid therapy was linked to increased mortality in patients having a viral infection like influenza and pneumonia. In these instances, to decreases, the incidences of COVID-19 leflunomide and steroids were stopped and hydroxychloroquine administration persisted owing to its potential antiviral activity, as well as its anti-rheumatic impact (Yao *et al.*, 2020, Song *et al.*, 2020).

CONCLUSION

This review provides an insight into the COVID-19 present situations and represents a picture of long-term complications associated with it. Future epidemiological studies and case records should elucidate the exact incidence of complications, pathogenesis with therapeutic options. This report of long-term complications of COVID-19 also provided an alarming signal to the patients of diabetes, central nervous system, respiratory disorders, hematological conditions, kidney disorder, and rheumatoid arthritis. These all diseased conditions are associated with an increased incidence of infections in case, if the symptoms persist to these patients they seek medical care in early stages only and follow the advice of healthcare professionals strictly.

ABBREVIATIONS

ACE2	Angiotensin-converting enzyme 2
ARDS	Acute respiratory distress syndrome
CBD	Cerebrovascular disease
CKD	Chronic kidney injury
CMV	Cytomegalovirus
COVID-19	Coronavirus epidemic 2019
CS	Coronary syndrome
CVD	Cardiovascular diseases
DIC	Disseminated intravascular coagulation
DM	Diabetes mellitus
FBG	Fibrinogen
GLP-1	Glucagon-like peptide 1
HSV	Herpes simplex virus
HTN	Hypertension
IL	Interleukin
MERS-CoV	Middle East Airborne Virus
PT	Prolonged prothrombin time
RA	Rheumatoid arthritis
SARS	Severe Acute Respiratory Syndrome
SIC	Sepsis-induced coagulopathy

TNF	Tumor necrosis factor
VZV	Varicella zoster

CONSENT FOR PUBLICATION

Not applicable.

CONFLICT OF INTEREST

The author declares no conflict of interest, financial or otherwise.

ACKNOWLEDGEMENTS

Declared none.

REFERENCES

Adapa, S, Chenna, A, Balla, M, Merugu, GP, Koduri, NM, Daggubati, SR, Gayam, V, Naramala, S & Konala, VM (2020) Covid-19 pandemic causing acute kidney injury and impact on patients with chronic kidney disease and renal transplantation. *J Clin Med Res,* 12, 352-61.
[http://dx.doi.org/10.14740/jocmr4200] [PMID: 32587651]

Ahmed, MU, Hanif, M, Ali, MJ, Haider, MA, Kherani, D, Memon, GM, Karim, AH & Sattar, A (2020) Neurological manifestations of COVID-19 (SARS-CoV-2): A review. *Front Neurol,* 11, 518.
[http://dx.doi.org/10.3389/fneur.2020.00518] [PMID: 32574248]

Antonio, GE, Wong, KT, Hui, DS, Wu, A, Lee, N, Yuen, EH, Leung, CB, Rainer, TH, Cameron, P, Chung, SS, Sung, JJ & Ahuja, AT (2003) Thin-section CT in patients with severe acute respiratory syndrome following hospital discharge: preliminary experience. *Radiology,* 228, 810-5.
[http://dx.doi.org/10.1148/radiol.2283030726] [PMID: 12805557]

Arentz, M, Yim, E, Klaff, L, Lokhandwala, S, Riedo, FX, Chong, M & Lee, M (2020) Characteristics and outcomes of 21 critically ill patients with Covid-19 in Washington State. *JAMA,* 323, 1612-4.
[http://dx.doi.org/10.1001/jama.2020.4326] [PMID: 32191259]

Arleevskaya, MI, Shafigullina, AZ, Filina, YV, Lemerle, J & Renaudineau, Y (2017) Associations between viral infection history symptoms, granulocyte reactive oxygen species activity, and active rheumatoid arthritis disease in untreated women at onset: results from a longitudinal cohort study of Tatarstan women. *Front Immunol,* 8, 1725.
[http://dx.doi.org/10.3389/fimmu.2017.01725] [PMID: 29259607]

Bernatsky, S, Hudson, M & Suissa, S (2007) Anti-rheumatic drug use and risk of serious infections in rheumatoid arthritis. *Rheumatology (Oxford),* 46, 1157-60.
[http://dx.doi.org/10.1093/rheumatology/kem076] [PMID: 17478469]

Bhatraju, PK, Ghassemieh, BJ, Nichols, M, Kim, R, Jerome, KR, Nalla, AK, Greninger, AL, Pipavath, S, Wurfel, MM, Evans, L, Kritek, PA, West, TE, Luks, A, Gerbino, A, Dale, CR, Goldman, JD, O'Mahony, S & Mikacenic, C (2020) 'Covid-19 in critically ill patients in the Seattle region—case series'. *N Engl J Med,* 382, 2012-22.
[http://dx.doi.org/10.1056/NEJMoa2004500] [PMID: 32227758]

Bloomgarden, ZT (2020) Diabetes and COVID-19. *J Diabetes,* 12, 347-8.
[http://dx.doi.org/10.1111/1753-0407.13027] [PMID: 32162476]

Blumentals, WA, Arreglado, A, Napalkov, P & Toovey, S (2012) Rheumatoid arthritis and the incidence of influenza and influenza-related complications: a retrospective cohort study. *BMC Musculoskelet Disord,* 13,

158.
[http://dx.doi.org/10.1186/1471-2474-13-158] [PMID: 22925480]

Bogdanos, DP, Smyk, DS, Invernizzi, P, Rigopoulou, EI, Blank, M, Pouria, S & Shoenfeld, Y (2013) Infectome: a platform to trace infectious triggers of autoimmunity. *Autoimmun Rev,* 12, 726-40.
[http://dx.doi.org/10.1016/j.autrev.2012.12.005] [PMID: 23266520]

Butler, MJ & Barrientos, RM (2020) The impact of nutrition on COVID-19 susceptibility and long-term consequences. *Brain Behav Immun,* 87, 53-4.
[http://dx.doi.org/10.1016/j.bbi.2020.04.040] [PMID: 32311498]

Chan, JF, Yuan, S, Kok, KH, To, KK, Chu, H, Yang, J, Xing, F, Liu, J, Yip, CC, Poon, RW, Tsoi, HW, Lo, SK, Chan, KH, Poon, VK, Chan, WM, Ip, JD, Cai, JP, Cheng, VC, Chen, H, Hui, CK & Yuen, KY (2020) A familial cluster of pneumonia associated with the 2019 novel coronavirus indicating person-to-person transmission: a study of a family cluster. *Lancet,* 395, 514-23.
[http://dx.doi.org/10.1016/S0140-6736(20)30154-9] [PMID: 31986261]

Chan, K, Zheng, J, Mok, Y, Li, Y, Liu, Y, Chu, C & Ip, M (2003) SARS: prognosis, outcome and sequelae. *Respirology,* 8 (Suppl.), S36-40.
[http://dx.doi.org/10.1046/j.1440-1843.2003.00522.x] [PMID: 15018132]

Cheng, A, Hu, L, Wang, Y, Huang, L, Zhao, L, Zhang, C, Liu, X, Xu, R, Liu, F & Li, J (2020) a 'Diagnostic performance of initial blood urea nitrogen combined with D-Dimer levels for predicting in-hospital mortality in Covid-19 patients'. *Int J Antimicrob Agents,* 56, 106-10.
[http://dx.doi.org/10.1016/j.ijantimicag.2020.106110]

Cheng, Y, Luo, R, Wang, K, Zhang, M, Wang, Z, Dong, L, Li, J, Yao, Y, Ge, S & Xu, G (2020) Kidney disease is associated with in-hospital death of patients with COVID-19. *Kidney Int,* 97, 829-38.
[http://dx.doi.org/10.1016/j.kint.2020.03.005] [PMID: 32247631]

Chu, KH, Tsang, WK, Tang, CS, Lam, MF, Lai, FM, To, KF, Fung, KS, Tang, HL, Yan, WW, Chan, HW, Lai, TS, Tong, KL & Lai, KN (2005) Acute renal impairment in coronavirus-associated severe acute respiratory syndrome. *Kidney Int,* 67, 698-705.
[http://dx.doi.org/10.1111/j.1523-1755.2005.67130.x] [PMID: 15673319]

Connaughton, RM, McMorrow, AM, McGillicuddy, FC, Lithander, FE & Roche, HM (2016) Impact of anti-inflammatory nutrients on obesity-associated metabolic-inflammation from childhood through to adulthood. *Proc Nutr Soc,* 75, 115-24.
[http://dx.doi.org/10.1017/S0029665116000070] [PMID: 26934951]

Cui, W, Fan, Y, Wu, W, Zhang, F, Wang, JY & Ni, AP (2003) Expression of lymphocytes and lymphocyte subsets in patients with severe acute respiratory syndrome. *Clin Infect Dis,* 37, 857-9.
[http://dx.doi.org/10.1086/378587] [PMID: 12955652]

Danser, AHJ, Epstein, M & Batlle, D (2020) Renin-angiotensin system blockers and the Covid-19 pandemic: At present, there is no evidence to abandon renin-angiotensin system blockers. *Hypertension,* 75, 1382-5.
[http://dx.doi.org/10.1161/HYPERTENSIONAHA.120.15082] [PMID: 32208987]

Davey, A, McAuley, DF & O'Kane, CM (2011) Matrix metalloproteinases in acute lung injury: mediators of injury and drivers of repair. *Eur Respir J,* 38, 959-70.
[http://dx.doi.org/10.1183/09031936.00032111] [PMID: 21565917]

Deng, Y, Liu, W, Liu, K, Fang, Y-Y, Shang, J, Zhou, L, Wang, K, Leng, F, Wei, S, Chen, L & Liu, HG (2020) Clinical characteristics of fatal and recovered cases of coronavirus disease 2019 in Wuhan, China: a retrospective study. *Chin Med J (Engl),* 133, 1261-7.
[http://dx.doi.org/10.1097/CM9.0000000000000824] [PMID: 32209890]

Ellul, M & Solomon, T (2018) Acute encephalitis - diagnosis and management. *Clin Med (Lond),* 18, 155-9.
[http://dx.doi.org/10.7861/clinmedicine.18-2-155] [PMID: 29626021]

Fan, BE, Chong, VCL, Chan, SSW, Lim, GH, Lim, KGE, Tan, GB, Mucheli, SS, Kuperan, P & Ong, KH (2020) Hematologic parameters in patients with COVID-19 infection. *Am J Hematol,* 95, E131-4.

[http://dx.doi.org/10.1002/ajh.25774] [PMID: 32129508]

Gangopadhyay, KK (2020) "Does having diabetes increase chances of contracting COVID-19 infection?". *Diabetes Metab Syndr,* 14, 765-6.
[http://dx.doi.org/10.1016/j.dsx.2020.05.048] [PMID: 32512520]

Geerlings, SE & Hoepelman, AI (1999) Immune dysfunction in patients with diabetes mellitus (DM). *FEMS Immunol Med Microbiol,* 26, 259-65.
[http://dx.doi.org/10.1111/j.1574-695X.1999.tb01397.x] [PMID: 10575137]

Guan, W-J, Ni, Z-Y, Hu, Y, Liang, W-H, Ou, C-Q, He, J-X, Liu, L, Shan, H, Lei, C-L, Hui, DSC, Du, B, Li, LJ, Zeng, G, Yuen, KY, Chen, RC, Tang, CL, Wang, T, Chen, PY, Xiang, J, Li, SY, Wang, JL, Liang, ZJ, Peng, YX, Wei, L, Liu, Y, Hu, YH, Peng, P, Wang, JM, Liu, JY, Chen, Z, Li, G, Zheng, ZJ, Qiu, SQ, Luo, J, Ye, CJ, Zhu, SY & Zhong, NS China Medical Treatment Expert Group for Covid-19 (2020) Clinical characteristics of coronavirus disease 2019 in china. *N Engl J Med,* 382, 1708-20.
[http://dx.doi.org/10.1056/NEJMoa2002032] [PMID: 32109013]

Guan, W, Ni, Z, Hu, Y, Liang, W, Ou, C, He, J, Liu, L, Shan, H, Lei, C & Hui, D (2019) China medical treatment expert group for Covid-19. *Clin Charact Corovirus Dis,* 1708-20.

Guo, T, Fan, Y, Chen, M, Wu, X, Zhang, L, He, T, Wang, H, Wan, J, Wang, X & Lu, Z (2020) 'Cardiovascular implications of fatal outcomes of patients with coronavirus disease 2019 (Covid-19)'. *JAMA Cardiol,* 5, 811-8.
[http://dx.doi.org/10.1001/jamacardio.2020.1017] [PMID: 32219356]

Guo, W, Li, M, Dong, Y, Zhou, H, Zhang, Z, Tian, C, Qin, R, Wang, H, Shen, Y, Du, K, Zhao, L, Fan, H, Luo, S & Hu, D (2020) Diabetes is a risk factor for the progression and prognosis of COVID-19. *Diabetes Metab Res Rev,* 36, e3319.
[http://dx.doi.org/10.1002/dmrr.3319] [PMID: 32233013]

Guo, Y-R, Cao, Q-D, Hong, Z-S, Tan, Y-Y, Chen, S-D, Jin, H-J, Tan, K-S, Wang, D-Y & Yan, Y (2020) The origin, transmission and clinical therapies on coronavirus disease 2019 (Covid-19) outbreak-An update on the status. *Mil Med Res,* 7, 1-10.
[http://dx.doi.org/10.1186/s40779-020-00240-0]

Harrison, C (2020) Coronavirus puts drug repurposing on the fast track. *Nat Biotechnol,* 38, 379-81.
[http://dx.doi.org/10.1038/d41587-020-00003-1] [PMID: 32205870]

Henry, BM & Lippi, G (2020) Chronic kidney disease is associated with severe coronavirus disease 2019 (COVID-19) infection. *Int Urol Nephrol,* 52, 1193-4.
[http://dx.doi.org/10.1007/s11255-020-02451-9] [PMID: 32222883]

Hussain, A, Bhowmik, B & do Vale Moreira, NC (2020) COVID-19 and diabetes: Knowledge in progress. *Diabetes Res Clin Pract,* 162, 108142.
[http://dx.doi.org/10.1016/j.diabres.2020.108142] [PMID: 32278764]

Iba, T, Arakawa, M, Di Nisio, M, Gando, S, Anan, H, Sato, K, Ueki, Y, Levy, JH & Thachil, J (2020) Newly proposed sepsis-induced coagulopathy precedes international society on thrombosis and haemostasis overt-disseminated intravascular coagulation and predicts high mortality. *J Intensive Care Med,* 35, 643-9.
[http://dx.doi.org/10.1177/0885066618773679] [PMID: 29720054]

Knapp, S (2013) Diabetes and infection: is there a link?--A mini-review. *Gerontology,* 59, 99-104.
[http://dx.doi.org/10.1159/000345107] [PMID: 23182884]

Koetz, K, Bryl, E, Spickschen, K, O'Fallon, WM, Goronzy, JJ & Weyand, CM (2000) T cell homeostasis in patients with rheumatoid arthritis. *Proc Natl Acad Sci USA,* 97, 9203-8.
[http://dx.doi.org/10.1073/pnas.97.16.9203] [PMID: 10922071]

Kohio, HP & Adamson, AL (2013) Glycolytic control of vacuolar-type ATPase activity: a mechanism to regulate influenza viral infection. *Virology,* 444, 301-9.
[http://dx.doi.org/10.1016/j.virol.2013.06.026] [PMID: 23876457]

Kuba, K, Imai, Y, Rao, S, Gao, H, Guo, F, Guan, B, Huan, Y, Yang, P, Zhang, Y, Deng, W, Bao, L, Zhang, B, Liu, G, Wang, Z, Chappell, M, Liu, Y, Zheng, D, Leibbrandt, A, Wada, T, Slutsky, AS, Liu, D, Qin, C, Jiang, C & Penninger, JM (2005) A crucial role of angiotensin converting enzyme 2 (ACE2) in SARS coronavirus-induced lung injury. *Nat Med,* 11, 875-9.
[http://dx.doi.org/10.1038/nm1267] [PMID: 16007097]

Kumar, A, Zarychanski, R, Pinto, R, Cook, DJ, Marshall, J, Lacroix, J, Stelfox, T, Bagshaw, S, Choong, K, Lamontagne, F, Turgeon, AF, Lapinsky, S, Ahern, SP, Smith, O, Siddiqui, F, Jouvet, P, Khwaja, K, McIntyre, L, Menon, K, Hutchison, J, Hornstein, D, Joffe, A, Lauzier, F, Singh, J, Karachi, T, Wiebe, K, Olafson, K, Ramsey, C, Sharma, S, Dodek, P, Meade, M, Hall, R & Fowler, RA Canadian critical care trials group H1N1 collaborative (2009) Critically ill patients with 2009 influenza A(H1N1) infection in Canada. *JAMA,* 302, 1872-9.
[http://dx.doi.org/10.1001/jama.2009.1496] [PMID: 19822627]

Lange, P, Groth, S, Kastrup, J, Mortensen, J, Appleyard, M, Nyboe, J, Jensen, G & Schnohr, P (1989) Diabetes mellitus, plasma glucose and lung function in a cross-sectional population study. *Eur Respir J,* 2, 14-9.
[PMID: 2651148]

Lazarian, G, Quinquenel, A, Bellal, M, Siavellis, J, Jacquy, C, Re, D, Merabet, F, Mekinian, A, Braun, T, Damaj, G, Delmer, A & Cymbalista, F (2020) Autoimmune haemolytic anaemia associated with COVID-19 infection. *Br J Haematol,* 190, 29-31.
[http://dx.doi.org/10.1111/bjh.16794] [PMID: 32374906]

Ledingham, J, Gullick, N, Irving, K, Gorodkin, R, Aris, M, Burke, J, Gordon, P, Christidis, D, Galloway, S, Hayes, E, Jeffries, A, Mercer, S, Mooney, J, van Leuven, S & Galloway, J BSR and BHPR Standards, Guidelines and Audit Working Group (2017) BSR and BHPR guideline for the prescription and monitoring of non-biologic disease-modifying anti-rheumatic drugs. *Rheumatology (Oxford),* 56, 865-8.
[http://dx.doi.org/10.1093/rheumatology/kew479] [PMID: 28339817]

Letko, M, Marzi, A & Munster, V (2020) Functional assessment of cell entry and receptor usage for SARS-CoV-2 and other lineage B betacoronaviruses. *Nat Microbiol,* 5, 562-9.
[http://dx.doi.org/10.1038/s41564-020-0688-y] [PMID: 32094589]

Li, G, He, X, Zhang, L, Ran, Q, Wang, J, Xiong, A, Wu, D, Chen, F, Sun, J & Chang, C (2020) Assessing ACE2 expression patterns in lung tissues in the pathogenesis of COVID-19. *J Autoimmun,* 112, 102463.
[http://dx.doi.org/10.1016/j.jaut.2020.102463] [PMID: 32303424]

Li, H, Liu, S-M, Yu, X-H, Tang, S-L & Tang, C-K (2020) Coronavirus disease 2019 (COVID-19): current status and future perspectives. *Int J Antimicrob Agents,* 55, 105951.
[http://dx.doi.org/10.1016/j.ijantimicag.2020.105951] [PMID: 32234466]

Li, T (2020) Diagnosis and clinical management of severe acute respiratory syndrome Coronavirus 2 (SARS-CoV-2) infection: an operational recommendation of Peking Union Medical College Hospital (V2.0). *Emerg Microbes Infect,* 9, 582-5.
[http://dx.doi.org/10.1080/22221751.2020.1735265] [PMID: 32172669]

Li, T, Lu, H & Zhang, W (2020) Clinical observation and management of COVID-19 patients. *Emerg Microbes Infect,* 9, 687-90.
[http://dx.doi.org/10.1080/22221751.2020.1741327] [PMID: 32208840]

Li, T, Qiu, Z, Zhang, L, Han, Y, He, W, Liu, Z, Ma, X, Fan, H, Lu, W, Xie, J, Wang, H, Deng, G & Wang, A (2004) Significant changes of peripheral T lymphocyte subsets in patients with severe acute respiratory syndrome. *J Infect Dis,* 189, 648-51.
[http://dx.doi.org/10.1086/381535] [PMID: 14767818]

Liao, D, Zhou, F, Luo, L, Xu, M, Wang, H, Xia, J, Gao, Y, Cai, L, Wang, Z, Yin, P, Wang, Y, Tang, L, Deng, J, Mei, H & Hu, Y (2020) Haematological characteristics and risk factors in the classification and prognosis evaluation of COVID-19: a retrospective cohort study. *Lancet Haematol,* 7, e671-8.
[http://dx.doi.org/10.1016/S2352-3026(20)30217-9] [PMID: 32659214]

Liao, Y-C, Liang, W-G, Chen, F-W, Hsu, J-H, Yang, J-J & Chang, M-S (2002) Il-19 induces production of il-6 and tnf-α and results in cell apoptosis through Tnf-A. *J Immunology,* 169, 4288-97.

Lima, CMAO (2020) Information about the new coronavirus disease (COVID-19). *Radiol Bras,* 53, V-VI.
[http://dx.doi.org/10.1590/0100-3984.2020.53.2e1] [PMID: 32336833]

Lin, L, Lu, L, Cao, W & Li, T (2020) Hypothesis for potential pathogenesis of SARS-CoV-2 infection-a review of immune changes in patients with viral pneumonia. *Emerg Microbes Infect,* 9, 727-32.
[http://dx.doi.org/10.1080/22221751.2020.1746199] [PMID: 32196410]

Llitjos, JF, Leclerc, M, Chochois, C, Monsallier, JM, Ramakers, M, Auvray, M & Merouani, K (2020) High incidence of venous thromboembolic events in anticoagulated severe COVID-19 patients. *J Thromb Haemost,* 18, 1743-6.
[http://dx.doi.org/10.1111/jth.14869] [PMID: 32320517]

Mao, L, Wang, M, Chen, S, He, Q, Chang, J, Hong, C, Zhou, Y, Wang, D, Miao, X, Li, Y & Hu, B (2020) Neurologic Manifestations of Hospitalized Patients With Coronavirus Disease 2019 in Wuhan, China. *AMA Neurol,* 77, 683-90.
[http://dx.doi.org/10.1001/jamaneurol.2020.1127] [PMID: 32275288]

Mathew, AJ & Ravindran, V (2014) Infections and arthritis. *Best Pract Res Clin Rheumatol,* 28, 935-59.
[http://dx.doi.org/10.1016/j.berh.2015.04.009] [PMID: 26096095]

Mercorelli, B, Palù, G & Loregian, A (2018) 'Drug repurposing for viral infectious diseases: How far are we? *Trends Microbiol,* 26, 865-76.
[http://dx.doi.org/10.1016/j.tim.2018.04.004] [PMID: 29759926]

Muniyappa, R & Gubbi, S (2020) COVID-19 pandemic, coronaviruses, and diabetes mellitus. *Am J Physiol Endocrinol Metab,* 318, E736-41.
[http://dx.doi.org/10.1152/ajpendo.00124.2020] [PMID: 32228322]

Nabirotchkin, S, Peluffo, AE, Bouaziz, J & Cohen, D (2020) Focusing on the unfolded protein response and autophagy-related pathways to reposition common approved drugs against Covid-19. *Preprints,* 2020, 2020030302.

Ni, Y-N, Chen, G, Sun, J, Liang, B-M & Liang, Z-A (2019) The effect of corticosteroids on mortality of patients with influenza pneumonia: a systematic review and meta-analysis. *Crit Care,* 23, 99.
[http://dx.doi.org/10.1186/s13054-019-2395-8] [PMID: 30917856]

Peiris, JSM, Chu, C-M, Cheng, VC-C, Chan, KS, Hung, IF, Poon, LL, Law, K-I, Tang, BS, Hon, TY, Chan, CS, Chan, KH, Ng, JS, Zheng, BJ, Ng, WL, Lai, RW, Guan, Y & Yuen, KY HKU/UCH SARS Study Group (2003) Clinical progression and viral load in a community outbreak of coronavirus-associated SARS pneumonia: a prospective study. *Lancet,* 361, 1767-72.
[http://dx.doi.org/10.1016/S0140-6736(03)13412-5] [PMID: 12781535]

Pennington, E (2020) Asthma increases risk of severity of Covid-19. *Cleve Clin J Med.*
[http://dx.doi.org/10.3949/ccjm.87a.ccc002] [PMID: 32371563]

Petrie, JR, Guzik, TJ & Touyz, RM (2018) Diabetes, hypertension, and cardiovascular disease: Clinical insights and vascular mechanisms. *Can J Cardiol,* 34, 575-84.
[http://dx.doi.org/10.1016/j.cjca.2017.12.005] [PMID: 29459239]

Popov, D & Simionescu, M (1997) Alterations of lung structure in experimental diabetes, and diabetes associated with hyperlipidaemia in hamsters. *Eur Respir J,* 10, 1850-8.
[http://dx.doi.org/10.1183/09031936.97.10081850] [PMID: 9272930]

Rao, S, Lau, A & So, H-C (2020) Exploring diseases/traits and blood proteins causally related to the expression of ACE2, the putative receptor of 2019-Ncov: A mendelian randomization analysis. *Diabetes Care,* 43, 1416-26.
[http://dx.doi.org/10.2337/dc20-0643] [PMID: 32430459]

Rosa, SGV & Santos, WC (2020) Clinical trials on drug repositioning for COVID-19 treatment. *Rev Panam*

Salud Publica, 44, e40.
[http://dx.doi.org/10.26633/RPSP.2020.40] [PMID: 32256547]

Schell-Chaple, HM, Puntillo, KA, Matthay, MA, Liu, KD, Wiedemann, HP & Arroliga, AC, Jr National Heart, Lung, and Blood Institute Acute Respiratory Distress Syndrome Network (2015) Body temperature and mortality in patients with acute respiratory distress syndrome. *Am J Crit Care,* 24, 15-23.
[http://dx.doi.org/10.4037/ajcc2015320] [PMID: 25554550]

Singh, S, Sharma, A & Arora, SK (2014) High producer haplotype (CAG) of -863C/A, -308G/A and -238G/A polymorphisms in the promoter region of TNF-α gene associate with enhanced apoptosis of lymphocytes in HIV-1 subtype C infected individuals from North India. *PLoS One,* 9, e98020.
[http://dx.doi.org/10.1371/journal.pone.0098020] [PMID: 24837009]

Singhal, T (2020) A review of coronavirus disease-2019 (Covid-19). *Indian J Pediatr,* 87, 281-6.
[http://dx.doi.org/10.1007/s12098-020-03263-6] [PMID: 32166607]

Snijders, D, Schoorl, M, Schoorl, M, Bartels, PC, van der Werf, TS & Boersma, WG (2012) D-dimer levels in assessing severity and clinical outcome in patients with community-acquired pneumonia. A secondary analysis of a randomised clinical trial. *Eur J Intern Med,* 23, 436-41.
[http://dx.doi.org/10.1016/j.ejim.2011.10.019] [PMID: 22726372]

Song, J, Kang, S, Choi, SW, Seo, KW, Lee, S, So, MW & Lim, DH (2020) Coronavirus disease 19 (COVID-19) complicated with pneumonia in a patient with rheumatoid arthritis receiving conventional disease-modifying antirheumatic drugs. *Rheumatol Int,* 40, 991-5.
[http://dx.doi.org/10.1007/s00296-020-04584-7] [PMID: 32314010]

Spiezia, L, Boscolo, A, Poletto, F, Cerruti, L, Tiberio, I, Campello, E, Navalesi, P & Simioni, P (2020) Covid-19-related severe hypercoagulability in patients admitted to intensive care unit for acute respiratory failure. *Thromb Haemost,* 120, 998-1000.
[http://dx.doi.org/10.1055/s-0040-1710018] [PMID: 32316063]

Tan, L, Wang, Q, Zhang, D, Ding, J, Huang, Q, Tang, Y-Q, Wang, Q & Miao, H (2020) Lymphopenia predicts disease severity of COVID-19: A descriptive and predictive study. *Signal Transduct Target Ther,* 5, 1-3.

Tang, N, Li, D, Wang, X & Sun, Z (2020) Abnormal coagulation parameters are associated with poor prognosis in patients with novel coronavirus pneumonia. *J Thromb Haemost,* 18, 844-7.
[http://dx.doi.org/10.1111/jth.14768] [PMID: 32073213]

Tauber, SC, Eiffert, H, Brück, W & Nau, R (2017) Septic encephalopathy and septic encephalitis. *Expert Rev Anti Infect Ther,* 15, 121-32.
[http://dx.doi.org/10.1080/14787210.2017.1265448] [PMID: 27885885]

Van Der Poll, T, van de Veerdonk, FL, Scicluna, BP & Netea, MG (2017) The immunopathology of sepsis and potential therapeutic targets. *Nat Rev Immunol,* 17, 407-20.
[http://dx.doi.org/10.1038/nri.2017.36] [PMID: 28436424]

Van Nieuwkoop, C (2020) COVID-19 associated pulmonary thrombosis. *Thromb Res,* 191, 151.
[http://dx.doi.org/10.1016/j.thromres.2020.04.042] [PMID: 32386985]

Vinogradova, Y, Hippisley-Cox, J & Coupland, C (2009) Identification of new risk factors for pneumonia: population-based case-control study. *Br J Gen Pract,* 59, e329-38.
[http://dx.doi.org/10.3399/bjgp09X472629] [PMID: 19843413]

Wang, D, Hu, B, Hu, C, Zhu, F, Liu, X, Zhang, J, Wang, B, Xiang, H, Cheng, Z, Xiong, Y, Zhao, Y, Li, Y, Wang, X & Peng, Z (2020) a 'Clinical characteristics of 138 hospitalized patients with 2019 novel coronavirus–infected pneumonia in Wuhan, China'. *JAMA,* 323, 1061-9.
[http://dx.doi.org/10.1001/jama.2020.1585] [PMID: 32031570]

Wang, Y, Wang, Y, Chen, Y & Qin, Q (2020) Unique epidemiological and clinical features of the emerging 2019 novel coronavirus pneumonia (COVID-19) implicate special control measures. *J Med Virol,* 92, 568-76.
[http://dx.doi.org/10.1002/jmv.25748] [PMID: 32134116]

Warren-Gash, C, Blackburn, R, Whitaker, H, McMenamin, J & Hayward, AC (2018) Laboratory-confirmed respiratory infections as triggers for acute myocardial infarction and stroke: a self-controlled case series analysis of national linked datasets from Scotland. *Eur Respir J,* 51, 1701794.
[http://dx.doi.org/10.1183/13993003.01794-2017] [PMID: 29563170]

Wösten-Van Asperen, RM, Bos, AP, Bem, RA, Dierdorp, BS, Dekker, T, van Goor, H, Kamilic, J, van der Loos, CM, van den Berg, E, Bruijn, M, van Woensel, JB & Lutter, R (2013) Imbalance between pulmonary angiotensin-converting enzyme and angiotensin-converting enzyme 2 activity in acute respiratory distress syndrome. *Pediatr Crit Care Med,* 14, e438-41.
[http://dx.doi.org/10.1097/PCC.0b013e3182a55735] [PMID: 24226567]

Wu, C, Chen, X, Cai, Y, Xia, J, Zhou, X, Xu, S, Huang, H, Zhang, L, Zhou, X, Du, C, Zhang, Y, Song, J, Wang, S, Chao, Y, Yang, Z, Xu, J, Zhou, X, Chen, D, Xiong, W, Xu, L, Zhou, F, Jiang, J, Bai, C, Zheng, J & Song, Y (2020) a 'Risk factors associated with acute respiratory distress syndrome and death in patients with coronavirus disease 2019 pneumonia in Wuhan, China. *JAMA Intern Med,* 180, 934-43.
[http://dx.doi.org/10.1001/jamainternmed.2020.0994] [PMID: 32167524]

Wu, Y, Xu, X, Chen, Z, Duan, J, Hashimoto, K, Yang, L, Liu, C & Yang, C (2020) Nervous system involvement after infection with COVID-19 and other coronaviruses. *Brain Behav Immun,* 87, 18-22.
[http://dx.doi.org/10.1016/j.bbi.2020.03.031] [PMID: 32240762]

Wu, Z & McGoogan, JM (2020) Characteristics of and important lessons from the coronavirus disease 2019 (covid-19) outbreak in china: summary of a report of 72 314 cases from the Chinese center for disease control and prevention. *JAMA,* 323, 1239-42.
[http://dx.doi.org/10.1001/jama.2020.2648] [PMID: 32091533]

Xiang, P, Xu, X, Gao, L, Wang, H, Xiong, H & Li, R (2020) First case of 2019 novel coronavirus disease with encephalitis. *Chinaxiv,* 202003, 00015.

Xu, H, Zhong, L, Deng, J, Peng, J, Dan, H, Zeng, X, Li, T & Chen, Q (2020) a 'High expression of ace2 receptor of 2019-ncov on the epithelial cells of oral mucosa'. *Int J Oral Sci,* 12, 1-5.
[http://dx.doi.org/10.1038/s41368-020-0074-x]

Xu, Z, Shi, L, Wang, Y, Zhang, J, Huang, L, Zhang, C, Liu, S, Zhao, P, Liu, H, Zhu, L, Tai, Y, Bai, C, Gao, T, Song, J, Xia, P, Dong, J, Zhao, J & Wang, FS (2020) Pathological findings of COVID-19 associated with acute respiratory distress syndrome. *Lancet Respir Med,* 8, 420-2.
[http://dx.doi.org/10.1016/S2213-2600(20)30076-X] [PMID: 32085846]

Yang, X, Yu, Y, Xu, J, Shu, H, Xia, J, Liu, H, Wu, Y, Zhang, L, Yu, Z, Fang, M, Yu, T, Wang, Y, Pan, S, Zou, X, Yuan, S & Shang, Y (2020) Clinical course and outcomes of critically ill patients with SARS-CoV-2 pneumonia in Wuhan, China: a single-centered, retrospective, observational study. *Lancet Respir Med,* 8, 475-81.
[http://dx.doi.org/10.1016/S2213-2600(20)30079-5] [PMID: 32105632]

Yao, X, Ye, F, Zhang, M, Cui, C, Huang, B, Niu, P, Liu, X, Zhao, L, Dong, E, Song, C, Zhan, S, Lu, R, Li, H, Tan, W & Liu, D (2020) In *vitro* antiviral activity and projection of optimized dosing design of hydroxychloroquine for the treatment of severe acute respiratory syndrome coronavirus 2 (sars-cov-2). *Clin Infect Dis,* 71, 732-9.
[http://dx.doi.org/10.1093/cid/ciaa237] [PMID: 32150618]

Zemans, RL, Colgan, SP & Downey, GP (2009) Transepithelial migration of neutrophils: mechanisms and implications for acute lung injury. *Am J Respir Cell Mol Biol,* 40, 519-35.
[http://dx.doi.org/10.1165/rcmb.2008-0348TR] [PMID: 18978300]

Zhang, J-J, Dong, X, Cao, Y-Y, Yuan, Y-D, Yang, Y-B, Yan, Y-Q, Akdis, CA & Gao, Y-D (2020) Clinical characteristics of 140 patients infected with SARS-CoV-2 in Wuhan, China. *Allergy,* 75, 1730-41.
[http://dx.doi.org/10.1111/all.14238] [PMID: 32077115]

Zhang, Y, Cui, Y, Shen, M, Zhang, J, Liu, B, Dai, M, Chen, L, Han, D, Fan, Y & Zeng, Y (2020) 'Comorbid diabetes mellitus was associated with poorer prognosis in patients with covid-19: a retrospective cohort study. *Medrxiv.*

Zheng, X-Y, Xu, Y-J, Guan, W-J & Lin, L-F (2018) Regional, age and respiratory-secretion-specific prevalence of respiratory viruses associated with asthma exacerbation: a literature review. *Arch Virol,* 163, 845-53.
[http://dx.doi.org/10.1007/s00705-017-3700-y] [PMID: 29327237]

Zheng, YY, Ma, YT, Zhang, JY & Xie, X (2020) COVID-19 and the cardiovascular system. *Nat Rev Cardiol,* 17, 259-60.
[http://dx.doi.org/10.1038/s41569-020-0360-5] [PMID: 32139904]

Zhou, F, Yu, T, Du, R, Fan, G, Liu, Y, Liu, Z, Xiang, J, Wang, Y, Song, B, Gu, X, Guan, L, Wei, Y, Li, H, Wu, X, Xu, J, Tu, S, Zhang, Y, Chen, H & Cao, B (2020) Clinical course and risk factors for mortality of adult inpatients with COVID-19 in Wuhan, China: a retrospective cohort study. *Lancet,* 395, 1054-62.
[http://dx.doi.org/10.1016/S0140-6736(20)30566-3] [PMID: 32171076]

Zhou, P, Yang, X-L, Wang, X-G, Hu, B, Zhang, L, Zhang, W, Si, H-R, Zhu, Y, Li, B, Huang, C-L, Chen, HD, Chen, J, Luo, Y, Guo, H, Jiang, RD, Liu, MQ, Chen, Y, Shen, XR, Wang, X, Zheng, XS, Zhao, K, Chen, QJ, Deng, F, Liu, LL, Yan, B, Zhan, FX, Wang, YY, Xiao, GF & Shi, ZL (2020) A pneumonia outbreak associated with a new coronavirus of probable bat origin. *Nature,* 579, 270-3.
[http://dx.doi.org/10.1038/s41586-020-2012-7] [PMID: 32015507]

Zhou, Y, Fu, B, Zheng, X, Wang, D, Zhao, C, Qi, Y, Sun, R, Tian, Z, Xu, X & Wei, H (2020) Pathogenic T-cells and inflammatory monocytes incite inflammatory storms in severe Covid-19 patients. *Natl Sci Rev,* 7, 998-1002.
[http://dx.doi.org/10.1093/nsr/nwaa041]

CHAPTER 5

Vaccine Development

Priya Sharma[1,#], **Shivani Joshi**[1,#], **Aishwarya Joshi**[1], **Nikunj Tandel**[1] and **Rajeev K. Tyagi**[2,*]

[1] *Institute of Science, Nirma University, Ahmedabad, Gujarat, India*

[2] *Biomedical Parasitology and Nano-immunology Lab, CSIR Institute of Microbial Technology (IMTECH), Chandigarh, India*

Abstract: The current COVID-19 pandemic is a wake-up call pointing towards the vulnerability of humankind as it has outstretched its arms to almost all the continents, sparing few socially isolated ones. The highly contagious nature, ultra-stable genetic makeup, novel modifications in open reading frame (ORF) region, air-born route of transmission, and ability to cross the species barrier prove the potential of COVID-19 to elicit the global pandemic situation. In current times, when even known antibiotics for combating several diseases are being rendered inefficacious owing to the rising multidrug resistance among pathogenic strains, the panacea to a wide array of diseases can be vaccination. A prominent characteristic for COVID-19 vaccine development is that numerous technologies from lipid nanoparticle (LNP)-encapsulation, dendritic cells (DCs)-based vaccines, antigen-presenting cells (artificial-APCs)-based vaccines, and DNA plasmid-based platforms to viral vector approaches are being evaluated for the cause. Certain vaccine development technologies may be better suited for some parts of the global population, while others may prove to be more efficacious for the other population subtypes. This may not only be arising due to geographical or ethnic distinctions, but also physiological differences such as the presence of comorbidities, immune profile of subjects, *etc*. In this chapter, we attempt to bring forth the various approaches or molecular platforms that have been taken up or proposed for the development of a vaccine against coronavirus disease. We also attempt to elaborate on the pros and cons associated with each of the approaches that may be feasible due to the distinctions in the various population subtypes.

Keywords: Air-borne transmission, Animal model, APCs-based vaccines, Artificial-APCs, Comorbidities, COVID-19, DCs-based vaccines, DNA plasmid-based platforms, Genetic makeup multidrug resistance, Global population, Immune profile, Lipid nanoparticle (LNP), Molecular platforms, Novel modifications, Pathogenic strains, Physiological differences, Population subtypes, Vaccine development, Viral vector approaches.

* **Corresponding author Rajeev K. Tyagi:** Biomedical Parasitology and Nano-immunology Lab, CSIR Institute of Microbial Technology (IMTECH), Chandigarh, India; Tel: 91-172-6665278;
E-mails: rajeevtyagi@imtech.res.in and rajeev.gru@gmail.com
# Equal Contribution

Neeraj Mittal, Sanjay Kumar Bhadada, O. P. Katare and Varun Garg (Eds.)

COVID-19: VACCINE DEVELOPMENT

Over the past decade, vaccine technology has undergone immense evolution, and different approaches for the development of vaccines against viruses and other pathogens have emerged. The advancement has enabled researchers to develop a wide range of vaccine candidates such as nucleic acid-based (DNA/RNA) vaccines, recombinant protein-based vaccines, and viral-vectored vaccines, *etc*. The rapid revelation of the genetic map of the SARS-CoV-2 viral genome has opened avenues facilitating several vaccine development programs against COVID-19 (Liu *et al.*, 2017). As of the current scenario, there is no antiviral drug available as a frontline treatment for the disease. To conquer the threat of COVID-19, urgent therapeutic intervention is the need of the hour, and therefore several strategies for vaccine development, besides drug development, have been initiated (Taghizadeh-Hesary and Akbari, 2020). As a result of these, there are currently 115 potential vaccine candidates across the globe, 78 of which are established as active projects; 5 among those candidates have already successfully crossed the pre-clinical stages (Grifoni *et al.*, 2020).

It is a remarkable feature of research & development for the COVID-19 vaccine that a wide assortment of platforms is being tried out. As mentioned earlier, platforms including nucleic acid-based vaccines, recombinant proteins, live attenuated virus, as well as inactivated virus-based approaches, alongside viral peptides, virus-like particles (VLPs), and replicating/non-replicating viral vectors are being explored for the development of SARS-CoV-2 vaccine. It is advantageous that several approaches have been taken up, especially concerning the fact that certain immunization technologies may be efficient for a specific group of population. This specific effectiveness relates not only in terms of age, ethnic, or epigenetic differences but also correlates to the physiological variances such as the presence of certain comorbidities (Grifoni *et al.*, 2020). The extensive study on the SARS-CoV-2 virus and its genome has revealed potential targets for vaccines and drug interventions. Bioinformatics and computational tools have a significant role to play in recognizing the most competent targets. A large number of databases have been created for easy and correct identification of potential vaccine targets (Taghizadeh-Hesary and Akbari, 2020). The characterization of the SARS-CoV-2 spike glycoprotein has enabled the researchers to identify precise immunogenic epitopes that can be taken into account for vaccine development. Their extensive analysis pointed out 13 and 3 epitopes for MHC-I & II respectively on the spike glycoprotein of the virus that can be incorporated in the formulation of a multi-epitopic peptide vaccine. Further, these candidate epitopes have been assessed for their effective immunogenicity through molecular docking with TLR-5; However, *in vitro* and *in vivo* validations are required to confirm the potential of this vaccine candidate. The fact that the SARS-CoV-2 virus is proximally related to MERS and SARS viruses which has allowed researchers to utilize structure-function comparisons to hasten the process of recognizing potential vaccine candidates (Taghizadeh-Hesary and Akbari, 2020).

Nevertheless, there are certain challenges associated with vaccine development. After the identification and *in silico* validation of a vaccine candidate, it is taken forward for a formulation, which itself is a long process. In the first phase, it passes through the rigorous tests for the efficacy and safety in animal models. It is safe to consider the fact that developing suitable animal models for SARS-CoV-2 may be a challenge in itself, as the virus is known to not propagate in wild-type mice; Further, this virus only induces a mild form of the disease in transgenic animals that are engineered to express human ACE2 (Liu *et al.*, 2017). However, even in the absence of animal models, it is not entirely impossible to assess the vaccine candidate. Serum obtained from the immunized animals can be further validated through *in vitro* testing *via* neutralization assays. The remaining part of this tier is to gauge the vaccine candidate for its safety in animals in a manner acquiescent to the GLP (Good Laboratory Practices) guidelines and usually lasts for a minimum period of 6 months. This is followed by the production of vaccine compliant to current good manufacturing practice (cGMP) that assures the quality and safety of the vaccine. The second tier that includes the clinical phase I (small trials to evaluate safety on humans), phase II (aimed at establishing dosages and formulations to substantiate efficacy in humans), and phase III trials (both efficacy and safety of the vaccine candidate should be validated in a larger population). However, in certain unexpected conditions, such as during the pandemic of COVID-19, the guidelines may be flexible, and the process for approval may be accelerated with necessary precautions taken.

COVID-19 VACCINE DEVELOPMENT: MODULATING THE HOST IMMUNE SYSTEM

To understand the mechanisms of immunization that can facilitate the modulation of the host immune system in response to SARS-CoV-2, it is substantial that we apprehend the natural manifestations that the host system gradually adapts to modulate the response to the viral infection. The virus can successfully invade the cells which express the ACE2 and TMPRSS2 (transmembrane protease serine 2) surface receptors. Once the cells get infected, the viral genome undergoes active replication followed by cascade steps and releases the copies of the packaged virus from the infected cell. It is followed by pyroptosis, a mechanism through which cells release the damage-associated molecular patterns (DAMPs). These DAMPs are recognized by surrounding cells such as epithelial cells, endothelial cells, and alveolar macrophages, which in turn trigger a pro-inflammatory condition in the milieu by inducing the generation of cytokines and chemokines, primarily IL-6, macrophage inflammatory protein (MIP)1α, MIP1β, interferon gamma-induced protein-10 (IP-10), and monocytes chemoattractant protein-1 (MCP-1). This conglomeration of pro-inflammatory cytokines stimulates the important players of the host-immune system to drive monocytes, macrophages, and T cells towards the site of infection. This results in the augmentation of inflammatory conditions, hence establishing a pro-inflammatory feedback loop (Tay *et al.*, 2020).

Both the branches of the host immune system, the innate and the adaptive immunity, are involved in response towards SARS. Due to the genomic resemblance of SARS-CoV-2 to SARS, a similar immune response is expected in the case of SARS-COV-2 (Taghizadeh-Hesary and Akbari, 2020). The innate wing of the immune response against a viral infection profoundly depends upon the type I-IFN and the subsequent cascade which induces appropriate immune responses. Nevertheless, the direct targeting of macrophages and T cells in the case of SARS and SARS-CoV-2 is yet to be determined. The innate immune sentinels should essentially recognize the viral invasion usually facilitated by PAMPs, in the form of genomic RNA or virus replication dsRNA intermediates. These virus-associated PAMPs are recognized by any of the receptors such as TLR 3 (toll-like receptor 3), TLR 7, RIG-I (retinoic acid-inducible gene I) & MDA 5 (melanoma differentiation-associated protein 5), and endosomal RNA receptors/cytosolic RNA sensors (Prompetchara *et al.*, 2020). This elicits a cascade of downstream signaling events resulting in the suppression of viral replication and propagation at an initial stage. In addition to this, the cascade which involves signaling-mediated activation and translocation of NF-κB (nuclear factor- kappa-B) and IRF 3 (Interferon regulatory transcription factor 3) towards the nucleus, facilitates the expression of pro-inflammatory cytokines, especially type I-IFN, which further conjunct with IFNAR (interferon α/β receptor), initiates the JAK-STAT signaling pathway, and activates the STAT1/2 proteins which form a complex with interferon regulatory factor-IRF 9. The cascade of this complex-formation signals the transcription of IFN-stimulated genes in the nucleus that enables the innate immune system to mount an efficacious response against the virus (Prompetchara *et al.*, 2020).

Adaptive immunity is specific in its nature of the action and is mediated majorly by T and B cells (Tay *et al.*, 2020). Typically, the central role in mediating adaptive immunity against virus infections is played by the Th1 cells (Prompetchara *et al.*, 2020). Th1 (T helper type 1 cells) cells mainly secrete IFN-γ, IL-2, and TNF-β (tumor necrosis factor β) cytokines, which further engage macrophages, hence involving the CMI (cell-mediated immunity) as well as inducing the response mechanisms dependent on phagocytic activity (Romagnani, 1999). Th1 subset is generally produced as a measure to combat intracellular bacterial and certain viral infections. Complementarily, another cell type, Th2 cells, are involved in the production of IL-4, IL-5, IL-10, and IL-13, which trigger a cognate-antibody production and stimulate the eosinophils, thus facilitating a phagocyte-independent immune response. It suggests that the Th2 subset is principally involved in generating immune responses against nematodes invading the gastrointestinal system (Romagnani, 1999). Alongside the Th cells that orchestrate the adaptive immunity, the cytotoxic T (Tc) cells majorly take part in identifying and eliminating the virus-infected host cells. Besides the role in mediating adaptive immunity, humoral mediated immunity (HMI) further comes into the picture at the later stage of the infection which is administered by B cells through the virus-specific antibody production. This results in the immediate neutralization of invading antigen and also generates the immunogenic memory which can eliminate the same antigen much rapidly during the relapse of infection.

In this regard, several studies based on structural proteome of various coronaviruses were conducted which also includes having the close resemblance to the SARS. The results of these studied have discovered several immunogenic epitopes which can further use as a potential vaccine candidates/components, given the feasibility of cross-reactivity with SARS-CoV-2 epitopes. As mentioned in the prior section, the approach of immunoinformatics and related computational tools can play a central role in facilitating the identification of such epitopes. For this purpose experts have utilized the database of IEDB (Immune epitope database and analysis resource), which is based upon the mathematical algorithm to fulfill the criteria in finding an appropriate epitopes for a given sequence. Another widely used repository in this regard is ViPR (virus pathogen resource) that offers data pertaining to viruses exhibiting human pathogenicity and encompasses genome/protein sequences, immunogenic epitopes and reveals the mechanism of host responses which might play a role for particular viral infections (Grifoni *et al.*, 2020). This study was the first attempted to define immunodominant regions within the SARS genome, wherein B cell epitopes derived from the genome were mapped back to a reference sequence using IEDB; following this, sequences of the SARS B cells epitope region were aligned against SARS-CoV-2 sequence to determine the similarities among the two regions. As a result, out of the 10 identified regions, six regions have showed an identity of more than 90% with SARS-CoV-2 sequences and another two have been matched with 80% to 89% identity (Grifoni *et al.*, 2020). Interestingly, their analysis depicted that the T cell epitopes hence recognized, show predominant association with the spike glycoprotein and the nucleoprotein. This study also sought to address identification of potential SARS-CoV-2 T cell-based epitopes *via* predictive algorithms that were used to map hundreds of human epitopes so as to account for HLA (human leukocyte antigen) polymorphism.

TYPES OF VACCINES AND THEIR CHARACTERISTICS

With the development and advances in the field of therapeutic interventions in last 200 years, vaccine development has emerged as one of the promising tools of medical technology to boost up the host immunity and/or to fight against a wide range of diseases (Rauch *et al.*, 2018). This section sheds light on the various major vaccine development approaches and their key features.

Live-attenuated Virus and Inactivated Whole Virus Vaccines

Live-attenuated vaccines are based upon direct mimicry of natural immune response that is elicited by the pathogens. This is the most primitive and the familiar approaches dating back to Edward Jenner's landmark work. These approaches, by and large, are centered on employing the disease-causative pathogen in an exterminated form or in a live, mitigated form (mitigation of the pathogenicity is achieved either through artificial means or through *in vitro* cell culture propagation). Such causative pathogen does not lead to clinical infection, but induces immunity at the same time (Loomis and Johnson, 2015). It has been reported that live-attenuated virus vaccines elicit strong HMI and CMI response by generating cognate B and T cells, respectively (Tse *et al.*, 2020). Overwhelming benefits of this approach that have been observed globally; for instance, MMR (mumps, measles and rubella) vaccine developed using this approach has helped in dampening the global load of mumps, measles and rubella (Loomis and Johnson, 2015). Nevertheless the design of this approach also has a few limitations that have urged researchers to venture into more advanced approaches. It is not necessarily feasible for all pathogens to be cultivated *in vitro;* it might not be possible to replicate certain conditions that support the culture of particular types of pathogen *in vitro*. Further, there is always a risk of inadequate practices that might lead to insufficient attenuation/inactivation, rendering the vaccine as lethal or detrimental as the pathogen itself. The possibility that an attenuated vaccine can elicit unwanted immune responses cannot be ruled out, indicating that these approaches might be extremely unsuitable for certain pathogens, especially those who demonstrate antigenic hypervariability; this might also hold true for pathogens that have a distinct intracellular phase in their pathophysiology (Rappuoli, 2004, Loomis and Johnson, 2015). In Beijing, Sinovac Biotech has developed two inactivated vaccines, one with alum as an adjuvant which is currently under Pre-clinical, Phase 1/2 stage trials. Similarly, Beijing Institute of Biological Products, China National Biotec Group, China has a candidate inactivate viral vaccine under phase 1/2 stage trial.

Subunit Vaccines

To tackle the diseases that cannot be challenged by the first generation vaccines, other technologies need to be ventured into. Subunit vaccines, as the name suggests, utilize only a part of the pathogen that is generally a conserved region and easily accessible/legible (in contrast to whole pathogen in the aforementioned section) which can elicit an appropriate immune response (Loomis and Johnson, 2015). Subunit vaccines are constructed on the basis of synthetic peptides or recombinant proteins which are specific in targeting well-defined neutralizing epitopes with enhanced efficacy or immunogenicity. Several vaccines for MERS and SARS have been developed with this approach. For both, the S protein has been regarded as a major candidate; not only the full-length S protein, but also its antigenic fragments such as the N-terminal domain (NTD), the C-terminal domain (CTD), S1 and S2 subunits can assume the role of potential targets for the subunit vaccine (Wang *et al.*, 2020). Nevertheless, though full-length S protein-based subunit vaccine could invoke a strong immune response, there are reports about certain antibodies triggered by these vaccines elevated the viral infection in *in vitro*, raising a red flag in the use of this approach. Further, as subunit vaccine candidates, the NTD fragment and the S2 fragment generate prompt immune responses. However less immunogenicity and generation of lower antibody titers are the major concerns associated with these vaccine candidates. Contrarily, a subunit vaccine constructed using the receptor-binding domain (RBD) of the virus consists of only the main neutralizing domain, and also elicits an apt immune response; besides other counterparts like S1 fragment, RBD can be considered as critical target for the development of a subunit vaccine, especially when the criteria of safety and efficacy are taken into consideration (Wang *et al.*, 2020). Besides the S protein, other candidates have also been considered as potential subunit vaccine targets for coronavirus diseases. The N protein of SARS and MERS viruses is unable to generate neutralizing antibodies which can hinder the virus-receptor interactions or nullify the infection. Although, the N protein might be able to induce cellular immune response as well as specific antibody response; several immunodominant epitopes for B and T cells, that are conserved among mice, non-human primates and humans, have been found in the N-proteins of both these viruses (Veit *et al.*, 2018, Wang *et al.*, 2020). Considering this, N-proteins might be used as an additional target, if not as the solitary target in a subunit vaccine.

There are several factors that affect the overall quality and the expression of the proteins that are used in the formation of subunit vaccines, especially in the case of the recombinant protein-based ones. A study carried out by Chang *et al.*, reported that incorporation of an intron splicing enhancer to S protein fragments resulted into the higher protein expression in mammalian cells with compare to the same using exon splicing enhancers in SARS subunit vaccine candidate (Chang *et al.*, 2006, Wang *et al.*, 2020). Besides molecular factors, other factors that affect the immunogenicity and efficacy of subunit vaccines might also come into play. For instance, the route of administration of the vaccine might affect the immunogenicity differently. Administration of adjuvants to stimulate higher Ig (immunoglobulin) titers and IFN-γ secretion is also a suitable approach to enhance the efficacy of subunit vaccines (Wang *et al.*, 2020).

Few groups of scientists designed subunit vaccine which failed since they either only used single protein or only CTL (cytotoxic T-lymphocytes) epitopes for vaccine design or neglected the importance of B-cell or helper T (Th) cell epitopes. Kalita *et al.*, (2020) constructed a subunit vaccine comprising of adjuvant, cytotoxic T cells (Tc), Th cells, and B cell epitopes connected with specific linkers. They retrieved the amino acid sequences of three SARS-CoV-2 proteins like nucleocapsid protein (N), membrane glycoprotein (M), and surface spike glycoprotein (S) from NCBI database, to ensure an optimal immune response since they are known to have an eminent role in host receptor recognition, pathogenicity and entry of the virus. 6 Th cells, 18 Tc cells, and 9 B-cell epitopes obtained from three proteins and human β-defensin as linker were used to construct the vaccine. Evaluation of the binding energy of vaccine with its TLR3 (Toll-like receptor) receptor was carried out with vaccine-receptor docking. The complex with lowest energy and -1491 kJ/mol binding energy was selected for MD simulation. Furthermore, the epitopes were checked for their potential toxicity. The subunit vaccine turned out thermostable, antigenic, and non-allergenic. Optimization of production process will lead to rapid testing and commercialization. Computational studies demonstrated good safety and protective efficacy of this multi-epitope vaccine against SARS-CoV-2 (Kalita *et al.*, 2020).

Vaccines Based on Virus-like Particles (VLPs)

The structural proteins of several viruses are capacitated such that they can direct the assembly of repetitive clusters or VLPs falling in the range of 22 to 150 nm (Grgacic and Anderson, 2006). Strikingly, these VLPs closely resemble to the viruses but are devoid of the ability to cause an infection as they lack the viral genetic material. These are attributed with greatly repetitive and high-density display of epitopes, which enables the vaccine design to prompt resilient host immune response. These virus-resembling particles induce not only the humoral arm, but also the cellular arm of the adaptive immunity. Moreover, the size range in which VLPs fall is optimal, as is the case with liposomes, for uptake by APCs such as dendritic cells (DCs) (Grgacic and Anderson, 2006). Because of this unique property, they do not require any additional adjuvants to stimulate the immune response. Their self-adjuvant attribute facilitates their uptake by DCs followed by the cascades of processing and MHC-II presentation. Further, exogenously designed and delivered VLPs can also be processed and presented *via* MHC-I pathway, leading to cross-presentation based activation of CD8[+] T cells (Tc cells). These properties give VLPs and edge over the more superseded approaches in the prospect of vaccine development. In fact, successful VLP vaccines against viral diseases like hepatitis B and human papilloma virus (HPV) have already been devised and licensed for human use (Grgacic and Anderson, 2006). However, viruses those pose a greater challenge to the immune system have certainly put this technology to test. Adaptations in their construct, in terms of factors like particle size and route of administration can be made in order to obtain optimal immune responses using this approach (Grgacic and Anderson, 2006). Assembling chimeric VLPs is a good tactic for incorporating those antigens in the construct, which cannot self-replicate in a particulate system; VLPs can be generated in various expression systems inclusive of mammalian, yeast and specific virus expression systems (Masavuli *et al.*, 2017). Utilizing adenoviral and lentivial vectors following BSL-2 practices, the pseudo-viral system was formed and used as experimental models to study the entry of enveloped viruses, including SARS-CoV-2 (Nie *et al.*, 2020, Ou *et al.*, 2020). A study on VLP-based vaccine construct reported that a chimeric construct incorporating SARS S protein plus MHV-CoV (mouse hepatitis coronavirus) E, M and N proteins stimulated higher production of antibodies specific to SARS (Zhang *et al.*, 2014, Lokugamage *et al.*, 2008). It is also regarded that vaccines designed with this approach tend to have abridged immunogenicity as compared to live attenuated vaccines or inactivated whole virus vaccines. To overcome this shortcoming, a handful of strategies can be utilized; for instance, molecules instigating APCs can be integrated to the VLP construct *via* genetic engineering protocols (Zhang *et al.*, 2014).

As an attainable relevant and safe substitute of naturally occurring viruses, there is a high demand of construction of SARS-CoV-2 VLPs for current fight against COVID-19. In a study carried out by Xu *et al.,* 2020, SARS-CoV-2 VLPs are efficiently constructed using mammalian expression system that helps the maintenance of protein glycosylation patterns. It revealed that out of four SARS-CoV-2 structural proteins, small envelope protein (E) and membrane protein (M) expression is critical for formation and release of SARS-CoV-2 VLPs (Xu *et al.*, 2020). M protein is found in abundance responsible for packaging of other structural proteins, just like in other members of *coronaviridae* family. E protein has also been found helpful for viral morphogenesis. The evaluation of SARS-CoV-2 VLPs morphology in Vero E6 cells showed increased incorporation of S glycoproteins on the surface. Thus the approach adopted by Xu *et al.,* 2020 confirmed the molecular and morphological resemblance between native virion particles and SARS-CoV-2 VLPs.

Viral Vector-based Vaccines

The viral vector-based vaccine is very distinct from the subunit or inactivated whole virus vaccines, the latter working as exogenous immunogens. On the contrary, a viral vector-construct utilizes the DNA carried by it that encodes immunogenic components in the host cell followed by their encoding for the antigenic peptide/protein, after which the antigen is expressed intracellularly. As a result it instigates the broad-spectrum of immunity that comprises of both, the HMI and CMI of the immune system. It is a lucrative approach because of the ease of development and the direct production of virus stock (Loomis and Johnson, 2015). In general, these vaccines are regarded as live vaccines, but due to their replication being diminished, they can be considered safe and used even for immunocompromised individuals (de Vries and Rimmelzwaan, 2016). The virus from which it is derived lays the platform for specific properties possessed by the vector and hence different viral vector-based vaccines have unique and distinctive set of advantages and limitations. However a major issue associated in general with this approach is the utmost requirement of assessment of safety and efficiency that covers several parameters of genotoxicity, replication insufficiency or the capacity of the vector to elude-pre-established immunity in the host (Ura *et al.*, 2014). Nevertheless, this approach is among the most popular ones in developing MERS vaccine; in fact two in three candidates for MERS vaccine making it to clinical trials are viral vector-based vaccines (Yong *et al.*, 2019). Among several viruses that are used to develop vaccines with this approach, vaccinia virus and MVA (modified vaccinia virus Ankara) are among the most extensively exploited ones. Particularly, these have been indicated in the development of influenza vaccines; though vaccinia virus vectors have exhibited great immunogenicity in animal models, frequent reports of substantial reactogenicity have also emerged. This makes it necessary to address the issue of reactogenicity by developing modified/engineered forms of this vaccinia virus vectors (de Vries and Rimmelzwaan, 2016). MVA is an attenuated form of the vaccinia virus that was developed by serial passaging of chorioallantoisvaccinia virus ankara in chicken embryo fibroblasts. This resulted into the deletions and alterations in the viral genome, helped in developing a viral vector that exhibited certain advantages over the original viral vector. It accounted for easy insertion of antigens in the vector genome, transient expression of heterologous antigens in *in-vivo* settings and subsequent stimulation of HIM and CMI in animal models and humans. To augment for favorable features offered by MVA viral vector, it also exhibited incapacity to elude the host immunity, and its safety was confirmed in immunodeficient mammals (de Vries and Rimmelzwaan, 2016). A study has also reported that MAIT cells (mucosal immunity-associated invariant T cells) might be playing a key role in the immunogenicity rendered by adenovirus vectors that are replication-deficient in nature. The activation of MAIT cells by this virus vector depicts requirement of transduction of monocytes for the production of IL-8, and pDCs (plasmacytoid dendritic cells) resulting in the generation and secretion of IFN-α (Provine *et al.*, 2019).

ChAdOx1 nCoV-19 is an adenovirus-vectored vaccine that encodes the spike protein of SARS-CoV-2. This candidate vaccine elicited a robust cell-mediated and humoral response and was found immunogenic in mice. The immunization with ChAdOx1 nCoV-19 (prime-only and prime-boost regimen) showed a balanced Th1/Th2 humoral and cellular response in rhesus macaques. Significant reduction in viral load of alveolar lavage was observed. Although, there was no difference in nasal shedding of vaccinated and control animals (Van Doremalen *et al.*, 2020).

DNA Vaccines

The approach of DNA vaccines gained popularity in the 1990s when the reports of intramuscular or intradermal delivery of plasmid DNA can induce antibody responses against viral/non-viral antigens. These vaccines are constructed using DNA coding sequences (that encode the candidate antigen protein) inserted in a suitable plasmid consist of a eukaryotic regulatory promoter. Other than the promoter, the plasmid should essentially possess a convenient cloning site for incorporating the gene of interest, a polyadenylation termination sequence, a prokaryotic origin of replication, and a selectable marker. The plus side of this approach is that DNA vaccines can be administered through various routes and a wide array of delivery mechanisms can be used; moreover, these can induce all-encompassing immune response inclusive of CD8$^+$ and CD4$^+$ T cells, and antibody production (Nichols and W. LeDuc, 2009). Additionally, the unmethylated DNA motifs in the vaccine can potentially prompt TLR-9 mediated innate immune responses (Kwissa *et al.*, 2007).

The conventional way of DNA vaccine delivery is mediated through intramuscular, intradermal or subcutaneous injection, majorly addressing the myocytes and keratinocytes, and the APCs in the surrounding milieu (Hobernik and Bros, 2018). Prior to internalization of DNA vaccine into the cell, it is translocated into the nucleus for transcription and subsequent translation into the cytoplasm. Henceforth, in the case of intradermal/subcutaneous route of administration, keratinocytes generate the specific antigen which is released by exosomes and internalized by APCs; the APCs present the antigen to CD4$^+$ T cells through MHC-II presentation. This leads to priming of B cells that mount an antibody response against the antigen. CD4$^+$ T cells also mediate complete activation of CD8$^+$ T cells (Hobernik and Bros, 2018, den Haan *et al.*, 2014). In the case of intramuscular delivery, the myocytes in which transfection has occurred successfully, undergo apoptosis and the apoptotic bodies are engulfed by APCs. The APCs cross-present the antigen (in the exogenous form) to CD8$^+$ T cells *via* MHC-I pathway (den Haan *et al.*, 2014, Lazzaro *et al.*, 2015).

Despite the positive outcomes of this approach, it still holds a question for its effectiveness, majorly because the success these exhibit at pre-clinical stages does not translate to the clinical stage as of yet. The major hindrance is the generation of mitigated immunogenicity in bigger animals and humans. This, in most probability, is due to the fact that upscale of the DNA amount used in smaller animals, for human system is a difficult process. To overcome this, certain measures can be taken up. These include optimization protocols such as the use of a hybrid promotor or of one exhibiting APC-specific activity; incorporation of immunostimulatory sequences, A/T rich sequences, nuclear localization sequences and so on. Other optimization protocols include adopting antigen specific modifications such as codon optimization, or combination of different Ags. Another approach that can be considered to address this challenge is to co-administer adjuvants such as the immunostimulatory CpG oligonucleotides (Hobernik and Bros, 2018).

Other means of DNA vaccine delivery such as gene gun-mediated delivery (Chen *et al.*, 1999), electroporation (Lee *et al.*, 2015) and nanoparticles mediated delivery, have been also assessed by several studies. Among these approaches, nanoparticle-based delivery holds great potential in enhancing immune response generated by DNA vaccines. The optimal size of the nanoparticles (<200 nm) facilitates their uptake by the host cells. Encapsulation of the DNA vaccine candidate in nanoparticles also prevents degradation of the nucleic acid which resulted in stabilizing the respective formulation (Shah *et al.*, 2014). Elastic liposomes entrapping a DNA vaccine candidate can easily undergo extravasation owing to their ultradeformability and enable us to overcome the challenges faced by conventional methods of transdermal immunization (Tyagi *et al.*, 2015).

Despite the promising approach that a DNA-based vaccine is, it cannot be neglected that its administration is not immunogenically inert. Genotoxicity arising from the integration of the DNA vaccine candidate into the genome, causing unsolicited mutations and subsequent adverse effects has always been in question. Another concern is that the administration of such formulations can generate the possible risk of producing anti-DNA antibodies by the host itself, a classic hallmark of several autoimmune disorders. In this regard, several studies are under pipeline over the years to assess the concerns of autoimmunity associated with DNA vaccines and a few studies have shown that DNA vaccines neither induce, nor worsen autoimmunity. However, their suitability and efficacy needs to be checked before taking them to the next stage.

NOVEL APPROACHES: USAGE OF MULTIDISCIPLINARY FIELDS

SARS-CoV-2 has turned out to be challenging which needs efforts of several disciplines to rejoin at the biggest platform to eliminate or to overcome from the dire condition. The pathophysiology of this infection has kept physicians and scientists under bleak condition where they have to search for every possible option to fight against the SARS-CoV-2. Therefore, several new options are explored and some of them are discussed below:

Serum Albumin Strategy

In addition to the existing approaches, adoption of a strategy which can target intracellular and extracellular viral particles is one of the prime priorities for the research. The drugs that can block the entry of viral particles or curb the intracellular viral component hold enormous potential (Kruse, 2020). Serum albumin is a multifunctional protein that interacts with a wide range of endogenous and exogenous compounds. Hence it can act as an efficient vehicle for wide range of targets such as viral protease, polymerase and RNA. Several clinical and experimental data suggests the correlation between the levels of albumin and inflammation where larger amount of albumin is taken by the cells, which are under the stress and inflamed condition (Don and Kaysen, 2004). Similarly, recent studies support the idea of albumin therapy in COVID-19 patients as there has been established a relationship between albumin and ACE-2 receptors which are responsible for virus entry in to human cells. Considering all above facts, a combinational therapy will be most beneficial where one component blocks the entry of virus and other targets internalized viral components. Furthermore, usage of serum albumin will aid the efficient internalization of drug and enhance pharmacological effects. A group of researchers proved that the use of epigallocatechingallate (EGCG) and curcumin is successful in neutralizing the range of viruses like hepatitis B, porcine circovirus type 2, influenza virus, zika and chikungunya (Chen *et al.*, 2010, Lai *et al.*, 2018, Li *et al.*, 2020). It was reported that EGCG and curcumin helps by inhibiting viral replication of SARS CoV-2 (Yang *et al.*, 2017, Siu *et al.*, 2019). If such drugs are internalized with the help of albumin in combination with molecules that inhibit the entry of virus in human cells, it will really help in improvement of patients' health.

Natural Product (Plant) Based Technology

Plant based vaccines have demonstrated great potential which even resulted in a few candidates being tested in clinical trials against swine flu, influenza, rabies, and hepatitis B (Rosales-Mendoza *et al.*, 2012). Hence plant based vaccines holds potential but the development process is very slow as of the novel approach in the field of therapeutic vaccines. History is suggestive of the fact that this technology can prove helpful in our quest for fighting COVID-19 pandemic. These vaccines are considered comparatively safe and their immunogenic characteristics were revealed through various *in vitro* assays which demonstrated positive outcome with no adverse effects. Plant based vaccine can serve a greater purpose of delivering cost effective alternative since they don't require any purification for antigen isolation. This technology can be used to trigger gut associated lymphoid tissue (GALT) with the help of plants that do not produce toxic metabolites (for example rice or corn transgenic lines or transplastomic lines) (Rosales-Mendoza and Salazar-Gonzalez, 2014). Additionally, it can overcome the usage of injection and risks associated with their invasive routes of administration. Few shortcomings like poor antigen stability and bioavailability pose concerns in development of plant based technology against COVID-19.

At present, accessible foreign protein expression methodologies in plants is dependent on nature of selected antigen. The use of VLPs is one of the most distinguished ways to develop plant based vaccine which can avoid shortcomings of attenuated or live vaccines however it attains the enough immunity to fight the infections. It has been observed that mice models injected with SARS CoV-2 VLPs subcutaneously show elevated titers of antibodies against SARS. Furthermore, cellular immunity was shown to be elicited with higher levels of cytokines IFN-γ and IL-4 (Lu *et al.*, 2007).

Another prominent approach is the development of multi-epitope based vaccines which will help us obtain rational vaccine design that can elicit robust immune response involving Th, B, and T cell epitopes. One noteworthy advantage of this approach is it can provide protection against the genetic variability (of virus) observed in SARS CoV-2. Given that, multi-epitope vaccine is successful translated in a plant system and the production of these vaccines will be highly feasible (Govea-Alonso *et al.*, 2013a). One of the several approach, is production of immune complexes (IC) which is comprise of antigens that are recognized by antibodies to form a complex and exposed to macromolecular entities which ultimately leads to antigen processing and presentation by APCs. This induces effective HMI and CMI based response. Plant cell machinery can be maneuvered as IC producing factories. Nonetheless, the major shortcoming faced here is requirement of defined antibodies targeting antigens which is not available for SARS CoV-2 yet.

Purification of antigens for injectable vaccines is a cumbersome and expensive process which can be overcome with the help of elastin-like polypeptide (ELP) fusions. ELPs possess a unique characteristic which precipitates the protein of interest by simply altering the temperature. For example, tobacco was used to express *M. tuberculosis* antigens Ag85B and ESAT-6 by fusing it with ELPs (Govea-Alonso *et al.*, 2013b, Phan *et al.*, 2013). Perhaps, the main challenge as faced by other candidate vaccines would be assessing their efficacy at larger stage of clinical trials and fulfilling all regulatory demands to assure safety. Although the motivating fact is a plant-made biopharmaceutical against influenza is under clinical trials with promising safety and efficacy.

Nanotechnology and Material Science

Spread of virus can be significantly attributed to air and surface contamination therefore recently the focus towards the development of anti-viral surfaces has opened a new area. It has been hypothesized that developing efficient air filtering system would highly contribute to dampen the viral load in environment and tackle the spreading of infections in health care workers due to the defective personal protective equipment (PPE) kits (Elias and Bar-Yam, 2020). This purpose can be served by using the approach of nanotechnology to design contamination-safe equipment. Antimicrobial properties of nanostructures copper, silver, and zinc species can be exploited. Release of copper ions and reactive oxygen species (ROS) leads to inactivation of SARS CoV-2 virus on copper and copper alloy surfaces (Van Doremalen *et al.*, 2020). Development of PPE kits can be accomplished using copper salt nanoparticles and/or solutions (chloride, iodide, sulfide, *etc.*) that render the virus ineffective. Sustained and controlled release can be obtained from metal nanoparticles acting as ion reservoirs. Noteworthy antimicrobial property has been observed on the metal-grafted graphene oxide (GO) used for non-woven tissues which is investigated for the treatment of PPE (Orłowski *et al.*, 2018). The anti-viral properties of nanoparticles are not fully explored, although silver nanoparticles (AgNPs) are well recognized for their anti-viral properties. It was reported that AgNPs interact with host receptors and blocks the entry of HIV-I (Kerry *et al.*, 2019). It has been established that metal NPs (<10 nm) can pierce through the cell membranes and curb viral replication. A nanotechnology-based solution containing titanium dioxide and silver ions was reportedly used to disinfect streets in Milan, Italy (Sportelli *et al.*, 2020). Nanomaterials based antiviral, packaging solutions, antiviral coatings, non-woven disposable products, synergistic/multifunctional surfaces, air-conditioning filters demand our prompt attention. Nanomaterials community has been encouraged to use their profound knowledge of Nanoscience that can be used to fight this pandemic (Sportelli *et al.*, 2020).

mRNA Based Approaches

One of the frontrunners in COVID-19 vaccine development program is mRNA based vaccines accounting to 18 potential candidate vaccines. Conventional vaccines developed with live or attenuated viruses or its antigens, require lengthy period for production and has limited manufacturing capacity. Meanwhile, mRNA based vaccines are a novel approach where antigen coding mRNA is introduced in an individual to trigger immune response as it gets expressed. This results in better immunogenicity, safety and efficacy as compared to traditional vaccines. mRNA vaccine candidate mRNA-1273 which encodes spike protein (S protein) of SARS-CoV-2, developed by Moderna is about to enter a Phase II study in Q2 2020.

There are two types of RNA vaccines exist; one is non-replicating mRNA vaccine and another is self-amplifying or replicon RNA vaccine (Iavarone *et al.*, 2017). The first step for exogenous mRNA to reach cytoplasm is to cross the lipid membrane barrier prior to getting translated in to protein (Midoux and Pichon, 2015). There are several factors that affect the mRNA delivery and organ distribution. Moreover, cellular selectivity is also observed. Irrespective of all the hurdles, mRNA vaccine is still holds enormous potential since it can be scaled up swiftly and does not pose any danger to the recipient. The hypothetical advantages of mRNA vaccines seem strong, although the factors affecting its stability and delivery cause concerns. The outcome of the phase I trial of the mRNA-1273 vaccine is still awaited.

ANIMAL MODELS TO TEST THE IMMUNOGENIC POTENTIAL OF CANDIDATE VACCINE ANTIGENS

Animal models are crucial in all facets of vaccine research and development. They are considered significant for predicting vaccine effectiveness and factors affecting their role as such include the robustness of the animal challenge model, the pathogen in question, and other known correlates of protection (Golding *et al.*, 2018). There are proof-of-concept (POC) studies that are carried out in small animal species, permitting the use of a large number of animals as well as multiple iterations of vaccine products. POC studies thus enable the identification of the optimal vaccine candidate, as well as the primary recognition of immunological end points (Golding *et al.*, 2018). Animal models can be developed to meet two resolutions: characterization of viral pathogenesis, and assessment of vaccines/anti-viral agents. Moreover, they play a significant role in comprehending the aforementioned in those infectious diseases for which carrying out clinical studies is not feasible. Animal models susceptible towards viral infection and exhibiting similarity with the clinical course are considered ideal. The straight-forwardness, ease of handling availability, generating statistically amenable data, and cost effectiveness are advantages with small laboratory animal models over larger ones (Sutton and Subbarao, 2015).

Animal Models Currently in Practice

Small animals such as mice are extensively used as a first-line screening of vaccine or a therapeutic candidate. Murine model is advantageous due to low genetic variability in inbred strains, and availability of a range of molecular biology and immunological reagents compatible for studies. The cost & effectiveness of murine models are also an added benefit for their use in R&D studies. However, one of the major shortcomings associated with these murine models lies in the fact that the viral pathogenesis observed in these animals, and the immunogenicity rendered by a vaccine in these models may not be extrapolated to humans in all cases. Another crucial drawback in using mice models is the limited blood volume sampling, and the need of several passages of viral load in the animal for an expedient infection (Ruiz *et al.*, 2017).

Several mouse models have been assessed for the study of infection by coronaviruses including SARS and MERS (Sutton and Subbarao, 2015). Balb/c murine models have been widely used for this purpose. A study reported that inoculation of Balb/c murine models with SARS, through the intranasal and oral routes simultaneously, resulted in replication of the virus in not only lung tissue, but also in the intestinal tissue (Wentworth *et al.*, 2004). The robust mouse models reiterating the pathogenesis of SARS-CoV-2 in humans have yet to be developed owing to incompatibility between the SARS-CoV-2 spike protein and the ACE2 receptor in mice (Wan *et al.*, 2020). However, transgenic mouse model (humanACE2-hACE2) has been developed for the study of SARS-CoV-2 pathogenicity. A study reported that transgenic hACE2 mice that were infected with the virus exhibited clinical infection symptoms like weight loss, besides viral replication in the lung tissue. Further, histopathological studies depicted interstitial pneumonia alongside classic immunological markers like infiltration of alveolar interstitium lymphocytes and monocytes, amassing of macrophages in alveolar cavities; viral antigens were also found in bronchial and alveolar epithilia. Moreover, these hallmarks were not exhibited in wild type mice with SARS-CoV-2 infection (Bao *et al.*, 2020). In another successful attempt ACE2 knockout mouse model (Imai *et al.*, 2005) and TMPRSS2 knockout (KO) mouse model (Iwata-Yoshikawa *et al.*, 2019) have been engineered, and these models were instrumental in unraveling the role of spike protein in SARS viral infection and development of pulmonary symptoms. Thus KO mice models may be utilized for evaluating the efficacy of proteins as vaccine/therapeutic targets. The knockout approach has also been extrapolated for various immunological proteins to facilitate various SARS studies. For instance, Stat1 KO models have been found to support SARS replication and allow progression of the disease in lungs; such a model was employed by a study to determine the effectiveness of a vaccine candidate which reports that the live, attenuated RNA virus vaccine provided protection to aged, immunocompromised mouse models (Graham *et al.*, 2012).

Small animals other than mice have also been commonly used as animal models for preclinical studies. The respiratory tract of ferrets is regarded as akin to that of humans, both, anatomically and histologically. Their larger size (when compared with mice) facilitates more frequent and larger blood samples. While these points pose ferrets as favorable animal models, there are drawbacks associated with their usage. They are outbred that might lead to inconsistent responses for a given parameter and to overcome this drawback greater numbers of animals should be incorporated in the study to obtain statistical significance. Additionally, transgenic ferrets are not accessible and molecular biology reagents compatible for their study are inadequate; admonitions arising with requirement of greater space and the tendency to exhibit aggressive behavior when procedures are repeated and other limitations associated with handling ferrets. Nevertheless, a ferret model of SARS-CoV-2 infection has been reported. Ferret models infected with the virus showed clinical signs of the disease such as elevated body temperature, alongside viral replication. Moreover, the study reported the infected ferret shed SARS-CoV-2 in nasal washes, saliva, and urine as well as in excreta for up-to 8 day post-infection. The study utilized the ferret model to address the transmission aspect of the disease; transmission in all naïve direct-contact ferrets at two days post-contract and in a few naïve indirect contact ferrets was reported. This suggests considerable recapitulation of the human disease in the model which advocated their use in R&D of SARS-CoV-2 therapeutics and vaccines (Kim *et al.*, 2020). Golden Syrian hamsters have also been recounted as highly permissive to SARS infection. A productive infection in these animals has been widely reported with the highest viral replication on 2-3 days post-infection in the nasal turbinates and the lungs. The pulmonary histology exhibited inflamed interstitial foci but the animals did not demonstrate explicit clinical disease or mortality (Sutton and Subbarao, 2015).

The next in line as animal models are non-human primates. These animals are genetically the most proximal species to humans; hence progression of disease and responses of the host immunity to the pathogen are closely in resemblance to those in humans. Though, ethical concerns and norms related to experimentation on non-human primates are the most stringent, dictating the study to be designed with utmost care and in a meticulous manner such that the smallest number of these animals is incorporated in the study (Ruiz *et al.*, 2017). Six non-human primates (african green monkeys, rhesus macaques, cynomolgus macaques, squirrel monkeys, the common marmoset, and mustached tamarins) have been assessed as models for SARS infection. All models but squirrel monkeys and mustached tamarins, were found to support SARS replication. Further, all species exhibited substantiations of interstitial pneumonia, though none among those were found to consistently reproduce clinical disease and none of the species exhibited mortality (Sutton and Subbarao, 2015). Studies using cynomolgus macaques have also been carried out to address comparisons of the three coronaviruses- SARS, MERS and SARS-CoV-2. The study reported absence of severe symptoms (that are observed in humans) in the models, but that the lung pathology that was observed in the models was similar to that in humans (Rockx *et al.*, 2020).

Humanized Mice Models

Small animal models have been the most effectual method for studying human afflictions, especially for that of certain human retroviruses. Currently available simian models are undoubtedly robust, but high expense and difficulty in maintaining those models is a major setback (Van Duyne *et al.*, 2009). There is a rising stipulation for effective models to facilitate experimental studies on human immune system and human hematopoietic system without putting individuals in danger. To overcome this challenge major breakthroughs have been made over the past few decades, beginning with the discovery of CB17-*Prkdc* (protein kinase, DNA-activated catalytic subunit) severe combined immunodeficiency (SCID) mice in 1983. These mice were successfully engrafted with human fetal tissue (regarded as SCID-Hu model) and peripheral blood mononuclear cells (Hu-PB--SCID model) for the first time in the year 1988. Subsequent breakthroughs in this field came with the development of NOD (Non-Obese Diabetic)/SCID mice and engrafting those with human hematolymphoid tissue in 1995. The NOD/SCID model has enhanced grafting capacity than the initial SCID-Hu mouse model. The next upgrade was brought about by developing an immunodeficient model *via* targeted mutation in IL-2 receptor common gamma chain in the early 2000s. This IL2rγ ^{null} mouse model reported significant engraftment increase and enhanced human hematolymphoid function even in comparison with NOD/SCID model (Pearson *et al.*, 2008).

For the purpose of vaccine development studies, the IL2rγ knockout model on NOD/SCID or Balb/c Rag2$^{-/-}$ background can be a remarkably useful platform. Findings have pointed out adequate purport for the suitability of engrafting human PBMCs (peripheral blood mononuclear cells), CBMCs (cord blood mononuclear cells) or CD34$^+$ cells along with target tissue (respective to the vaccine candidate) in the aforesaid model construct, so as to obtain a unique human-like entity to test for the efficacy of vaccines. Despite being the most permissive host for human tissue engraftment, the SCID-IL2R$\gamma^{-/-}$ knockout model holds substantial scope for improvisation in order to further promote its application in research and development. Transgenic mice can be engineered to carry human HLA I and II. This can confer the model with the capability of human-like MHC presentation in their tissues, and can prove an indispensible asset for evaluating the effects of various therapies/formulations with refined and clinically relevant human resemblance (Koo *et al.*, 2009).

A study reported that K18 mice engineered for transgenic expression of hACE2 in the respiratory and other epithelial tissue developed a lethal infection post intranasal inoculation of SARS strain infecting humans. Their findings show macrophage and lymphocyte infiltration lung tissue post infection, as well as upregulation of proinflammatory cytokines in the lungs and brain, suggesting the usefulness of this model in pathophysiology studies and for antiviral R&D (Soo *et al.*, 2009). Recently, a Russian study group has reported a proposal to create a humanized mouse model for the application in SARS-CoV-2 research. They have designed the model to comprise *hACE2* and *hTMPRSS2* by introducing the genes in the mouse genome *via* CRISPR/cas9 technology. This will enable the model to be successfully infected by SARS-CoV-2 virus, as well as render the pathophysiology in close resemblance to that in humans (Soldatov *et al.*, 2020). In a major advancement, a recent study has reported a humanized lung-only mouse model. Bone marrow liver thymic (BLT) mice were implanted with human lung tissue, comprising of up-to 40 distinct cell types. The model has been demonstrated to facilitate replication of clinically relevant human viruses, and exhibits robust antigen-specific HMI & CMI responses (Wahl *et al.*, 2019).

With the robust advancement in the development of humanized models, several hurdles in the fight against the SARS-CoV-2 can be overcome and direct the research towards an efficient and safe vaccine/anti-viral intervention.

Novel Approach of Using Zebrafish (Their Advantages)

Animal models mimicking various human diseases have proven revolutionary in identifying and then screening of leading drug candidates for developing specific therapeutic targets. Among the choice list of researcher's, murine model stands on first however, a more convenient vertebrate model, is surfacing as a better substitute (Callaway, 2020). Scientifically named as *Daniorerio,* the zebrafish is a prominent vertebrate model organism in research for more than a century (Sullivan and Kim, 2008). Notably, zebrafish exist as an exceptionally important tool for research in genomics, genetics, embryology and immunology (Santoriello and Zon, 2012). What makes zebrafish distinct from presently available testing models is; it's easy maintenance, reproduction and morphological attributes. Owing to the simplicity of their natural habitat and versatile nature, these organisms are robust and easy to uphold and provides scope for maintaining them in laboratory at ease than other existing mammalian models. Small size and petite generation time of 3–5 months shortens the overall experiment duration making their culturing cost-effective (Saleem and Kannan, 2018) and ideal for mutant and transgenic cell line production. Additionally, these fish undergo external fertilization, making it simpler for studying early embryonic development which is difficult in rodent models due to the internal mode of fertilization (Dooley and Zon, 2000). Reports suggest that embryos are pretty malleable to genetic manipulation by morpholino antisense oligonucleotide, transgenes, mRNAs and genome editing techniques like CRISPR-Cas9, TALENS (Hwang *et al.*, 2013, Schmid and Haass, 2013, Hisano *et al.*, 2014). One noteworthy advantage of working with zebrafish is its embryos with unrivalled optical clarity, permitting visualization of body physiology and genes individually throughout the course of development, using low power microscope, fluorescent imaging or by using non-invasive imaging techniques which can then prove boon in studying mutations and genetic manipulations (Lieschke and Currie, 2007). As a matter of fact, despite the physiological differences, humans share 70% of genes and 84% disease-related genetic factor with zebrafish (McKie, 2013, Howe *et al.*, 2013). Having high genome homology with humans, it's not strange that zebrafish shows same major tissue and organs alike human counterparts. Their blood, muscle, eyes and kidney share many lineaments with human systems. In recent years, zebrafish animal model is gaining lot of popularity in the scientific community, in reference to assets it has, especially as a model for human disease. It has been used extensively in research for alzheimer's disease, different types of cancer, cardiac disease, kidney disorder, hematopoiesis and obesity (Dooley and Zon, 2000). Accompanying to this, zebrafish is also used widely as a means for study of host-pathogen interactions and infectious diseases of fungal, viral or bacterial origin (Varela *et al.*, 2017). The pathogensis of tuberculosis is a sensible example to discuss, were *Mycobacterium marinum* (a close relative of *Mycobacterium tuberculosis* which infects human) was used to establish infection in zebrafish larvae, mimicking model of mycobacteria infecting humans and were later screened (Takaki *et al.*, 2013). Statistic data revels, countries with more the inhabitants tested for SARS-CoV-2 tend to have least number of deaths from COVID-19 and thus WHO also recommends for mass scale testing of native population but dearth of rapid testing kits posse a big hurdle in this task achievement. In direction of identifying new alternatives for rapid testing, Charlie-silva and his group proposed a novel strategy to develop a quick COVID-19 infected patient detection and tracking kit using zebrafish as animal model. According to the idea, viral peptides will be dosed into female zebrafish at an interval of a week as per two immunization sections with a target of generating plasma antibodies. Transfer of antibodies passively to eggs occurs naturally as stated by Wang and their colleagues (Wang *et al.*, 2012). After successful immunization, female fishes will be motivated to mate and generate the eggs with desired antibodies, which can then be isolated, filtered and introduced in a test strip (Charlie-Silva, 2020). Regardless of how serious the effect of COVID-19 might be, promising and progressive ventures between research organizations with advance zebrafish facilities under the leadership of top scientists globally, the application of the above-discussed zebrafish techniques could offer novel results soon.

CURRENT STATUS OF VACCINE DEVELOPMENT

SARS-CoV-2 genetic sequence was published on January 11, 2020 by researchers (Wan *et al.*, 2020) creating a ripple in global R&D activity for vaccine development against the disease. New generation vaccine technology through novel paradigms is driven by economic and humanitarian impact of COVID-19 pandemic in order to speed up the vaccine development. The first candidate vaccine entered clinical trials with striking swiftness on 16 March 2020. This chapter will include vaccine development programs reported by WHO's authoritative as well as other ongoing projects retrieved from proprietary sources.

A commendable feature of the vaccine development program for COVID-19 is the variety of technology platforms being explored. At present under the Global Vaccine Development Program (GVDP) there are 115 candidate vaccines are there and out of which 78 are active while 37 are unconfirmed (WHO, 2020). Currently, 73 vaccine candidates from active ones are at preclinical stage meanwhile the most advanced candidate vaccines are under clinical development which involves Ad5-nCoV from CanSino Biologics, mRNA-1273 from Moderna, INO-4800 from Inovio and LV-SMENP-DC as well as pathogen specific aAPC from Shenzhen Geno-Immune Medical Institute.

Candidate vaccines mentioned in Table **1** include novel platforms based on DNA or mRNA that will offer great liberty to scientists for antigen manipulation which will aid the speed of development. Indeed after 2 months of publishing COVID-19 gene sequence, Moderna started clinical trials of its mRNA-based vaccine mRNA-1273 (ClinicalTrials.gov: NCT04283461). Viral vector based vaccines express high levels of proteins, offer stability for long duration along with strong immune response following vaccination. These candidates can also advantage from pre-existing scale-up process.

Table 1. The list of clinical-phase vaccine candidates for COVID-19 (Source: Regulatory Affairs Professional Society-last updated on August 27, 2020).

Sr. No.	Candidate Vaccine	Phase Status	Outcome	Other Information	Location
1.	Inactivated vaccine	III	• Results of phase I/II have shown the promising results in terms of appropriate neutralizing Ab responses • Phase III study is ongoing in Morocco, United Arab Emirates and Peru	Randomized, double-blind (ChiCTR2000031809)	Funded by Ministry of Science & Technology, China
2.	CoronaVac (PiCoVacc)	III	Results of phase I/II has depicted the safety & immunogenicity Phase III study is underway in collaboration with InstitutoButantan in Brazil	Enrolled 743 healthy volunteers & received two dosage of vaccines/placebo Phase I-143 Patients (NCT04352608) Phase II-600 Patients (NCT04383574)	Sinovac Research & Development Co.Ltd, China
3.	mRNA-1273	III	Results of phase I study shown the production of neutralizing Abs (dose of 25/100 µg) Phase III study involves almost 30,000 patients who are at the higher risk of COVID-19 infection and receive 100 µg of dose/ placebo followed up to 2 yrs (NCT04470427)	Phase I-120 Patients (NCT04283461) Phase II-600 Patients (NCT04405076) (Evaluated 50 & 100 µg dose level) All are healthy individuals	Moderna, Inc. USA

(Table 1) cont.....

Sr. No.	Candidate Vaccine	Phase Status	Outcome	Other Information	Location
4.	Ad5-nCoV	III	Results of phase I study have confirmed its humoral and immunogenic response and in phase II neutralizing Ab and IFN-γ based immune responses was observed The Central Military Commission of China has approved the use of Ad5-nCoV for the initial period of 1 year and phase III study is ongoing in Saudi Arabia	A recombinant novel coronavirus vaccine includes adenovirus types 5 vector (Ad5) Phase I have 108 participants and received low, medium and high dose (ChiCTR2000030906; NCT04313127) and followed by Phase II (ChiCTR2000031781)	CanSino Biologics, China
5.	AZD1222/Covishield	II/III	Results of the I/II study have confirmed its safety at acceptable level and noticed the Ab production after 1st dose in almost all patients and after two doses all the participants have shown Ab generation Phase II/III study will shortly begin in India	A chimpanzee adenovirus vaccine vector AZD1222 (ChAdOx1) is a candidate Phase I/II (NCT04324606), a single-blinded, multi-centric study enrolled 1090 healthy volunteers having four regimen of treatment	The University of Oxford, Ministry of Health, UK & BARDA
6.	BNT162	II/III	Results of phase I/II have confirmed their usage for phase II/III (on the basis of their available data of immune response and tolerability) The modRNA candidate (BNT162b2) was finally selected for advanced phase II/III study	Initially there were four vaccine candidates; two consist of nucleoside modified mRNA-based (modRNA), one is uridine containing mRNA (uRNA) and the last one is self-amplifying mRNA-based (saRNA)	Pfizer and BioNTech

(Table 1) cont.....

Sr. No.	Candidate Vaccine	Phase Status	Outcome	Other Information	Location
7.	NVX-CoV2373	IIb	Results of phase I have shown the development of Abs after multiple dosages and also cross the safety level Phase IIb trial is ongoing in South Africa	It is a perfusion protein nanoparticle vaccine candidate used in randomized, observed-blinded trial included 130 healthy volunteers (NCT04368988)	Novavax, Department of Defence, USA
8.	Adjuvant recombinant vaccine	II	Phase II is underway	Phase I results will be expected in September	Anhui ZhifeiLongcom Biopharma. & Institute of Microbiology of the Chinese Academy of Science
9.	ZyCoV-D	II	The enrolment for the phase II trial was begun	It is a plasmid DNA vaccine candidate which targets the entry of viral membrane protein of the virus Phase I was accomplished in the month of August	ZydusCadila, Gujarat, India
10.	Covaxin	II	The results of the candidate vaccines was found to be encouraging and as per Indian Council of Medical Research (ICMR) it has entered in phase II	It is inactivated vaccine candidate	Bharat Biotech, National Institute of Virology, India
11.	BBIBP-CorV	I/II	The results of the phase I have confirmed its higher efficiency and its potential in rhesus macques It is currently in phase II (ChiCTR2000032459)	It is inactivated vaccine candidate which is formulated with Beijing Institute of Biological Products	Ministry of Science & Technology, China
12.	GRAd-COV2	I/II	They have expected the completion of phase I in 3 months before their phase II at multinational level	A DNA vaccine candidate used in randomized 190 healthy participants	Genexine, South Korea

(Table 1) cont.....

Sr. No.	Candidate Vaccine	Phase Status	Outcome	Other Information	Location
13.	Sputnik V	I/II	The Ministry have a target of covering more than 40,000 people from 45 different medical centers which would be consider equivalent to phase III	It is a non-replicating viral vector candidate & it has been declared as the first vaccine for COVID-19. In phase I/II 38 participants received the vaccines (NCT04436471)	Gamaleya Research Institute of Epidemiology and Microbiology, Health Ministry of Russian Federation
14.	Self-amplifying RNA vaccine	I/II	Animal testing is ongoing Phase I/II will enroll around 300 individuals followed by efficacy trial in October	The vaccine has been developed within 14 days after the sequenced received from the China	UK Secretary of State for Health (Imperial College of London)
15.	LUNAR-COV19	I/II	Pre-clinical study have shown the adaptive (CD8+) and balanced (Th1/Th2) immune response. Phase I/II will be initiated in Singapore	It is the combination of self-replicating RNA and nanoparticle non-viral delivery system.	Arcturus, Duke-NUS Medical School, Singapore
16.	INO-4800	I/II	Results of early phase I study have confirmed the immune responses in all the patients and it also inhibits the replication of SARS-CoV-2 in mice The phase I/II will be conducted in coordination with Korea National Institute of Health (KNIH)	It is a DNA based vaccine and it is given by intradermal route through device In phase I (NCT04336410) 40 healthy participants were enrolled in a non-randomized trial In pre-clinical study (in mice and guinea pigs) neutralizing Abs and humoral and T cell responses were observed	Inovio-Pharmaceutical

(Table 1) cont.....

Sr. No.	Candidate Vaccine	Phase Status	Outcome	Other Information	Location
17.	Ad26.COV2-S	I/II	Earlier study have confirmed the neutralizing Ab responses as well as the complete or mostly-complete protection in challenge study The phase III will be enrolled up-to 60,000 participants from international level and USA (NCT04505722)	It consists of AdVac and PER.C6 system which were earlier used to develop Ebola vaccine. It is a double-blind, randomized, placebo-controlled study of phase I include 1045 healthy individuals of US and Belgium (NCT04436276)	Johnson & Johnson
18.	mRNA based Vaccine	I	Results of pre-clinical studies have shown the titer of neutralizing Abs and T-cell responses.	It is mRNA based vaccine which will work by using the nucleotides which are modified non-chemically for appropriate immune responses	CureVac, German federal government
19.	SCB-2019	I	The results of the phase I study will be expected in the August.	It uses the combination of Trimer platform of Clover's, AS03 adjuvant from GSK's and CpG 1018 adjuvant of Dynavax's The phase I study (NCT04405908) has around 108 participants	CEPI
20.	COVAX-19	I	The expected results includes the formation of neutralizing Ab formation and T cell responses against the spike protein of COVID-19.	It is monovalent recombinant protein vaccine developed by Vaxin Pty Ltd. and phase I (NCT04453852) is a randomized placebo controlled trails having 40 healthy adults. Two doses will be given at the interval of three weeks.	NIAID

(Table 1) cont.....

Sr. No.	Candidate Vaccine	Phase Status	Outcome	Other Information	Location
21.	Plant-based adjuvant COVID-19 vaccine candidate.	I	The animal study confirms the positive Ab responses within the 10 days Phase I study is ongoing and phase II will be start in the month of October 2020.	It has been developed by Medicago who has developed the VLP-influenza vaccine and the candidate vaccine has been tested alongside the two additional adjuvants from GSK and Dynavax.	Medicago
22.	Molecular clamp vaccine	I	The earlier results have confirmed the formation of neutralizing Abs Phase I is ongoing and if the clinical trial have the successful results than it can be available by the end of 2021.	This vaccine candidate helps in identification of protein on virus Phase I has 120 individuals and the university has collaborated with CSL and CEPI (Coalition for Epidemic Preparedness Innovations).	The university of Queensland
23.	V590	I	The phase I is currently recruiting participants at both the centers (NCT04497298).	It is based on the Merck's rVSV (recombinant vesicular stomatitis virus) technology used for Ebola vaccine.	Merck and BARD (Biomedical Advanced Research and Development Authority).
24.	GRAd-CoV2	I	Phase I is underway in Italy	It is adenovirus based vaccine.	ReiThera (Italy), Leukocare (Germany) and Univercells (Belgium)
25.	AdimrSC-2f	I	Earlier animal studies have shown the positive results and now they are planning randomized phase I study (NCT04522089).	This vaccine candidate targets spike protein of SARS-CoV-2.	Adimmune (Taiwanese)
26.	bacTRL-spike	Pre-clinical	Currently it is being tested in phase I (NCT04334980) having 84 healthy individuals with various dosages.	It is a bifidobacteria monovalent DNA based oral vaccine.	Symvivo Corporation, Canada

(Table 1) cont.....

Sr. No.	Candidate Vaccine	Phase Status	Outcome	Other Information	Location
27.	PittCoVacc	Pre-clinical	Animal studies in mice have shown an effective results delivered *via* a fingertrip patch.	UPMC has recently received the fund from CEPI to develop this vaccine candidate.	University of Pittsburgh School of Medicine (UPMC).
28.	V591	Pre-clinical	Animal studies in mice have shown the promising results.	UPMC, Themis Biosciences and Institute Pasteur alongside Merck will develop the vaccine candidate.	Merck
29.	Ii-Key peptide COVID-19 vaccine	Pre-clinical	The vaccine development program is underway which can develop and tested in humans in 90 days.	-	Generex
30.	Recombinant vaccine	Pre-clinical	Earlier animal studies have shown the SARS-CoV-2 Abs after the 1st and 2nd dose The phase I study will initiate in the second half of 2020.	It is a oral recombinant vaccine candidate.	Vaxart
31.	LineaDNA	Pre-clinical	Earlier pre-clinical studies have shown the strong Ab and T-cell responses The human trials will be begin in fall.	It is a DNA based vaccine mainly produced by Takis Biotech and Applied DNA science.	Takis Biotech
32.	AdCOVID	Pre-clinical	Animal studies have shown the neutralizing activity, strong Ab response and potent mucosal immunity The clinical trials will be expected in the fourth quarter of 2020.	The technology used for COVID-19 vaccine is similar to used for influenza vaccine (NasoVAX). It can be injected through intranasal route to activate the entire immune response (humoral, cellular and mucosal).	Altimmune

(Table 1) cont.....

Sr. No.	Candidate Vaccine	Phase Status	Outcome	Other Information	Location
33.	T-COVIDTM	Pre-clinical	Despite the same mechanism for vaccine development, it works through different mechanism.	The technology used for COVID-19 vaccine is similar to used for influenza vaccine (NasoVAX). It can be injected through intranasal route to activate the entire immune response (humoral, cellular and mucosal).	Altimmune
34.	Protein subunit vaccine	Pre-clinical	Early studies have shown the generation of immune response. Animal studies is ongoing.	The international vaccine center and the university of Saskatchewan's Vaccine is developing this vaccine based candidate.	-
35.	Adenovirus-based vaccine	Pre-clinical	Animal studies have shown the generation of CD4$^+$and CD8$^+$T-cell which are Ag specific.	It is adenovirus based vaccine which can taerget spike and nucleocaspid DNA in SARS-CoV-2.	ImmunityBio&NantKwest
36.	AAVCOVID	Pre-clinical	-	It is a gene based candidate vaccine.	Wyc-Grousbeck
37.	Recombinat vaccine	Pre-clinical	Early non-human studies have confirmed the generation of immune response The phase I/II will begin in the month of September.	It is designed on the basis of rDNA technology which was earlier used for the SARS vaccine.	Sanofi and Translate Bio
38.	Halovax	Pre-clinical	Two different sets of this candidate is currently under animal studies	The candidate vaccine will be designed using the Self-Assembling Vaccine (SAV) platform.	Voltron Therapeutics and Hoth Therapeutics
39.	mRNA-based vaccine	Pre-clinical	Animal studies in monkeys and mice have shown the successful Ab response The clinical trial will begin in the month of September.	This particular vaccine candidate is similar to the mRNA based vaccine of Moderna.	University's Center of Excellence in Vaccine Research & Development, Thailand

(Table 1) cont.....

Sr. No.	Candidate Vaccine	Phase Status	Outcome	Other Information	Location
40.	HDT-301	Pre-clinical	The animal studies have demonstrated the robust Ab responses in mice and primates. At the earliest, the phase I trial will begin.	It is a replicon RNA vaccine candidate.	University of Washington, National Institute of Health Rocky Mountain Laboratories & HDT Bio Corp.
41.	gp96-based vaccine	Pre-clinical	The animal studies have confirmed the immune response Especially the latest report suggest that it can generate human-HLA-restricted T-cells against the immunodominant epitope of SARS-CoV-2 spike protein.	It uses the gp96 heat shock protein in the designing of the vaccine.	Heat Biologics
42.	ChAd-SARS-CoV-2	Pre-clinical	Pre-clinical studies in animals have shown the strong immune response in terms of formation of neutralizing Abs specifically in upper and lower respiratory track. At the earliest non-human primate and human clinical study will be initiated.	It is based on the chimpanzee adenovirus vectored vaccine. The route will be intranasal and targets the spike protein of the virus.	Washington University School of Medicine in St.Louis.
43.	mRNA lipid nanoparticle vaccine.	Early-phase	The time line for this candidate vaccine has not been disclosed.	It uses the Precision Nanosystem's RNA vaccine platform.	CanSino Biologics & Precision Nanosystem.

For some vaccine candidates, adjuvants would strengthen the immunogenicity and enhance the viability of lower doses (Le *et al.*, 2020), thereby avoiding the risk of compromised protection of individuals. Developers like GlaxoSmithKline, Seqirus and Dynavax have indicated plans of delivering adjuvants AS03, MF59 and CpG 1018, respectively which will be used for manufacturing COVID-19 vaccine supplemented with adjuvants. A huge number multinational pharmaceuticals like Janssen, Sanofi, Pfizer and GlaxoSmithKline have engaged in COVID-19 vaccine development, still lead developers involve small or inexperienced vaccine manufacturers in large-scale production hence, co-ordination will be critical to meet the supply demand.

The worldwide vaccine R&D in response to the COVID-19 pandemic is unmatched in terms of scale and speed. It has been indicated that by early 2021, vaccine for emergency use or under likewise protocols will be made available. This would speak to an essential advance change from the customary immunization improvement pathway which takes on an average 10 years, even if we compare the first fastest delivery of Ebola vaccine which took 5 years. Hence, COVID-19 vaccine would demand extraordinary scale-up manufacturing and innovative regulatory process to ensure safety and eliminate involved risks.

BENCH TO BEDSIDE: OBSTACLES AND OUTCOMES

Immunization has extraordinarily diminished the weight of irresistible infections. Absurdly, an intense demand for vaccine development thrives regardless of undeniable achievement of immunization programs against in the past fearsome diseases that are now rare in evolved countries. Studies on contagious disease and its pattern of infectivity, especially in industrialized countries gave evidences for a successive decline in pre-reproductive mortality since 19th century's end, and this lowering in cases of death from previous thought 'incurable diseases' was due to development of 'concept of immunization'. Apart from enhancement in sanitation, housing and nutrition facilities, vaccination has also played an indisputable role in laying strong foundation stone on which mankind stands today. Death rate prior to vaccination phase during previously encountered pandemics of smallpox and measles were devastating, were half of the population was cleared and a bit less lethal for population affected from measles (Greenwood, 2014).

The problem of vaccine acceptance has been dwelling in the society. The only possible route to answer this issue is by providing data that is scientifically validated but unfortunately, it's far easy to say than to execute on real ground because the major demerit of the game humans are playing is that, it is not governed by the rules that generally exist in field of science and justifiably, public attention is more inclined towards vaccine safety then its effectiveness, but clinical observations and data has verified that vaccines designed are far safer and secure than restorative medicines till date (Vaccines *et al.*, 2012, Andre *et al.*, 2008).

Vaccine, does not aim to prevent the disease but instead goal to safeguard the vaccinated population from the risk of future re-encounter. The level we target the vaccination program tells us the expected output, like at individual scale it may help to modify or prevent the infection while at population scale, the intension is to cease the spread of disease in mass. As thought, knowledge of personal protection and grip on epidemicity will definitely eradicate the causative pathogen. Yet, any vaccine effectiveness is governed by some crucial factors enlisted (Graham, 2013).

- Understanding and identifying the challenge at biological front and developing strategies to overcome.
- Technological advancements that can aid to solve small and large scale operational hurdles.
- Political and social consent of local institutions, communities and governing bodies.
- Other environmental parameters like resources, genetic buildup, demographic localizations *etc.*

Microbiological evidences stand as another determinant to narrate about the load or incidences of pathogenicity. To explain the point, nothing can be better than HPV vaccine licensing, which was developed not to prevent the infection but on contrary to save the patient from cervical neoplasia (Garland *et al.*, 2007). Another example, HIV and HSV vaccines were formulated to aim for complete viral clearance, but these viruses posed some major obstructions for the vaccinologists in achieving abortive infection or sterilizing immunity after the infection rather than treatment for any physiological symptoms attributed to their ability to establishing latency, evading host's natural immune-surveillance and clearance with high risk of relapse and recurrence in time-independent manner.

Looking at their genetic framework designed for establishing latency, evading body's natural immune-surveillance and clearance, altogether with high risk of relapse and recurrence were the issues vaccinologists were answerable for. The role assigned to any therapeutic vaccine candidate, is to aid in rapid clearing of both virus and virus infected cells so as to avoid the chance of infection persistence rather than actually inducing sterilizing kind of immunity. VZV (varicella Zoster Virus) vaccine works on the similar principle of avoiding persistent infection from natural wild strain in children and cases of HSZ and postherpetic neuralgia in adults, then to avert the pathology (Oxman *et al.*, 2005). A new concept of charitable vaccine proposed, designed to protect from transmission then benefiting on individual level, though none vaccine formulation fits in the definition, yet few have been developed for diseases prevention *via* passive immunization, RSV (respiratory syncytial virus), congenital rubella syndrome and CMV (cytomegalovirus) are on the list.

Lessons from Previous Vaccine Development

Complete eradication of virus from a population stands as sign of success for the vaccine. CMI and HMI are key-role players during adaptive immunological response and have a characteristic marker of memory formation. Antibodies are equipped with the ability to catch a virus before it can enter the cell, in association with peculiarity for target specificity and high avidity, thus making them an ideal candidate for vaccine development (Graham, 2013). Antibody works on any of the three major mechanism in general; immobilization or aggregation of viral particle, blocking of viral attachment facilitating proteins and receptors on host cell, and lastly, post-attaching neutralizing reaction tendency. Cytotoxic T cell mediated response is primly concerned with recognizing and clearing cells infected with virus.

In recent times, both vaccine industry and scientific community have been asked to quickly reciprocate to global pandemics of H1N1 influenza (2009), Ebola (2013-2016), Zika (2015-2016), and currently ongoing SARS-CoV-2. Vaccine for H1N1 influenza was commercialized in very less time owing to previously gathered knowledge and strategies on the paradigm of cell-based platforms, as getting licensed was easy and profitable. Although, northern hemispheric countries had to wait for the monovalent H1N1 vaccine, but soon the remedy was commercially available in addition to the seasonal flu-vaccines. Antagonistic to this route, vaccines for Zika and SARS were not into existence by the time epidemic got under border and thus central funding agencies were forced to reallocate funds that were committed for respective vaccine research and development, leaving a void in financial gain and setting back vaccine programs operating in parallel.

Ebola vaccine production was kept on hold between 2013-2016 by the Public Health Agency of Canada, which was then funded by the USA and transferred to private sector company, Merck. The company kept the production on even after the virus was almost uprooted from the infected demographic area generating huge stockpiles. CEPI (coalition for epidemic preparedness innovation) additionally favors development of new platforms for "Disease-X" -like some novel epidemic, one being COVID-19. Of all those concepts under trial for vaccine design, the utmost promises are of RNA and DNA- based programs and then the leading candidates are recombinant-subunit vaccines. One prime advantage of RNA and DNA-based vaccines is, synthesis independent of fermentation or cell culture procedures making it ideal choice for oncology vaccines as personalized medicine. No licensed RNA-vaccine exists till now but many of them are already under clinical trials and seem to have promising results in near future. Recent advancements like, next generation sequencing (NGS) and reverse genetics using the ground of genomics and proteomics and link with phylogenic relationship may facilitate to cut down the development time, which was a major challenge for conventional vaccines.

Even with such innovative platform, designing a correct vaccine for SARS-CoV-2 is still a challenging task, attributed to elements such as;

- Area for targeting the viral spike protein, receptor domain or whole length protein using adjuvants or other subunit type.
- Absence of reliable animal model for testing and assurance
- Lessons from SARS and MERS epidemics where intensified cases of lung severity, as a cause of direct of antibody medicated implication was witnessed
- Th2 medicated CMI response which can be more damaging then benefiting
- Lack of experimentally validated data from immunopathological front
- Insufficient data on dosing pattern, mode and duration of immunity furnished as correlated with SARS and MERS epidemics scenarios

To introduce a vaccine for mankind, it necessitates many years of intensive research with N number of candidates having high conflicting opinions on its efficacy and long lasting impact on wider scale with high financial input and uncertainty of failures (Gouglas *et al.*, 2018). These risks force the manufactures to follow a linear sequence of development with ample of halts and step-to-step data evaluation which in longer run slows down the development process considerably. As a solution, carrying out phase I clinical trial simultaneously with animal studies can benefit to certain extend but again this will heighten the risk of financial losses to a next level. However, looking at current pandemic crisis, this huge time investment seems likely to be unaffordable and thus a novel paradigm with multi-dimensional planning is the need of the hour.

LIST OF ABBREVIATIONS

AgNps	Sliver nanoparticles
CMI	Cell-mediated immunity
CTD	C-terminal domain
CTL	Cytotoxic T-lymphocytes
DAMPs	Damage-associated molecular patterns
DCs	Dendritic cells
EGCG	Epigallocatechingallate
ELP	Elastin-like polypeptide
GALT	Gut associated lymphoid tissue
GO	Graphene oxide
HLA	Human leukocyte antigen
HMI	Humoral mediated immunity

HPV	Human papilloma virus
IC	Immune complex
IEDB	Immune epitope database and analysis resource
IRF 3	Interferon regulatory transcription factor 3
KO	Knockout
LNPs	Lipid nanoparticles
MDA 5	Melanoma differentiation-associated protein 5
MHC	Major histocompatibility complex
MMR	Mumps, measles and rubella
NF-Kb	Nuclear factor- kappa-B
NOD	Non-Obese Diabetic
NTD	N-terminal domain
ORF	Open reading frame
PBMCs	Peripheral blood mononuclear cells
pDCs	plasmacytoid dendritic cells
PPE	Personal protective equipment
RBD	Receptor-binding domain
RIG-I	Retinoic acid-inducible gene I
SCID	Severe combined immunodeficiency
TLR	Toll like receptor
ViPR	Virus pathogen resource
VLPs	Virus like particles

CONSENT FOR PUBLICATION

Not applicable.

CONFLICT OF INTEREST

The author declares no conflict of interest, financial or otherwise.

ACKNOWLEDGEMENTS

The instrumentation facility of CSIR-IMTECH and Nirma University is duly acknowledged. Authors express their gratitude towards the funding agencies, CSIR, New Delhi and DBT, New Delhi for supporting this study. Nikunj Tandel thanks the Indian Council of Medical Research (ICMR), New Delhi, Gov. of India for providing fellowship for his research (ICMR-SRF No.: 2020-7623/CM--BMS.

REFERENCES

Andre, FE, Booy, R, Bock, HL, Clemens, J, Datta, SK, John, TJ, Lee, BW, Lolekha, S, Peltola, H, Ruff, TA, Santosham, M & Schmitt, HJ (2008) Vaccination greatly reduces disease, disability, death and inequity worldwide. *Bull World Health Organ,* 86, 140-6.
[http://dx.doi.org/10.2471/BLT.07.040089] [PMID: 18297169]

Bao, L, Deng, W, Huang, B, Gao, H, Liu, J, Ren, L, Wei, Q, Yu, P, Xu, Y, Qi, F, Qu, Y, Li, F, Lv, Q, Wang, W, Xue, J, Gong, S, Liu, M, Wang, G, Wang, S, Song, Z, Zhao, L, Liu, P, Zhao, L, Ye, F, Wang, H, Zhou, W, Zhu, N, Zhen, W, Yu, H, Zhang, X, Guo, L, Chen, L, Wang, C, Wang, Y, Wang, X, Xiao, Y, Sun, Q, Liu, H, Zhu, F, Ma, C, Yan, L, Yang, M, Han, J, Xu, W, Tan, W, Peng, X, Jin, Q, Wu, G & Qin, C (2020) The pathogenicity of SARS-CoV-2 in hACE2 transgenic mice. *Nature,* 583, 830-3.
[http://dx.doi.org/10.1038/s41586-020-2312-y] [PMID: 32380511]

Callaway, E (2020) Labs rush to study coronavirus in transgenic animals - some are in short supply. *Nature,* 579, 183-3.
[http://dx.doi.org/10.1038/d41586-020-00698-x] [PMID: 32152596]

Chang, CY, Hong, WW, Chong, P & Wu, SC (2006) Influence of intron and exon splicing enhancers on mammalian cell expression of a truncated spike protein of SARS-CoV and its implication for subunit vaccine development. *Vaccine,* 24, 1132-41.
[http://dx.doi.org/10.1016/j.vaccine.2005.09.011] [PMID: 16194584]

Charlie-Silva, I (2020) Zebrafish model in the development of COVID-19 rapid test. *Ars Veterinaria,* 36, 03-5.
[http://dx.doi.org/10.15361/2175-0106.2020v36n1p03-05]

Chen, CH, Ji, H, Suh, KW, Choti, MA, Pardoll, DM & Wu, TC (1999) Gene gun-mediated DNA vaccination induces antitumor immunity against human papillomavirus type 16 E7-expressing murine tumor metastases in the liver and lungs. *Gene Ther,* 6, 1972-81.
[http://dx.doi.org/10.1038/sj.gt.3301067] [PMID: 10637448]

Chen, DY, Shien, JH, Tiley, L, Chiou, SS, Wang, SY, Chang, TJ, Lee, YJ, Chan, KW & Hsu, WL (2010) Curcumin inhibits influenza virus infection and haemagglutination activity. *Food Chem,* 119, 1346-51.
[http://dx.doi.org/10.1016/j.foodchem.2009.09.011]

de Vries, RD & Rimmelzwaan, GF (2016) Viral vector-based influenza vaccines. *Hum Vaccin Immunother,* 12, 2881-901.
[http://dx.doi.org/10.1080/21645515.2016.1210729] [PMID: 27455345]

den Haan, JM, Arens, R & van Zelm, MC (2014) The activation of the adaptive immune system: cross-talk between antigen-presenting cells, T cells and B cells. *Immunol Lett,* 162, 103-12.
[http://dx.doi.org/10.1016/j.imlet.2014.10.011] [PMID: 25455596]

Don, BR & Kaysen, G (2004) Poor nutritional status and inflammation: Serum albumin: relationship to inflammation and nutrition. *Seminars in Dialysis,* Wiley Online Library 432-7.
[http://dx.doi.org/10.1111/j.0894-0959.2004.17603.x]

Dooley, K & Zon, LI (2000) Zebrafish: a model system for the study of human disease. *Curr Opin Genet Dev,* 10, 252-6.
[http://dx.doi.org/10.1016/S0959-437X(00)00074-5] [PMID: 10826982]

Elias, B & Bar-Yam, Y (2000) Could air filtration reduce COVID-19 severity and spread. Cambridge, MA, New England Complex Systems Institute 1-4.

Garland, SM, Hernandez-Avila, M, Wheeler, CM, Perez, G, Harper, DM, Leodolter, S, Tang, GW, Ferris, DG, Steben, M, Bryan, J, Taddeo, FJ, Railkar, R, Esser, MT, Sings, HL, Nelson, M, Boslego, J, Sattler, C, Barr, E & Koutsky, LA Females United to Unilaterally Reduce Endo/Ectocervical Disease (FUTURE) I Investigators (2007) Quadrivalent vaccine against human papillomavirus to prevent anogenital diseases. *N Engl J Med,* 356, 1928-43.
[http://dx.doi.org/10.1056/NEJMoa061760] [PMID: 17494926]

Golding, H, Khurana, S & Zaitseva, M (2018) What is the predictive value of animal models for vaccine efficacy in humans? the importance of bridging studies and species-independent correlates of protection. *Cold Spring Harb Perspect Biol,* 10, a028902.
[http://dx.doi.org/10.1101/cshperspect.a028902] [PMID: 28348035]

Gouglas, D, Thanh Le, T, Henderson, K, Kaloudis, A, Danielsen, T, Hammersland, NC, Robinson, JM, Heaton, PM & Røttingen, J-A (2018) Estimating the cost of vaccine development against epidemic infectious diseases: a cost minimisation study. *Lancet Glob Health,* 6, e1386-96.
[http://dx.doi.org/10.1016/S2214-109X(18)30346-2] [PMID: 30342925]

Govea-Alonso, DO, Gómez-Cardona, EE, Rubio-Infante, N, García-Hernández, AL, Varona-Santos, JT, Salgado-Bustamante, M, Korban, SS, Moreno-Fierros, L & Rosales-Mendoza, S (2013) Production of an antigenic C4 (V3) 6 multiepitopic HIV protein in bacterial and plant systems. *Plant Cell Tissue Organ Cult,* 113, 73-9.
[http://dx.doi.org/10.1007/s11240-012-0252-4]

Govea-Alonso, DO, Rubio-Infante, N, García-Hernández, AL, Varona-Santos, JT, Korban, SS, Moreno-Fierros, L & Rosales-Mendoza, S (2013) Immunogenic properties of a lettuce-derived C4(V3)6 multiepitopic HIV protein. *Planta,* 238, 785-92.
[http://dx.doi.org/10.1007/s00425-013-1932-y] [PMID: 23897297]

Graham, BS (2013) Advances in antiviral vaccine development. *Immunol Rev,* 255, 230-42.
[http://dx.doi.org/10.1111/imr.12098] [PMID: 23947359]

Graham, RL, Becker, MM, Eckerle, LD, Bolles, M, Denison, MR & Baric, RS (2012) A live, impaired-fidelity coronavirus vaccine protects in an aged, immunocompromised mouse model of lethal disease. *Nat Med,* 18, 1820-6.
[http://dx.doi.org/10.1038/nm.2972] [PMID: 23142821]

Greenwood, B (2014) The contribution of vaccination to global health: past, present and future. *Philos Trans R Soc Lond B Biol Sci,* 369, 20130433.
[http://dx.doi.org/10.1098/rstb.2013.0433] [PMID: 24821919]

Grgacic, EV & Anderson, DA (2006) Virus-like particles: passport to immune recognition. *Methods,* 40, 60-5.
[http://dx.doi.org/10.1016/j.ymeth.2006.07.018] [PMID: 16997714]

Grifoni, A, Sidney, J, Zhang, Y, Scheuermann, RH, Peters, B & Sette, A (2020) A sequence homology and bioinformatic approach can predict candidate targets for immune responses to SARS-CoV-2. *Cell Host Microbe,* 27, 671-680.e2.
[http://dx.doi.org/10.1016/j.chom.2020.03.002] [PMID: 32183941]

Hisano, Y, Ota, S & Kawahara, A (2014) Genome editing using artificial site-specific nucleases in zebrafish. *Dev Growth Differ,* 56, 26-33.
[http://dx.doi.org/10.1111/dgd.12094] [PMID: 24117409]

Hobernik, D & Bros, M (2018) DNA vaccines—how far from clinical use? *Int J Mol Sci,* 19, 3605.
[http://dx.doi.org/10.3390/ijms19113605] [PMID: 30445702]

Howe, K, Clark, MD, Torroja, CF, Torrance, J, Berthelot, C, Muffato, M, Collins, JE, Humphray, S, McLaren, K, Matthews, L, McLaren, S, Sealy, I, Caccamo, M, Churcher, C, Scott, C, Barrett, JC, Koch, R, Rauch, GJ, White, S, Chow, W, Kilian, B, Quintais, LT, Guerra-Assunção, JA, Zhou, Y, Gu, Y, Yen, J, Vogel, JH, Eyre, T, Redmond, S, Banerjee, R, Chi, J, Fu, B, Langley, E, Maguire, SF, Laird, GK, Lloyd, D, Kenyon, E, Donaldson, S, Sehra, H, Almeida-King, J, Loveland, J, Trevanion, S, Jones, M, Quail, M, Willey, D, Hunt, A, Burton, J, Sims, S, McLay, K, Plumb, B, Davis, J, Clee, C, Oliver, K, Clark, R, Riddle, C, Elliot, D, Threadgold, G, Harden, G, Ware, D, Begum, S, Mortimore, B, Kerry, G, Heath, P, Phillimore, B, Tracey, A, Corby, N, Dunn, M, Johnson, C, Wood, J, Clark, S, Pelan, S, Griffiths, G, Smith, M, Glithero, R, Howden, P, Barker, N, Lloyd, C, Stevens, C, Harley, J, Holt, K, Panagiotidis, G, Lovell, J, Beasley, H, Henderson, C, Gordon, D, Auger, K, Wright, D, Collins, J, Raisen, C, Dyer, L, Leung, K, Robertson, L, Ambridge, K, Leongamornlert, D, McGuire, S, Gilderthorp, R, Griffiths, C, Manthravadi, D, Nichol, S, Barker, G,

Whitehead, S, Kay, M, Brown, J, Murnane, C, Gray, E, Humphries, M, Sycamore, N, Barker, D, Saunders, D, Wallis, J, Babbage, A, Hammond, S, Mashreghi-Mohammadi, M, Barr, L, Martin, S, Wray, P, Ellington, A, Matthews, N, Ellwood, M, Woodmansey, R, Clark, G, Cooper, J, Tromans, A, Grafham, D, Skuce, C, Pandian, R, Andrews, R, Harrison, E, Kimberley, A, Garnett, J, Fosker, N, Hall, R, Garner, P, Kelly, D, Bird, C, Palmer, S, Gehring, I, Berger, A, Dooley, CM, Ersan-Ürün, Z, Eser, C, Geiger, H, Geisler, M, Karotki, L, Kirn, A, Konantz, J, Konantz, M, Oberländer, M, Rudolph-Geiger, S, Teucke, M, Lanz, C, Raddatz, G, Osoegawa, K, Zhu, B, Rapp, A, Widaa, S, Langford, C, Yang, F, Schuster, SC, Carter, NP, Harrow, J, Ning, Z, Herrero, J, Searle, SM, Enright, A, Geisler, R, Plasterk, RH, Lee, C, Westerfield, M, de Jong, PJ, Zon, LI, Postlethwait, JH, Nüsslein-Volhard, C, Hubbard, TJ, Roest Crollius, H, Rogers, J & Stemple, DL (2013) The zebrafish reference genome sequence and its relationship to the human genome. *Nature,* 496, 498-503.
[http://dx.doi.org/10.1038/nature12111] [PMID: 23594743]

Hwang, WY, Fu, Y, Reyon, D, Maeder, ML, Tsai, SQ, Sander, JD, Peterson, RT, Yeh, JR & Joung, JK (2013) Efficient genome editing in zebrafish using a CRISPR-Cas system. *Nat Biotechnol,* 31, 227-9.
[http://dx.doi.org/10.1038/nbt.2501] [PMID: 23360964]

Iavarone, C, O'hagan, DT, Yu, D, Delahaye, NF & Ulmer, JB (2017) Mechanism of action of mRNA-based vaccines. *Expert Rev Vaccines,* 16, 871-81.
[http://dx.doi.org/10.1080/14760584.2017.1355245] [PMID: 28701102]

Imai, Y, Kuba, K, Rao, S, Huan, Y, Guo, F, Guan, B, Yang, P, Sarao, R, Wada, T, Leong-Poi, H, Crackower, MA, Fukamizu, A, Hui, CC, Hein, L, Uhlig, S, Slutsky, AS, Jiang, C & Penninger, JM (2005) Angiotensin-converting enzyme 2 protects from severe acute lung failure. *Nature,* 436, 112-6.
[http://dx.doi.org/10.1038/nature03712] [PMID: 16001071]

Iwata-Yoshikawa, N, Okamura, T, Shimizu, Y, Hasegawa, H, Takeda, M & Nagata, N (2019) TMPRSS2 contributes to virus spread and immunopathology in the airways of murine models after coronavirus infection. *J Virol,* 93, e01815-8.
[http://dx.doi.org/10.1128/JVI.01815-18] [PMID: 30626688]

Kalita, P, Padhi, AK, Zhang, KYJ & Tripathi, T (2020) Design of a peptide-based subunit vaccine against novel coronavirus SARS-CoV-2. *Microb Pathog,* 145, 104236.
[http://dx.doi.org/10.1016/j.micpath.2020.104236] [PMID: 32376359]

Kerry, RG, Malik, S, Redda, YT, Sahoo, S, Patra, JK & Majhi, S (2019) Nano-based approach to combat emerging viral (NIPAH virus) infection. *Nanomedicine (Lond),* 18, 196-220.
[http://dx.doi.org/10.1016/j.nano.2019.03.004] [PMID: 30904587]

Kim, Y-I, Kim, S-G, Kim, S-M, Kim, E-H, Park, S-J, Yu, K-M, Chang, J-H, Kim, EJ, Lee, S, Casel, MAB, Um, J, Song, MS, Jeong, HW, Lai, VD, Kim, Y, Chin, BS, Park, JS, Chung, KH, Foo, SS, Poo, H, Mo, IP, Lee, OJ, Webby, RJ, Jung, JU & Choi, YK (2020) Infection and rapid transmission of SARS-CoV-2 in ferrets. *Cell Host Microbe,* 27, 704-709.e2.
[http://dx.doi.org/10.1016/j.chom.2020.03.023] [PMID: 32259477]

Koo, GC, Hasan, A & O'Reilly, RJ (2009) Use of humanized severe combined immunodeficient mice for human vaccine development. *Expert Rev Vaccines,* 8, 113-20.
[http://dx.doi.org/10.1586/14760584.8.1.113] [PMID: 19093778]

Kruse, RL (2020) Therapeutic strategies in an outbreak scenario to treat the novel coronavirus originating in Wuhan, China. *F1000 Res,* 9, 72.
[http://dx.doi.org/10.12688/f1000research.22211.2] [PMID: 32117569]

Kwissa, M, Amara, RR, Robinson, HL, Moss, B, Alkan, S, Jabbar, A, Villinger, F & Pulendran, B (2007) Adjuvanting a DNA vaccine with a TLR9 ligand plus Flt3 ligand results in enhanced cellular immunity against the simian immunodeficiency virus. *J Exp Med,* 204, 2733-46.
[http://dx.doi.org/10.1084/jem.20071211] [PMID: 17954572]

Lai, Y-H, Sun, C-P, Huang, H-C, Chen, J-C, Liu, H-K & Huang, C (2018) Epigallocatechin gallate inhibits hepatitis B virus infection in human liver chimeric mice. *BMC Complement Altern Med,* 18, 248.
[http://dx.doi.org/10.1186/s12906-018-2316-4] [PMID: 30189898]

Lazzaro, S, Giovani, C, Mangiavacchi, S, Magini, D, Maione, D, Baudner, B, Geall, AJ, De Gregorio, E, D'Oro, U & Buonsanti, C (2015) CD8 T-cell priming upon mRNA vaccination is restricted to bone-marro--derived antigen-presenting cells and may involve antigen transfer from myocytes. *Immunology,* 146, 312-26.
[http://dx.doi.org/10.1111/imm.12505] [PMID: 26173587]

Lee, TT, Andreadakis, Z, Kumar, A, Gómez Román, R, Tollefsen, S, Saville, M & Mayhew, S (2020) The COVID-19 vaccine development landscape. *Nat Rev Drug Discov,* 19, 305-6.
[http://dx.doi.org/10.1038/d41573-020-00073-5] [PMID: 32273591]

Lee, S-H, Danishmalik, SN & Sin, J-I (2015) DNA vaccines, electroporation and their applications in cancer treatment. *Hum Vaccin Immunother,* 11, 1889-900.
[http://dx.doi.org/10.1080/21645515.2015.1035502] [PMID: 25984993]

Li, J, Song, D, Wang, S, Dai, Y, Zhou, J & Gu, J (2020) Antiviral effect of epigallocatechin gallate *via* impairing porcine circovirus type 2 attachment to host cell receptor. *Viruses,* 12, 176.
[http://dx.doi.org/10.3390/v12020176] [PMID: 32033244]

Lieschke, GJ & Currie, PD (2007) Animal models of human disease: zebrafish swim into view. *Nat Rev Genet,* 8, 353-67.
[http://dx.doi.org/10.1038/nrg2091] [PMID: 17440532]

Liu, WJ, Zhao, M, Liu, K, Xu, K, Wong, G, Tan, W & Gao, GF (2017) T-cell immunity of SARS-CoV: Implications for vaccine development against MERS-CoV. *Antiviral Res,* 137, 82-92.
[http://dx.doi.org/10.1016/j.antiviral.2016.11.006] [PMID: 27840203]

Lokugamage, KG, Yoshikawa-Iwata, N, Ito, N, Watts, DM, Wyde, PR, Wang, N, Newman, P, Kent Tseng, CT, Peters, CJ & Makino, S (2008) Chimeric coronavirus-like particles carrying severe acute respiratory syndrome coronavirus (SCoV) S protein protect mice against challenge with SCoV. *Vaccine,* 26, 797-808.
[http://dx.doi.org/10.1016/j.vaccine.2007.11.092] [PMID: 18191004]

Loomis, RJ & Johnson, PR (2015) Emerging vaccine technologies. *Vaccines (Basel),* 3, 429-47.
[http://dx.doi.org/10.3390/vaccines3020429] [PMID: 26343196]

Lu, X, Chen, Y, Bai, B, Hu, H, Tao, L, Yang, J, Chen, J, Chen, Z, Hu, Z & Wang, H (2007) Immune responses against severe acute respiratory syndrome coronavirus induced by virus-like particles in mice. *Immunology,* 122, 496-502.
[http://dx.doi.org/10.1111/j.1365-2567.2007.02676.x] [PMID: 17680799]

Masavuli, MG, Wijesundara, DK, Torresi, J, Gowans, EJ & Grubor-Bauk, B (2017) Preclinical development and production of virus-like particles as vaccine candidates for hepatitis C. *Front Microbiol,* 8, 2413.
[http://dx.doi.org/10.3389/fmicb.2017.02413] [PMID: 29259601]

McKie, R (2013) How the diminutive zebrafish is having a big impact on medical research. *The Guardian/The Observer.*

Midoux, P & Pichon, C (2015) Lipid-based mRNA vaccine delivery systems. *Expert Rev Vaccines,* 14, 221-34.
[http://dx.doi.org/10.1586/14760584.2015.986104] [PMID: 25540984]

Nie, J, Li, Q, Wu, J, Zhao, C, Hao, H, Liu, H, Zhang, L, Nie, L, Qin, H, Wang, M, Lu, Q, Li, X, Sun, Q, Liu, J, Fan, C, Huang, W, Xu, M & Wang, Y (2020) Establishment and validation of a pseudovirus neutralization assay for SARS-CoV-2. *Emerg Microbes Infect,* 9, 680-6.
[http://dx.doi.org/10.1080/22221751.2020.1743767] [PMID: 32207377]

Orłowski, P, Kowalczyk, A, Tomaszewska, E, Ranoszek-Soliwoda, K, Węgrzyn, A, Grzesiak, J, Celichowski, G, Grobelny, J, Eriksson, K & Krzyzowska, M (2018) Antiviral activity of tannic acid modified silver nanoparticles: potential to activate immune response in herpes genitalis. *Viruses,* 10, 524.
[http://dx.doi.org/10.3390/v10100524] [PMID: 30261662]

Ou, X, Liu, Y, Lei, X, Li, P, Mi, D, Ren, L, Guo, L, Guo, R, Chen, T, Hu, J, Xiang, Z, Mu, Z, Chen, X, Chen, J, Hu, K, Jin, Q, Wang, J & Qian, Z (2020) Characterization of spike glycoprotein of SARS-CoV-2 on virus entry and its immune cross-reactivity with SARS-CoV. *Nat Commun,* 11, 1620.

[http://dx.doi.org/10.1038/s41467-020-15562-9] [PMID: 32221306]

Oxman, MN, Levin, MJ, Johnson, GR, Schmader, KE, Straus, SE, Gelb, LD, Arbeit, RD, Simberkoff, MS, Gershon, AA, Davis, LE, Weinberg, A, Boardman, KD, Williams, HM, Zhang, JH, Peduzzi, PN, Beisel, CE, Morrison, VA, Guatelli, JC, Brooks, PA, Kauffman, CA, Pachucki, CT, Neuzil, KM, Betts, RF, Wright, PF, Griffin, MR, Brunell, P, Soto, NE, Marques, AR, Keay, SK, Goodman, RP, Cotton, DJ, Gnann, JW, Jr, Loutit, J, Holodniy, M, Keitel, WA, Crawford, GE, Yeh, SS, Lobo, Z, Toney, JF, Greenberg, RN, Keller, PM, Harbecke, R, Hayward, AR, Irwin, MR, Kyriakides, TC, Chan, CY, Chan, IS, Wang, WW, Annunziato, PW & Silber, JL Shingles Prevention Study Group (2005) A vaccine to prevent herpes zoster and postherpetic neuralgia in older adults. *N Engl J Med,* 352, 2271-84.
[http://dx.doi.org/10.1056/NEJMoa051016] [PMID: 15930418]

Pearson, T, Greiner, DL & Shultz, LD (2008) Humanized SCID mouse models for biomedical research. *Curr Top Microbiol Immunol,* 324, 25-51.
[http://dx.doi.org/10.1007/978-3-540-75647-7_2] [PMID: 18481451]

Phan, HT, Pohl, J, Floss, DM, Rabenstein, F, Veits, J, Le, BT, Chu, HH, Hause, G, Mettenleiter, T & Conrad, U (2013) ELPylated haemagglutinins produced in tobacco plants induce potentially neutralizing antibodies against H5N1 viruses in mice. *Plant Biotechnol J,* 11, 582-93.
[http://dx.doi.org/10.1111/pbi.12049] [PMID: 23398695]

Prompetchara, E, Ketloy, C & Palaga, T (2020) Immune responses in COVID-19 and potential vaccines: Lessons learned from SARS and MERS epidemic. *Asian Pac J Allergy Immunol,* 38, 1-9.
[PMID: 32105090]

Provine, NM, Amini, A, Garner, LC, Dold, C, Hutchings, C, FitzPatrick, ME, Reyes, LS, Chinnakannan, S, Oguti, B & Raymond, M (2019) Activation of MAIT cells plays a critical role in viral vector vaccine immunogenicity. *bioRxiv,* 661397.

Rappuoli, R (2004) From Pasteur to genomics: progress and challenges in infectious diseases. *Nat Med,* 10, 1177-85.
[http://dx.doi.org/10.1038/nm1129] [PMID: 15516917]

Rauch, S, Jasny, E, Schmidt, KE & Petsch, B (2018) New vaccine technologies to combat outbreak situations. *Front Immunol,* 9, 1963.
[http://dx.doi.org/10.3389/fimmu.2018.01963] [PMID: 30283434]

Rockx, B, Kuiken, T, Herfst, S, Bestebroer, T, Lamers, MM, Oude Munnink, BB, de Meulder, D, van Amerongen, G, van den Brand, J, Okba, NMA, Schipper, D, van Run, P, Leijten, L, Sikkema, R, Verschoor, E, Verstrepen, B, Bogers, W, Langermans, J, Drosten, C, Fentener van Vlissingen, M, Fouchier, R, de Swart, R, Koopmans, M & Haagmans, BL (2020) Comparative pathogenesis of COVID-19, MERS, and SARS in a nonhuman primate model. *Science,* 368, 1012-5.
[http://dx.doi.org/10.1126/science.abb7314] [PMID: 32303590]

Romagnani, S (1999) Th1/Th2 cells. *Inflamm Bowel Dis,* 5, 285-94.
[http://dx.doi.org/10.1097/00054725-199911000-00009] [PMID: 10579123]

Rosales-Mendoza, S, Govea-Alonso, DO, Monreal-Escalante, E, Fragoso, G & Sciutto, E (2012) Developing plant-based vaccines against neglected tropical diseases: where are we? *Vaccine,* 31, 40-8.
[http://dx.doi.org/10.1016/j.vaccine.2012.10.094] [PMID: 23142588]

Rosales-Mendoza, S & Salazar-González, JA (2014) Immunological aspects of using plant cells as delivery vehicles for oral vaccines. *Expert Rev Vaccines,* 13, 737-49.
[http://dx.doi.org/10.1586/14760584.2014.913483] [PMID: 24766405]

Ruiz, SI, Zumbrun, EE & Nalca, A (2017) Animal models of human viral diseases. In: Conn, P.M., (Ed.), *Animal Models for the Study of Human Disease* Elsevier 853-901.
[http://dx.doi.org/10.1016/B978-0-12-809468-6.00033-4]

Saleem, S & Kannan, RR (2018) Zebrafish: an emerging real-time model system to study Alzheimer's disease and neurospecific drug discovery. *Cell Death Discov,* 4, 45.

[http://dx.doi.org/10.1038/s41420-018-0109-7] [PMID: 30302279]

Santoriello, C & Zon, LI (2012) Hooked! Modeling human disease in zebrafish. *J Clin Invest,* 122, 2337-43. [http://dx.doi.org/10.1172/JCI60434] [PMID: 22751109]

Schmid, B & Haass, C (2013) Genomic editing opens new avenues for zebrafish as a model for neurodegeneration. *J Neurochem,* 127, 461-70. [http://dx.doi.org/10.1111/jnc.12460] [PMID: 24117801]

Shah, MAA, He, N, Li, Z, Ali, Z & Zhang, L (2014) Nanoparticles for DNA vaccine delivery. *J Biomed Nanotechnol,* 10, 2332-49. [http://dx.doi.org/10.1166/jbn.2014.1981] [PMID: 25992460]

Siu, KL, Yuen, KS, Castaño-Rodriguez, C, Ye, ZW, Yeung, ML, Fung, SY, Yuan, S, Chan, CP, Yuen, KY, Enjuanes, L & Jin, DY (2019) Severe acute respiratory syndrome coronavirus ORF3a protein activates the NLRP3 inflammasome by promoting TRAF3-dependent ubiquitination of ASC. *FASEB J,* 33, 8865-77. [http://dx.doi.org/10.1096/fj.201802418R] [PMID: 31034780]

Soldatov, VO, Kubekina, MV, Silaeva, YY, Bruter, AV & Deykin, AV (2020) On the way from SARS-Co--sensitive mice to murine COVID-19 model. *Res Results Pharmacol,* 6, 1-7. [http://dx.doi.org/10.3897/rrpharmacology.6.53633]

Soo, P-C, Horng, Y-T, Chang, K-C, Wang, J-Y, Hsueh, P-R, Chuang, C-Y, Lu, C-C & Lai, H-C (2009) A simple gold nanoparticle probes assay for identification of *Mycobacterium tuberculosis* and *Mycobacterium tuberculosis* complex from clinical specimens. *Mol Cell Probes,* 23, 240-6. [http://dx.doi.org/10.1016/j.mcp.2009.04.006] [PMID: 19463945]

Sportelli, MC, Izzi, M, Kukushkina, EA, Hossain, SI, Picca, RA, Ditaranto, N & Cioffi, N (2020) Can Nanotechnology and Materials Science Help the Fight against SARS-CoV-2? *Nanomaterials (Basel),* 10, 802. [http://dx.doi.org/10.3390/nano10040802] [PMID: 32326343]

Sullivan, C & Kim, CH (2008) Zebrafish as a model for infectious disease and immune function. *Fish Shellfish Immunol,* 25, 341-50. [http://dx.doi.org/10.1016/j.fsi.2008.05.005] [PMID: 18640057]

Sutton, TC & Subbarao, K (2015) Development of animal models against emerging coronaviruses: From SARS to MERS coronavirus. *Virology,* 479-480, 247-58. [http://dx.doi.org/10.1016/j.virol.2015.02.030] [PMID: 25791336]

Taghizadeh-Hesary, F & Akbari, H (2020) The powerful immune system against powerful COVID-19: A hypothesis. *Med Hypotheses,* 140, 109762. [http://dx.doi.org/10.1016/j.mehy.2020.109762] [PMID: 32388390]

Takaki, K, Davis, JM, Winglee, K & Ramakrishnan, L (2013) Evaluation of the pathogenesis and treatment of Mycobacterium marinum infection in zebrafish. *Nat Protoc,* 8, 1114-24. [http://dx.doi.org/10.1038/nprot.2013.068] [PMID: 23680983]

Tay, MZ, Poh, CM, Rénia, L, MacAry, PA & Ng, LFP (2020) The trinity of COVID-19: immunity, inflammation and intervention. *Nat Rev Immunol,* 20, 363-74. [http://dx.doi.org/10.1038/s41577-020-0311-8] [PMID: 32346093]

Tse, LV, Meganck, RM, Graham, RL & Baric, RS (2020) The current and future state of vaccines, antivirals and gene therapies against emerging coronaviruses. *Front Microbiol,* 11, 658. [http://dx.doi.org/10.3389/fmicb.2020.00658] [PMID: 32390971]

Tyagi, RK, Garg, NK, Jadon, R, Sahu, T, Katare, OP, Dalai, SK, Awasthi, A & Marepally, SK (2015) Elastic liposome-mediated transdermal immunization enhanced the immunogenicity of P. falciparum surface antigen, MSP-119. *Vaccine,* 33, 4630-8. [http://dx.doi.org/10.1016/j.vaccine.2015.06.054] [PMID: 26141014]

Ura, T, Okuda, K & Shimada, M (2014) Developments in viral vector-based vaccines. *Vaccines (Basel),* 2, 624-41.

[http://dx.doi.org/10.3390/vaccines2030624] [PMID: 26344749]

Vaccines, IoMCtRAEo, Stratton, KR & Clayton, EW (2012) *Adverse Effects of Vaccines: Evidence and Causality.*National Academies Press Washington, DC.

Van Doremalen, N, Bushmaker, T, Morris, DH, Holbrook, MG, Gamble, A, Williamson, BN, Tamin, A, Harcourt, JL, Thornburg, NJ, Gerber, SI, Lloyd-Smith, JO, de Wit, E & Munster, VJ (2020) Aerosol and surface stability of SARS-CoV-2 as compared with SARS-CoV-1. *N Engl J Med,* 382, 1564-7.
[http://dx.doi.org/10.1056/NEJMc2004973] [PMID: 32182409]

Van Duyne, R, Pedati, C, Guendel, I, Carpio, L, Kehn-Hall, K, Saifuddin, M & Kashanchi, F (2009) The utilization of humanized mouse models for the study of human retroviral infections. *Retrovirology,* 6, 76.
[http://dx.doi.org/10.1186/1742-4690-6-76] [PMID: 19674458]

Varela, M, Figueras, A & Novoa, B (2017) Modelling viral infections using zebrafish: Innate immune response and antiviral research. *Antiviral Res,* 139, 59-68.
[http://dx.doi.org/10.1016/j.antiviral.2016.12.013] [PMID: 28025085]

Veit, S, Jany, S, Fux, R, Sutter, G & Volz, A (2018) CD8+ T cells responding to the middle east respiratory syndrome coronavirus nucleocapsid protein delivered by vaccinia virus MVA in mice. *Viruses,* 10, 718.
[http://dx.doi.org/10.3390/v10120718] [PMID: 30558354]

Wahl, A, De, C, Abad Fernandez, M, Lenarcic, EM, Xu, Y, Cockrell, AS, Cleary, RA, Johnson, CE, Schramm, NJ, Rank, LM, Newsome, IG, Vincent, HA, Sanders, W, Aguilera-Sandoval, CR, Boone, A, Hildebrand, WH, Dayton, PA, Baric, RS, Pickles, RJ, Braunstein, M, Moorman, NJ, Goonetilleke, N & Victor Garcia, J (2019) Precision mouse models with expanded tropism for human pathogens. *Nat Biotechnol,* 37, 1163-73.
[http://dx.doi.org/10.1038/s41587-019-0225-9] [PMID: 31451733]

Wan, Y, Shang, J, Graham, R, Baric, RS & Li, F (2020) Receptor recognition by the novel coronavirus from Wuhan: an analysis based on decade-long structural studies of SARS coronavirus. *J Virol,* 94, e00127-20.
[http://dx.doi.org/10.1128/JVI.00127-20] [PMID: 31996437]

Wang, H, Ji, D, Shao, J & Zhang, S (2012) Maternal transfer and protective role of antibodies in zebrafish Danio rerio. *Mol Immunol,* 51, 332-6.
[http://dx.doi.org/10.1016/j.molimm.2012.04.003] [PMID: 22551698]

Wang, N, Shang, J, Jiang, S & Du, L (2020) Subunit vaccines against emerging pathogenic human coronaviruses. *Front Microbiol,* 11, 298.
[http://dx.doi.org/10.3389/fmicb.2020.00298] [PMID: 32265848]

Wentworth, DE, Gillim-Ross, L, Espina, N & Bernard, KA (2004) Mice susceptible to SARS coronavirus. *Emerg Infect Dis,* 10, 1293-6.
[http://dx.doi.org/10.3201/eid1007.031119] [PMID: 15324552]

WHO (2020) DRAFT landscape of COVID-19 candidate vaccines. *WORLD.*

Xu, R, Shi, M, Li, J, Song, P & Li, N (2020) Construction of SARS-CoV-2 Virus-Like Particles by Mammalian Expression System. *Front Bioeng Biotechnol,* 8, 862.
[http://dx.doi.org/10.3389/fbioe.2020.00862] [PMID: 32850726]

Yang, C-W, Lee, Y-Z, Hsu, H-Y, Shih, C, Chao, Y-S, Chang, H-Y & Lee, S-J (2017) Targeting coronaviral replication and cellular JAK2 mediated dominant NF-κB activation for comprehensive and ultimate inhibition of coronaviral activity. *Sci Rep,* 7, 1-13.
[http://dx.doi.org/10.1038/s41598-017-04203-9]

Yong, CY, Ong, HK, Yeap, SK, Ho, KL & Tan, WS (2019) Recent advances in the vaccine development against Middle East respiratory syndrome-coronavirus. *Front Microbiol,* 10, 1781.
[http://dx.doi.org/10.3389/fmicb.2019.01781] [PMID: 31428074]

Zhang, N, Jiang, S & Du, L (2014) Current advancements and potential strategies in the development of MERS-CoV vaccines. *Expert Rev Vaccines,* 13, 761-74.
[http://dx.doi.org/10.1586/14760584.2014.912134] [PMID: 24766432]

CHAPTER 6

The Future of COVID-19 Treatment

Sahil Arora[1,#], **Manvendra Kumar**[1,#], **Gaurav Joshi**[1,*] and **Raj Kumar**[1,*]

[1] *Department of Pharmaceutical Sciences and Natural Products, Central University of Punjab, Bathinda, 151001, India*

Abstract: Severe Acute Respiratory Syndrome Coronavirus 2 (SARS-CoV-2) or coronavirus disease or COVID-19 is a disease that has led to colossal mortality worldwide. The fast spread of this disease has caused havoc and panic among individuals, which has further worsened with the unavailability of vaccines or some proven drug regime. To date, only 12 new antiviral drugs have been approved by the FDA (8 against hepatitis C virus (2 in combinations for HIV). Thus, it becomes of utmost importance to identify drugs for new and re-emerging viruses, including the coronavirus. Considering the quest, we have put forth this book chapter to update readers about current repurposed and experimental drugs for this novel coronavirus. The viral lifecycle assisted in providing vital potential targets for drug therapy. The present chapter also deals with the existing mechanism of action of the drugs, their category, and clinical data reported.

Keywords: ACE2 inhibitors, Antiarrhythmic, Antibacterial, Anticancer, Anticoagulants, Antidiabetic, Antifungal, Anti-inflammatory, Antimalarial, Antioxidant, Antiparasitic, Antiprotozoal, Antiviral, Chelating agents, COVID-19, Drug repurposing, Natural products, Psychotropics, RAAS-ACE-ARBs inhibitors, SARS-CoV-2.

INTRODUCTION

Considering the COVID-19 pandemic, it becomes of utmost importance to identify drugs that possess potential and efficacy in treating COVID-19 disease (Mercorelli *et al.*, 2018, Cupertino *et al.*, 2020). The COVID-19 disease is notably marked with attacks at the lower respiratory system that leads to viral pneumonia along with affecting kidney, liver, heart, central nervous system, and gastrointestinal system leading to multiple organ failure responsible for high morbidity (Su *et al.*, 2016, Zhu *et al.*, 2020). Recently, drug target validation in

---

[*] **Corresponding authors Gaurav Joshi and Raj Kumar:** Department of Pharmaceutical Sciences and Natural Products, Central University of Punjab, Bathinda, 151001, India;
E-mails: garvpharma29@gmail.com and raj.khunger@gmail.com; raj.khunger@cup.edu.in
[#] Both, the authors, contributed equally

Neeraj Mittal, Sanjay Kumar Bhadada, O. P. Katare and Varun Garg (Eds.)

SAR-CoV-2 has led to the identification of newer targets for therapeutic development (Mani *et al.*, 2019). To date, (June 4, 2020) 53 targets have been identified.

The important one includes non-structural proteins, spike proteins, membrane protein, nucleocapsid proteins, *etc.* The identified targets/proteins possess enzymatic activities and catalyze the virus-cell cycle by hijacking the host cells.

The virus division cycle (Fig. **1**) consists of six phases, which include attachment of virus with the host cell receptors, allowing its entry, followed by translation, replication, and release, and the subsequent damage resulting from the compromised immune system.

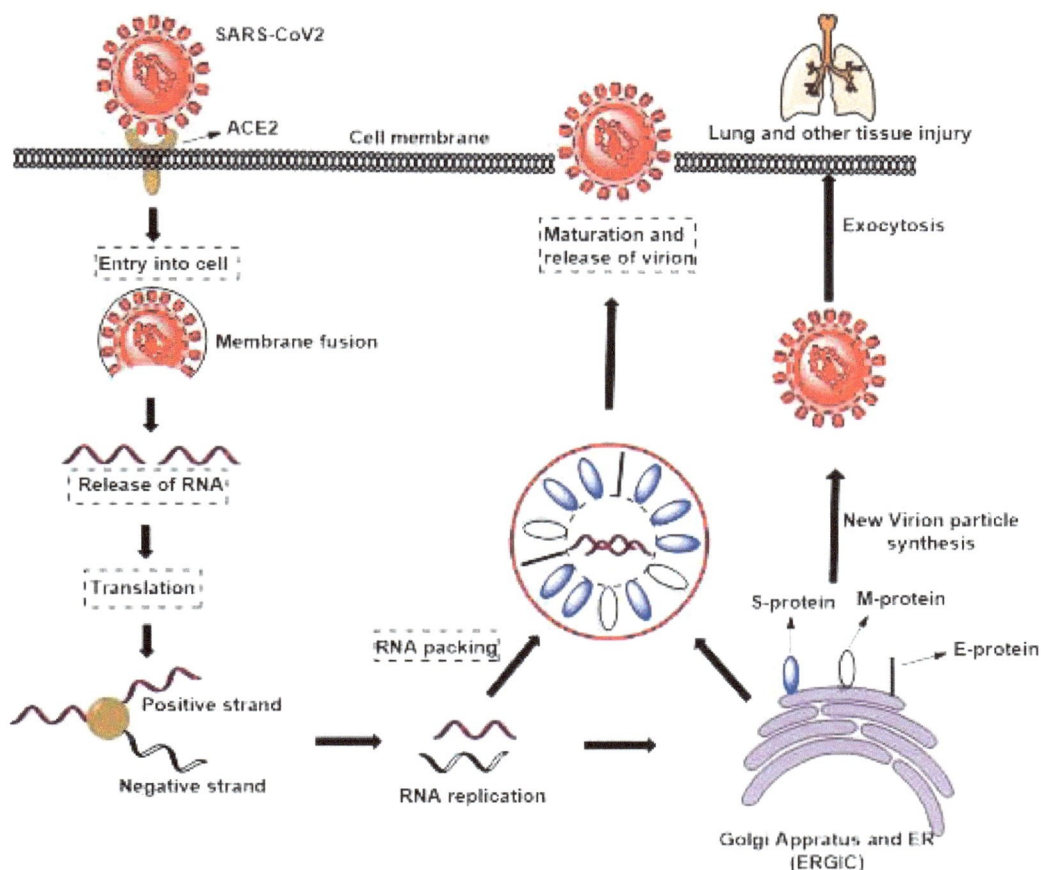

Fig. (1). SARS-CoV-2 life cycle in the host cell. The cycle consists of critical phases starting from the attachment of the virus with host cell receptors, endocytosis, proteolysis, translation, replication, maturation, and release of mature virions that ultimately are shredded, leading to subsequent damage of the organ system resulting from the compromised immune system.

Taking into account the reported interaction pattern of the virus with the host cell, many drugs have been repurposed so far. The drugs are currently under various clinical trials, and their efficacy and potential are still awaited. Drug repurposing characterizes a practical drug discovery approach from already known drugs (for different therapeutic use). It could minimize the time and decrease the cost associated with the *de novo* drug discovery (Zhou *et al.*, 2020b). This practice has been gaining popularity in recent years (Aubé, 2012). The approved drug requires regulatory approval for novel therapeutic applications which were already optimized for efficacy and safety in a particular disease (Chong *et al.*, 2007). The strategy used for drug repurposing involves identification of ligand for an indication of interest, drug assessment in preclinical models by mechanistic interpretation, efficacy evaluation in phase II clinical trials. There are various approaches used for drug repurposing, such as computational and experimental approaches. Computational approaches include molecular docking (Kitchen *et al.*, 2004), signature matching (Hieronymus *et al.*, 2006), pathway mapping(Smith *et al.*, 2012), genetic association (Sanseau *et al.*, 2012), novel data sources (Althouse *et al.*, 2015), and retrospective clinical analysis (Hurle *et al.*, 2013). Experimental approaches, such as phenotypic screening (Moffat *et al.*, 2017) and binding assays, are involved in the identification of relevant target interactions (Molina *et al.*, 2013). Some of the success stories of drug repurposing in other diseases include the use of paromomycin (from antibiotic in acute and chronic intestinal amebiasis to visceral and cutaneous leishmaniasis) (Ben Salah *et al.*, 2013), doxycycline (from bacteriostatic to antimalarial) (Tan *et al.*, 2011), miltefosine (from cancer to leishmaniasis) (Dorlo *et al.*, 2012), allopurinol (from cancer to gout) (Yasuda *et al.*, 2008), amantadine (from antiviral to tremors) (Gironell *et al.*, 2006), atomoxetine (from antidepressant to attention deficit hyperactivity disorder) (Turgay, 2005), colchicine (from gout to post-pericardiotomy syndrome) (Imazio *et al.*, 2010), and bromocriptine (from Parkinson's disease to type 2 diabetes) (Shaughnessy, 2011). Some examples of repurposed drugs used for the previous counterpart of SARS-CoV-2, *i.e.*, SARS and Middle East Respiratory Syndrome (MERS), include nitazoxanide (Rossignol, 2016), hydroxychloroquine (Zhou *et al.*, 2020a), emetine (Sharif-Yakan *et al.*, 2014), terconazole (Omrani *et al.*, 2015), lopinavir (Chan *et al.*, 2015), ritonavir (Chan *et al.*, 2015), ribavirin (Khalili *et al.*, 2020), homoharringtonine (Mustafa *et al.*, 2018), *etc.* The drugs for repurposing for the treatment of COVID-19 disease fall into multiple categories possessing various essential mechanisms. The essential categories include antivirals, anticancer, Angiotensin Converting Enzyme-Renin–Angiotensin–Aldosterone system (ACE-RAAS) inhibitors, anti-inflammatory, immune modulators, antibiotics, antirheumatics, *etc.* Besides this, some of the herbal drugs and nutraceuticals have also exhibited significant inhibitory potential against SARS-CoV-2 (Khan *et al.*, 2020, Liu *et al.*, 2020b).

The fast spread of this disease has caused havoc and panic among individuals, which has further worsened with the unavailability of vaccines or some proven drug regime. Considering the quest, we have put forth this book chapter to update readers about current repurposed and experimental drugs for this novel coronavirus. The viral lifecycle has assisted in providing vital potential targets for drug therapy. In the present chapter, we have focused primarily on small molecules (< 900 Daltons molecular weight) as drug candidates for COVID-19, along with their classification, mechanism of action, categories, preclinical and clinical evidence. It is to be noted that detailed discussion on vaccine development and current treatment is out of the scope of the present chapter as it is dealt with separately.

DRUGS AFFECTING VIRAL REPLICATION AND TRANSLATION IN COVID-19 DISEASE

Many antivirals, such as ribavirin, lopinavir/ritonavir, and arbidol are incorporated for the prevention and treatment of COVID-19 disease (Dong *et al.*, 2020). They inhibit the $3CL^{pro}$ protease of SARS-CoV-2, which plays a crucial role in the viral replication cycle. Another drug, umifenovir, blocks the fusion of the viral membrane with the endosome after endocytosis. NS3/4A protease is having an essential function in viral replication. Danoprevir plays a crucial role in inhibiting NS3/4A protease and decreases the host response against viral infection. It also reduces the hyperactivation of the host immune system.

For the replication and transcription, SARS-CoV-2 relies chiefly on the RNA-dependent RNA polymerase (RdRp). Drugs, including remdesivir, and favipiravir (nucleoside analog), inhibit RNA polymerase, and terminate the RNA transcription (Agostini *et al.*, 2018, Chen *et al.*, 2020). Remdesivir is a nucleoside analog prodrug, for which USFDA issued emergency use authorization for the treatment of COVID-19 on May 1, 2020, based on two Phase III clinical trials (Zheng *et al.*, 2020). Another trial conducted by Gilead's global SIMPLE trial (NCT04292899) found that remdesivir-treated patients were discharged in less than a week overcoming COVID-19 symptoms. According to the USFDA, remdesivir is administered intravenously to treat suspected or confirmed severe COVID-19 cases requiring intensive breathing support. However, some trials failed to show any benefit of remdesivir in patients with severe COVID-19 (Wang *et al.*, 2020b). Still, 19 clinical trials are in several phases for remdesivir that are investigating its efficacy and safety. Remdesivir is the part of WHO's SOLIDARITY trial for COVID-19.

Another drug, galidesivir attaches to a viral RNA polymerase in place of the natural nucleotide. As a result, there is a structural alteration in the viral enzyme because of restructured electrostatic interactions. Interruption of viral RNA polymerase function leads to premature termination of the elongating RNA strand (Westover *et al.*, 2018). Emtricitabine inhibits the reverse transcriptase, which results in the reduction of viral load, thereby preventing the entry of virus RNA into human DNA (Orkin *et al.*, 2018).

Interestingly, non-steroidal anti-inflammatory agents (NSAIDs) such as indomethacin a potential cyclooxygenase (COX) inhibitor, are found to affect viral replication and translation by blocking viral RNA synthesis and anticipated to be useful in the management of COVID-19 disease (Amici *et al.*, 2006). Further, antirheumatic drugs such as leflunomide inhibit virus replication and thus inhibit the development of activated autoimmune lymphocytes through blocking the cell cycle progression (Zhong *et al.*, 2020).

In the category of antidiabetic drugs, dapagliflozin, which is a sodium-glucose cotransporter-2 (SGLT2) inhibitor, is recently found to inhibit sodium–hydrogen exchanger-1(NHE) directly (Ye *et al.*, 2018). Dapagliflozin results in the lowering of increased lactate levels, which occurs due to increased LDH (Lactic Acid Dehydrogenase) levels by cell destruction in COVID-19 infection (Cure *et al.*, 2020). Thus, the drug helps lower cytosolic pH and reduces the viral load in the COVID-19 disease. Considering antiarrhythmic drugs such as amiodarone, block voltage-gated calcium and potassium channels, and thereby block viral entry. Amiodarone has also been reported to interfere with the endocytic pathway and inhibits virus replication (Yang *et al.*, 2020). A report by Zhang *et al.* further disclosed that calcium channel blockers might extensively reduce the post-entry replication of SARS-CoV-2 (Zhang *et al.*, 2020b). All the drugs which affect viral replication and translation with their NCT (National Clinical Trial Number) (if any) are collected in Table **1**, and their chemical structures are given in Fig. (**2**).

Table 1. List of repurposed drugs affecting viral replication and translation in COVID-19 disease.

Repurposed Drug (Trade Name) /NCT No.[a]	Clinical Trial Phase	Class	Target	Mechanism of Action
Umifenovir (Arbidol) NCT04260594	Phase 4	Antiviral	Viral glycoprotein	Block the entry of viral membrane by inhibiting endocytosis.
Darunavir (Prezcobix) NCT04252274	Phase 3	Antiviral	Gag-Pol	Inhibits cleavage of Gag-Pol, an encoded viral protein.
TMC-310911	Preclinical	Antiviral		

(Table 1) cont.....

Repurposed Drug (Trade Name) /NCT No.[a]	Clinical Trial Phase	Class	Target	Mechanism of Action
Ritonavir (Norvir) + Lopinavir (Kaletra) NCT04295551	Unknown	Antiviral	3CL1[pro]	Inhibit the 3CL1[pro] protease activity thus blocking the formation of polyproteins.
Ribavirin (Rebetol) + Ritonavir + Lopinavir (Kaletra) NCT04276688	Phase 2	Antiviral	-	-
Favipiravir (Avigan) NCT04336904	Phase 3	Antiviral	RNA-dependent RNA polymerase (RdRp)	Inhibit viral replication by blocking RdRp
Remdesivir (Captisol) NCT04365725 NCT04292899	Phase 3			
Levovir (Clevudine) NCT04347915	Phase 2			
Galidesivir (BCX4430) NCT03891420	Phase 1	Antiviral	Nucleoside RNA polymerase (antimetabolite)	Structural alteration in the viral RNA polymerase enzyme
Emtricitabine NCT04334928	Phase 3	Antiviral	Non-nucleotide reverse transcriptase	Inhibition of reverse transcriptase and blocks the viral transcription
Ribavirin (Rebetol) NCT04276688	Phase 2	Antiviral	RNA-dependent RNA polymerase	Inhibit viral replication by blocking RdRp
Naproxen (aleve) NCT04325633	Phase 3	NSAID	blocks viral RNA replication	Interferes with the RNA replication process
Indomethacin (indocid) NCT04344457	Phase 2	NSAID		
Leflunomide (Arava) NCT04361214	Phase 1	Antirheumatic	mitochondrial enzyme dihydroorotate dehydrogenase	inhibits the development of activated autoimmune lymphocytes through blocking the cell cycle progression.
Dapagliflozin (farxiga) NCT04350593	Phase 3	Antidiabetic	SGLT2	Lowers cytosolic pH and reducing the viral load
Amiodarone (Nexterone) NCT04351763	Phase 2	Antiarrhythmic	endosome	Blocks virus replication

(Table 1) cont.....

Repurposed Drug (Trade Name) /NCT No.[a]	Clinical Trial Phase	Class	Target	Mechanism of Action
Nicardipine (cardene) NCT04330300	Phase 4	Calcium channel blockers	Calcium channel	Activator of autophagy
Nimodipine (Nimotop)	Phase 4			
Nifedipine (Adalat)	Phase 4			
Felodipine (Plendil)	Phase 4			
Diltiazem (Cardizem)	Phase 3			

[a] National Clinical trial (NCT) number retrieved from https://clinicaltrials.gov

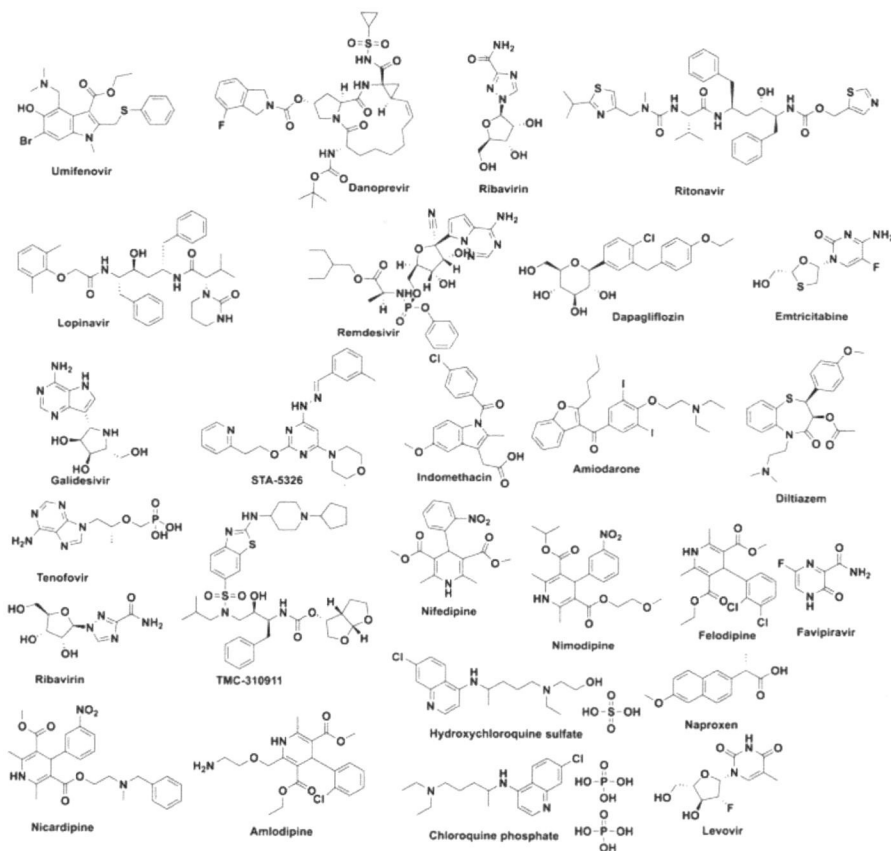

Fig. (2). Chemical structures of drugs affecting viral replication and translation.

DRUGS INTERFERING WITH INFLAMMATION AND OVERCOMING CYTOKINE STORM IN COVID-19 DISEASE

Due to the host inflammatory response, there is lung damage and subsequent mortality during the treatment of severe cases of COVID-19. As visualized in COVID-19 disease, Calcitonin gene-related peptide (CGRP) is recognized for the increased cytokine-dependent Il-6 production; (Sakuta *et al.*, 1995). Therefore, drugs used in migraine treatments that block the CGRP pathway, *e.g.*, vazegepant, a nasal spray, is found to show its mark in hyperinflammatory response in COVID-19 patients (Robertson, 2020). Further, it is also evidenced that during the progression of COVID-19 disease, substance P interacts with neurokinin-1 (NK-1) receptor resulting in severe lung parenchymal injury and a viral infection where tradipitant has found to be a suitable candidate in overcoming NK-1 mediated interaction (Sanders *et al.*, 2020, Jean *et al.*, 2020). Further, inhalational anaesthetics are also found useful in reducing lung inflammation and dilate airways *via* γ-aminobutyric acid (GABA) type A receptors (Forkuo *et al.*, 2018, Fortis *et al.*, 2012). Another class of drugs such as antioxidants like vitamin C quenches free reactive oxygen species and free radicals. It may show beneficial effects in viral infected patients by increasing α/β interferon production and downregulating pro-inflammatory cytokines production (Frei, 1994, Carr *et al.*, 2017, Kim *et al.*, 2013). Recently, vitamin C is shown to assist in the growth and maturation of T lymphocytes and NK (natural killer) cells against viral agents by enhancing immune response. Also, it aids in the modulation of the cytokine network typical of systemic inflammatory syndrome (Klein *et al.*, 2018). Many psychotropics agents such as valproic acid and haloperidol are newly added to a list of repurposed medications with the possibility for action against COVID-19 after they exhibited anti-inflammatory and mild intrinsic antiviral effect *in vitro* (O'Meara *et al.*). Drugs like fluvoxamine have shown their potential to overcome the cytokine storm by reducing the development of inflammatory response during sepsis (Rosen *et al.*, 2019). Melatonin is also known to exhibit antioxidant and anti-inflammatory properties (Li *et al.*, 2020a). Another category of drugs belonging to anticoagulants is anticipated to play a vital role in COVID-19 disease; for example, camostat, a serine protease inhibitors (Yamaya *et al.*, 2015), blocks the mechanism of SARS-CoV-2, which uses TMPRSS2 (serine protease) for docking to the ACE2(Bittmann *et al.*, 2020, Hoffmann *et al.*, 2020). This hampers the binding of the spike protein of the virus to the host cell. The drug is also found to affect inflammatory pathways mediating *via* NF-κB on the host cell membrane by inhibiting Toll-like receptors and significantly increasing the expression of the **MYD88** gene (Totura *et al.*, 2015). This alternatively could facilitate a decrease in lung infection and improve the survival of COVID-19 patients. Also, antihyperlipidemic agents have demonstrated that statins stabilize MYD88 levels after a pro-inflammatory trigger, such as hypoxia (Yuan *et al.*, 2014). Considering antipsychotic drugs, chlorpromazine (CPZ) has shown anticholinergic, antihistaminic effects that may assist in overcoming inflammation in COVID-19 disease(Baller *et al.*, 2020). Another drug, fingolimod, which is a

Sphingosine 1-phosphate receptor (S1P) analogue, and develops lung endothelial cell integrity, has been found to manage the vascular permeability. As a high level of cytokines was observed in COVID-19 patients, so the immunomodulatory effect of fingolimod is a better therapeutic option. Another example includes tacrolimus, which upon binding with host immunophilin FKBP-12, decreases peptidyl-prolyl isomerase and forms a new FKBP12-FK506 complex that inhibits the T-lymphocyte signal transduction and IL-2 transcription. Table **2** summarizes the list of drugs interfering with inflammation and overcoming cytokine storm in COVID-19 disease, whereas their chemical structures are compiled in Fig. (**3**).

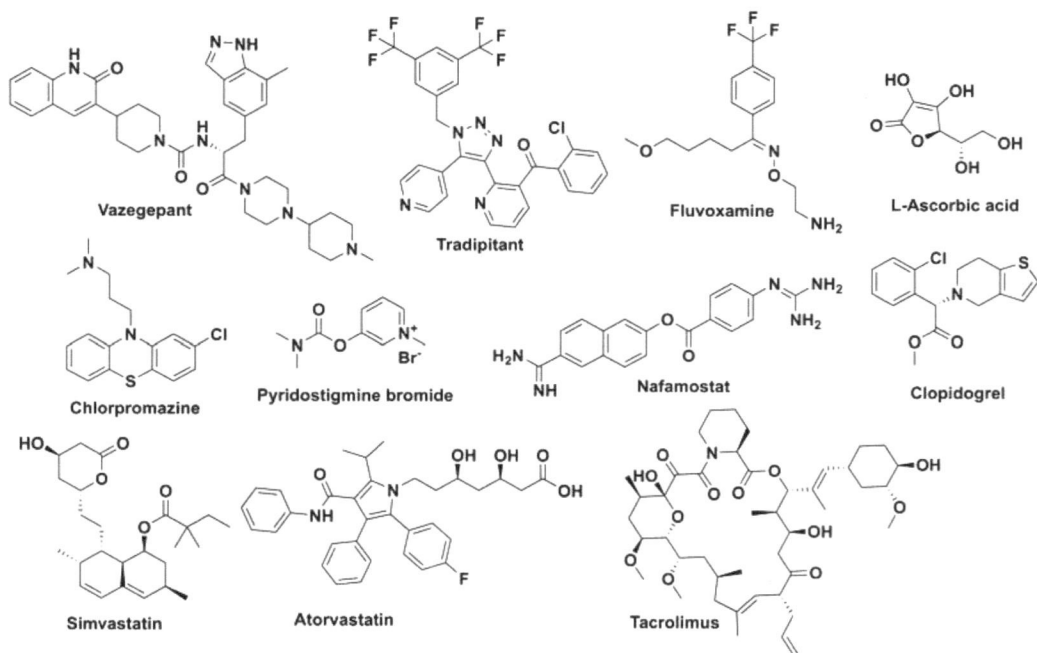

Fig. (3). Chemical structures of drugs interfering with inflammation and overcoming cytokine storm in COVID-19 disease.

Table 2. Drugs interfering with inflammation and overcoming cytokine storm in COVID-19 disease.

Drug (Trade Name)/NCT No. [a]	Clinical Trial Phase	Class	Target	Mechanism of Action
Vazegepant (BHV-3500) NCT04346615	Phase 2	Antimigraine	Calcitonin gene-related peptide receptor	Blocks CGRP receptor-mediated effects.
Tradipitant NCT04326426	Phase 3	neurokinin 1 antagonist (experimental)	neurokinin-1 receptor (NK-1R)	Blocks signaling of substance P.
Sevoflurane (sojourn) NCT04359862	Phase 4	Anesthetic agent	GABA A receptor; NMDA receptor	Overcome acute respiratory distress syndrome (ARDS) by vascular dilation, improves oxygenation in ventilator patients.
L-ascorbic acid (vitamin C) NCT04363216	Phase 2	Antioxidant	NK (natural killer) cells	able to scavenge damaging reactive oxygen species and increases the immune function.
Fluvoxamine (Luvox) NCT04342663	Phase 2	antidepressant	sigma-1 receptor	Prevents cytokine storms
Enoxaparin (Lovenox) NCT04366960	Phase 3	Anticoagulant	Antithrombin-III, Coagulation factor X	Inhibits viral attachment
Camostat NCT04353284	Phase 2	Anticoagulant	TMPRSS2	Inhibits serine protease TMPRSS2, preventing the priming of the viral spike protein
Chlorpromazine (Thorazine) NCT04366739	Phase 3	Antipsychotic	postsynaptic dopamine receptors	Inhibits viral replication
Pyridostigmine Bromide (Mestinon) NCT04343963	Phase 2	Cholinesterase inhibitor	AChE receptor	Diminishes T cell activation and proliferation, as well as increase the anti-inflammatory cytokine IL-10 and decrease the pro-inflammatory cytokine IFN-gamma
Simvastatin (Zocor) NCT04343001	Phase 3	Antihyperlipidemic agents	HMG-CoA reductase	Decreases IL levels by inhibiting MYD88 pathway
Atorvastatin (Lipitor) NCT04343001	Phase 3			

(Table 2) cont.....

Drug (Trade Name)/NCT No. [a]	Clinical Trial Phase	Class	Target	Mechanism of Action
Fingolimod (gilenya) NCT04280588	Phase 2	Immunomodulators	Sphingosine 1-phosphate receptor 5	Reduce lymphocyte circulation thereby overcoming inflammation
Tacrolimus (Prograf) NCT04341038	Phase 3	Immunosuppressant	Calcineurin	Inhibits viral replication and maturation by inhibiting T lymphocyte activation and proliferation in response to antigenic and cytokine.

[a] National Clinical trial (NCT) number retrieved from https://clinicaltrials.gov

ANTICANCER DRUGS IN THE TREATMENT OF COVID-19 DISEASE

The entry of the virus results in the activation of the innate and adaptive immune system to release numerous cytokines and chemokines, including IL-6. Activation of adaptive immunity results in the release of T- and B-cells for antiviral action and promote the activation of inflammatory cytokines. The release of these pro-inflammatory factors leads to an increase in vascular permeability and ultimately causes dyspnoea and even respiratory failure (Zhang *et al.*, 2020a). These activations of cytokines, including IL-6, are through the Janus kinase (JAK) signaling. The JAKs were encoded as the crucial facilitator of cytokines. From the uncountable research, it is clear that JAK-STAT signaling is one of the major causes of inflammatory responses (Liu *et al.*, 2020a). The potential use of JAK inhibitors for suppressing the hyperactivation of the immune system by targeting IL-6 and cytokines through JAK dependent signaling pathways is one of the many approaches to control the extreme level of cytokine signaling (Spinelli *et al.*, 2020). For the inflammation chiefly mediated *via* JAK pathways, JAK inhibitors such as siltuximab, ruxolitinib, baricitinib are found to possess a critical role in preventing elevated levels of cytokines (including interferon-γ), which significantly mediate signaling *via* JAK-STAT pathways(Stebbing *et al.*, 2020, Huang *et al.*, 2020). Ruxolitinib, apart from inhibition of JAK-STAT also inhibits interleukins, IFN-(α, β, γ), and growth factors (GM-CSF, TGF-β, erythropoietin, and thrombopoietin) (Virtanen *et al.*, 2019). Cardama *et al.* assessed JAK1 and JAK2 potential of ruxolitinib in cell and enzyme-based assays and testified their IC_{50} values 3.3 ± 1.2 and 2.8 ± 1.2 µM, respectively (Quintás-Cardama *et al.*, 2010). The drug has also shown good results in inhibition of phosphorylated STAT3 following stimulation with IL-6 (JAK1 prototype cytokine signal) or TPO (JAK2 cytokine signal) in whole blood assays with IC_{50} in nanomolar range (300 nM) (Quintás-Cardama *et al.*, 2010).

Further, Bruton's tyrosine kinase (BTK) inhibitors are analyzed for their capability to suppress the hyperactivation of cytokine release positively seen in COVID-19 patients. Treon and associates reported that the BTK inhibitors impart in the protection of lungs from various injuries in COVID-19 patients (Treon *et al.*, 2020). SARS-CoV-2 is coded with viroporins. These viroporins promote the immune signaling receptor NLRP3 through lysosomal disruption, which results in the release of cytokines (IL-1β and IL-6), tumor necrosis factor (TNF), triggering inflammation. Thus, the NLRP3 inhibitors were found to be effective and promising approaches in the treatment of COVID-19 (Shah, 2020). Table **3** summarizes the list of anticancer agents that are under investigation as COVID-19 therapeutics, whereas their chemical structures are compiled in Fig. (**4**).

Table 3. Anticancer agents in the treatment of COVID-19 disease.

Drug (Trade Name)/NCT No. [a]	Clinical Trial Phase	Class	Target	Mechanism of Action
Ruxolitinib (Jakafi) NCT04354714	Phase 2 (Withdrawn)	Anticancer	JAK-STAT pathway	Inhibits Janus associated kinases 1 and 2 and modulates their signaling pathways *via* reducing phosphorylation and activating STATs resulting in inhibition of cytokine and chemokine transcription Suppress the immune-hyperactivation.
Baricitinib (Olumiant) NCT04358614	Phase 2			
Selinexor (Xpovio) NCT04349098	Phase 2			
Acalabrutinib (Calquence) NCT04346199	Phase 2	BTK inhibitor Anticancer	BTK pathway	
Ibrutinib (Imbruvica) NCT04356690	Phase 2			
Nintedanib (Vargatef) NCT04338802	Phase 2	TNF-α and VEGR	EGFR	
Colchicine (Colcrys) NCT04322565	Phase 2	Anticancer	NALP3	Decreases IL-1beta activation and it blocks the inflammasome complex in both neutrophils and monocytes.
Thalidomide (Thalomid) NCT04273581	Phase 2	Anticancer	NLRP3 inflammasome	Decreases the synthesis of TNF-alpha.
Lenalidomide (Revlimid) NCT04361643	Phase 4	Anticancer	ubiquitin E3 ligase	Stimulates or regulate host cell immune.

[a] National Clinical trial (NCT) number retrieved from https://clinicaltrials.gov

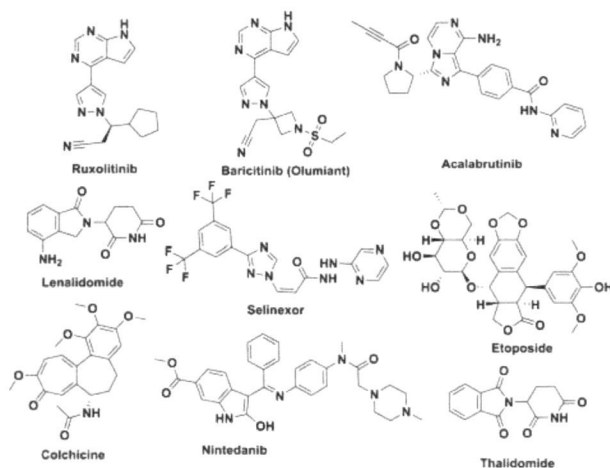

Fig. (4). Chemical structures for anticancer drugs repurposed for COVID-19 disease.

ANTIPARASITIC, ANTIPROTOZOAL, AND ANTIFUNGAL DRUGS IN THE TREATMENT OF COVID-19 DISEASE

Antiparasitic drugs such as nitazoxanide and niclosamide are among FDA-approved drugs that inhibit the expression of the viral N protein and consequently block viral replication. Nitazoxanide blocks TMEM16A ion channels, causing bronchodilation (Wang *et al.*, 2020a). It exhibits an antiviral mechanism by amplifying cytoplasmic RNA sensing and type IFN pathways and also upregulates host cellular defense mechanisms (Jasenosky *et al.*, 2019). Antimalarial drugs, including hydroxychloroquine (HCQ) and chloroquine, alter the pH of endosomes and inhibits entry of the virus into the host cell, thereby inhibiting endocytosis of the virus within the host cell (Devaux *et al.*, 2020, Olofsson *et al.*, 2005). Also, these drugs inhibit the addition of sialic acid moiety and the intracellular glycosylation of the ACE2 (trafficking), resulting in inhibition of virus fusion and its subsequent entry into the host cell (Savarino *et al.*, 2006). HCQ has also been explored in autoimmune diseases, including lupus erythematosus and rheumatoid arthritis, immunomodulator and viral diseases such as H1N1, Zika, hepatitis B, and HIV (D'Alessandro *et al.*, 2020, Browning, 2014). Recently, HCQ made its way back to the headlines in the middle of the COVID-19 disease (Downes *et al.*, 2020). USFDA issued guidelines for the emergency use of CQ/HCQ on March 28, 2020 (Food *et al.*, 2020). Findings from studies revealed HCQ to be more efficacious than CQ with *in vitro* IC_{50} of 5.47 µM. Further, there have been limited *in vivo* studies of HCQ to elucidate the mechanism. *In vivo,* clinical results were first disclosed in February 2020, by the Chinese government, where it was revealed significant improvement in pneumonia and lung imaging along with the reduction in the span of illness in

COVID-19 patients (Gao *et al.*, 2020). Another Chinese study involving 62 patients disclosed that HCQ could reduce the time of clinical recovery (Chen *et al.*). National Institute for the Infectious Diseases "L. Spallanzani" IRCCS in Italy published its recommendations for the use of HCQ (400 mg/day) for treatment of COVID-19 in combination with other antiviral drugs (Nicastri *et al.*, 2020). These encouraging results further assisted the Indian Council of Medical Research (ICMR) to recommend the use of HCQ for chemoprophylaxis on March 22, 2020. The guidelines recommended the use of HCQ by asymptomatic health workers (400 mg twice on day one, followed by 400 mg once every week for seven weeks) or household contacts of positive patients (400 mg twice on day 1, followed by 400 mg once every week for three weeks). However, few reports did not support the use of HCQ for treatment of COVID-19 disease. One of the reports by Ferner and Aronson disclosed disparity between laboratory and clinical experiments due to complex pharmacokinetics that would makes it difficult to extrapolate drug concentrations in culture media to human doses (Ferner *et al.*, 2020). Further, Molina and co-researchers emphasized on lack of evidence in support of the efficacy of a combination of HCQ and azithromycin in patients with severe COVID-19 infection (Molina *et al.*, 2020). The study by Lane and group on the use of HCQ alone or in combination evidenced an increase in QT interval prolongation leading to cardiovascular adverse events and death (Lane *et al.*, 2020). Another study by Mehra *et al.* (retracted) denied the beneficial effect of CQ/HCQ when used alone or in combination with a macrolide (Mehra *et al.*, 2020). However, the study was retracted owing to the shortcomings and expression of concern raised interrogating the accuracy of data and demanding a third-party review (Lancet, 2020). Considering these flaws, USFDA revoked authorized use of HCQ/CQ recently on June 15, 2020. Nevertheless, there is much debate on whether to use these drugs for COVID-19 or not.

Further, antifungal agents such as sirolimus act as an effective inhibitor of mTOR and have displayed significant outcome H1N1 pneumonia patients with acute respiratory failure (Wang *et al.*, 2014). Details of drugs are compiled in Table **4** and Fig. (**5**).

Table 4. Antiparasitic, antiprotozoal, and antifungal drugs in the treatment of COVID-19 disease.

Drug (Trade Name)/NCT No. [a]	Clinical Trial Phase	Class	Target	Mechanism of Action
Nitazoxanide (Alina) NCT04348409	Not Known	Antiprotozoal	viral transcription factor immediate-early 2 (IE2) and eukaryotic translation initiation factor 2α	Inhibit expression of the viral, N protein, and viral replication. Also blocks TMEM16A ion channels, causing bronchodilation.

(Table 4) cont.....

Drug (Trade Name)/NCT No. [a]	Clinical Trial Phase	Class	Target	Mechanism of Action
Ivermectin (stromectol) NCT04373824	Phase 2	Antiparasitic	IMPα/β1 heterodimer	It dissociates the IMPα/β1 heterodimer, and it is accountable for nuclear transport of viral protein.
Levamisole (ergamisol) NCT04360122	Phase 3	Antiprotozoal	Inhibits PL$_{pro}$ of SARS-CoV-2	Decrease level of TNF α and IL-6 and virus shedding.
Sirolimus (Rapamune) NCT04371640	Phase 1	Antifungal	mTOR	Efficiently restrict the expression of viral protein and virion release.
Carrimycin (Bite) NCT04286503	Phase 4	Antibacterial	Ribosomal protein subunit of the host cell and Furin protein	Involved in the inhibition of viral fusion with the targeted membrane.
Azithromycin (Zithromax) NCT04359316	Phase 4			
Chloroquine phosphate (Aralen phosphate) NCT04344951	Phase 2	Antimalarial	Endosomes of host cells cellular receptors of SARS-CoV	Decreases the viral copy amount of the cell supernatant and viral infection.
Hydroxychloroquine sulfate (Plaquenil sulfate) NCT04303507	Withdrawn			Increasing the pH of endosome which inhibits the viral entry in the host cell.

[a] National Clinical trial (NCT) number retrieved from https://clinicaltrials.gov

DRUGS AFFECTING THE RENIN-ANGIOTENSIN-ALDOSTERONE SYSTEM IN COVID-19

The Renin-Angiotensin-Aldosterone System (RAAS) exhibits a crucial role in maintaining blood volume that affects the cardiac output. SARS-CoV-2 interacts with the RAAS due to ACE2, a protein that physiologically promotes the activation of RAAS. It is identified as a functional receptor for SARS-CoV-1 and 2 (Vaduganathan *et al.*, 2020). It is also responsible for viral entry for SARS-CoV-2. With the last shreds of evidence, it is clear that ACE2 has a prolonged function in the pathogenesis of SARS-CoV-2 (Patel *et al.*, 2020). The SARS-CoV-2 codes spike S protein-containing receptor-binding domain (RBD), which is attached with the host ACE2, and leads to membrane fusion and acceptances of the SARS-CoV-2 into target cells (lung) through endocytosis, which commands the host cells for the activation of protein synthesis mechanism for the synthesis of viral proteins and viral replication. As RAAS emerged as a central part of COVID-19, so hitting the essential component(s) of RAAS might be suitable for the treatment. In RAAS, renin (kidney) helps in cleaving angiotensinogen (liver) to produce angiotensin I. Angiotensin I is further cleaved by ACE to give angiotensin II. The feasible pathway for COVID-19 therapy would be to hit the RAAS (Table **5**). Conventional pulmonary vasodilators such as an inhaled nitric oxide (iNO) (Alessandri *et al.*, 2018, Vickers, 2017, Khan *et al.*, 2009) reduce mean pulmonary artery pressure and enhance oxygenation in COVID-19 patients with acute respiratory distress syndrome (ARDS) (Åkerström *et al.*, 2005). Another category, such as vitamins, including β-carotene, retinol, and retinoic acid, is a group of fat-soluble compounds useful in the immune function system and lowers infection susceptibility (Huang *et al.*, 2018). Vitamin A and isotretinoin help in the down-regulation of ACE 2 (Sinha *et al.*, 2020).

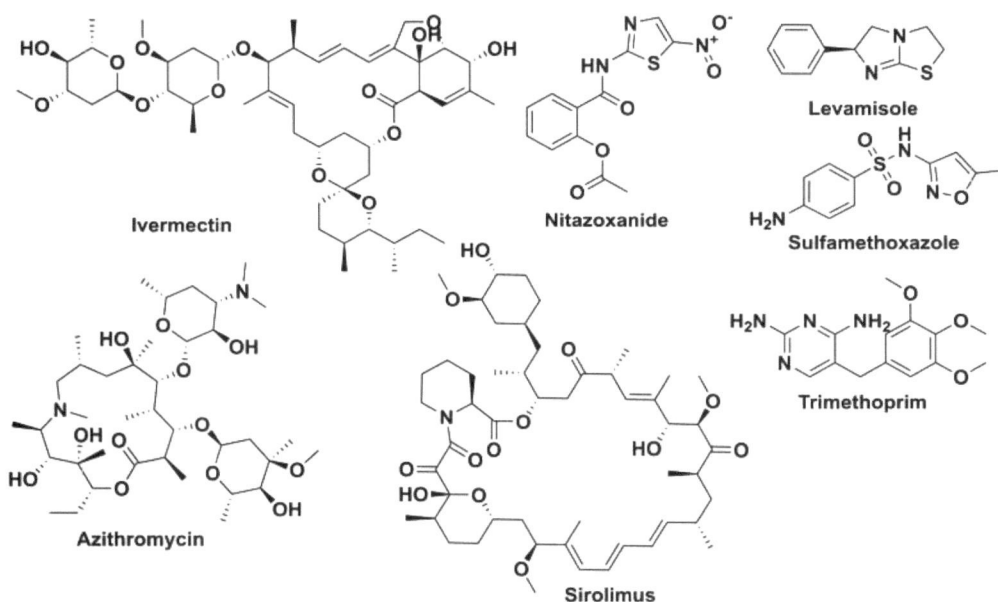

Fig. (5). Antiparasitic, antiprotozoal, antifungal, and antibacterial drugs in the treatment of COVID-19 disease.

Table 5. Drugs affecting renin-angiotensin-aldosterone system in COVID-19.

Drug (Trade Name)/NCT No. [a]	Clinical Trial Phase	Class	Target	Mechanism of Action
NORS (Nitric Oxide Releasing Solution) NCT04337918	Phase 2	Gasotransmitters	Endothelium-derived relaxing factor (EDRF)	Inhibits *S*-nitrosylation of viral proteins thus inhibiting viral protein and RNA synthesis.
Nitric oxide Gas (Inomax) NCT04338828	Phase 2			

[a] National Clinical trial (NCT) number retrieved from https://clinicaltrials.gov

MISCELLANEOUS

Endogenous protease plasmin of the host cell acts on the SARS-CoV-2 virus, thus cleaving a furin site in the S protein of the virus that results in viral infection (Mittal *et al.*, 2020). Patients with various diseases such as hypertension, diabetes, coronary artery disease, cerebrovascular illness, lung disease, and kidney dysfunction commonly have higher amounts of plasmin/plasminogen. Therefore, drugs that reduce the conversion of plasminogen to plasmin, such as tranexamic acid, might be useful (Paumgartten *et al.*, 2020). Chelating agents such as deferoxamine can be administered as an antidote for the management of chronic iron overload and acute iron toxicity. In systemic toxicity inversion, deferoxamine could remove extra iron from tissues and plasma (Yuen *et al.*, 2019) and act as a useful supportive agent in the management of the viral infection (Ghasemiyeh *et al.*).

Further, methylprednisolone an immunosuppressive drug that helps in the delay of pneumonia progression, has been found sufficient to overcome acute respiratory distress syndrome (ARDS) associated with COVID-19 disease. In the recent study, Wu *et al.* demonstrated a reduced risk of death (up to 62%) by administrating methylprednisolone in 201 participants with COVID-19 infection having severe ARDS conditions (Wu *et al.*, 2020, Veronese *et al.*, 2020, Huang *et al.*, 2020).

Further, memantine is used for the treatment of cognitive dysfunction, Parkinson, and alleviates fatigue and might be protective against COVID-19 by targeting the NMDA receptor (Rejdak *et al.*, 2020). Natural thyroid hormones block viral infection and affect the activation of p38 mitogen-activated protein kinase (MAPK). MAPK plays a crucial role in the replication of SARS-CoV-2. Also, it protects tissue from injury and shows antiapoptotic action with promising effects on the immune system and viral load in infected tissue (Velavan *et al.*, 2020, Paumgartten *et al.*, 2020). The phosphodiesterase-5 (PDE-5) inhibitor, such as sildenafil citrate, is a vasodilator used for treating erectile dysfunction (Scaglione *et al.*, 2017) has recently shown indication for pulmonary arterial hypertension (PAH) (Galiè *et al.*, 2005). Sildenafil may be useful in idiopathic pulmonary fibrosis (Rogosnitzky *et al.*, 2020) and renoprotective in interstitial lung disease (Webb *et al.*, 2015). It is currently under phase 3 clinical trial to treat patients with COVID-19 (NCT04304313). Another category, such as bronchodilators, including formoterol, is used in the management of chronic obstructive pulmonary disease (COPD) and asthma and also relaxes muscles in the airways to improve breathing (Arya *et al.*, 2020). A detailed list of various drugs with their mechanism is compiled in Table **6**, however, their chemical structures are collected in Fig. (**6**).

DISCUSSION AND CONCLUSION

There has been tremendous research going on to find a putative lead to treat COVID-19. To date, a total of 315 small molecules falling in the categories of antiviral, antimalarial, anticancer, anti-infective, anti-inflammatory, and many more are under consideration for the treatment of COVID-19 disease. Further, there have been many advancements in the development of robust *in vitro* and *in vivo* models to assess anti-SARS-CoV-2 drug candidates. The important *in vitro* models include human airway epithelial cells, vero E6 cells (both wild type and TMPRSS2 overexpressing), caco-2 cells, calu-3 cells, HEK293T cells, and Huh7 cells. Considering the *in vivo* studies, various animal models comprising mice, Syrian hamsters, ferrets, cats, cynomolgus macaques, rhesus macaques are being used for testing drug candidates (Li *et al.*, 2020b).

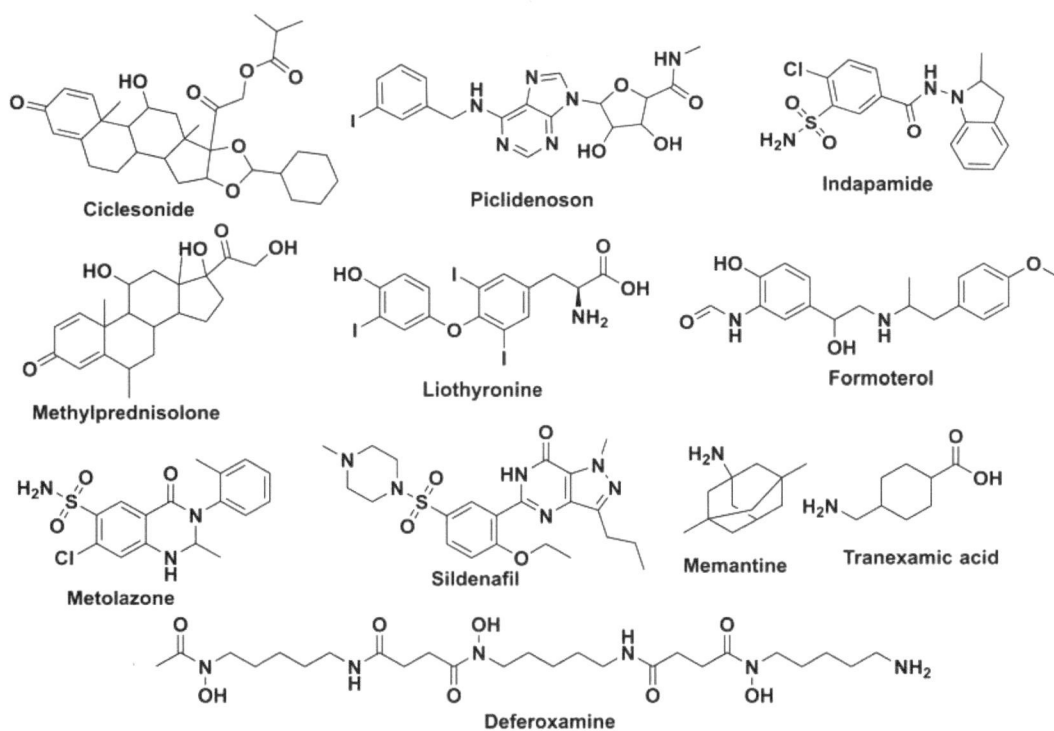

Fig. (6). Miscellaneous drugs used for the treatment of COVID-19.

Table 6. Miscellaneous drugs are being used for the management of COVID-19 disease.

Drug (Trade Name)/NCT no.[a]	Clinical Trial Phase	Class	Target	Mechanism of Action
Ciclesonide (Alvesco) NCT04381364	Phase 2	Anti-inflammatory	Nsp-15	Inhibit Nsp-15 thereby affecting viral replication.
Methylprednisolone (Medrol) NCT04374071	Study Completed	Anti-inflammatory, immunomodulator	NF-κB and TNF	Decreases circulating lymphocytes thereby inhibiting TNF-α expression and NF-κB by activating reformed gene expression *via* activating specific nuclear receptors
Sildenafil (Viagra) NCT04304313	Phase 3	Phosphodiesterase (PDE) inhibitors	PDE5	Blocks PDE5, thus restoring cGMP levels *via* the release of nitric oxide (NO), causing dilation of the blood vessels in the lungs
Formoterol (Atock) NCT04331470	Phase 2	Bronchodilators	β2-adrenergic agonist	reduces the activation of hypersensitivity mediators (*e.g.*, histamine, leukotrienes)
Liothyronine (Cytomel) NCT04348513	Phase 2	A synthetic derivative of a natural thyroid hormone	p38 MAPK activation	Improves the immune system and decrease viral load in infected tissue.
Tranexamic acid (Cyklokapron) NCT04338126	Phase 2	Antifibrinolytic	Plasminogen inhibitor	Inhibits plasmin, which acts on coronavirus and cleaves the newly inserted furin site at the S protein portion.
Memantine (Axura)	Not Known	Anti-Alzheimer	Cathepsin L	Inhibits cathepsin L, a lysosomal protease involved in SARS-CoV-2 entry to cells

[a] National Clinical trial (NCT) number retrieved from https://clinicaltrials.gov

Further, to overcome the ethical issues in *in vivo* drug monitoring, various 3D models are being developed. The important one includes organoid technology, which comprises human bronchial organoids, human lung organoids, human kidney organoids, human liver ductal organoids, human intestinal organoids, and human blood vessel organoids (Takayama, 2020, Jeon *et al.*, 2020, Touret *et al.*, 2020). Besides this, technologies such as bioprinting, single-cell analysis, and bio-fabrication are coming up to test drug candidates for COVID-19 disease.

As per data assessed for the clinical trial for COVID-19 (https://clinicaltrials.gov/) on July 7, 2020, at 14:00 Hrs IST), around 2427 clinical trials are reported. The data suggested (Fig. **7**) that among all the studies 25 are undergoing at preclinical phase, 141 in Phase 1, 539 in Phase 2, 327 in Phase 3, and 71 in Phase 4. Further, data also indicated that among all the studies, 182 had been completed, 1421 are either ongoing/recruiting/active, not recruiting/enrolling by invitation, whereas 41 have been either suspended/terminated or withdrawn, while remaining have unknown status.

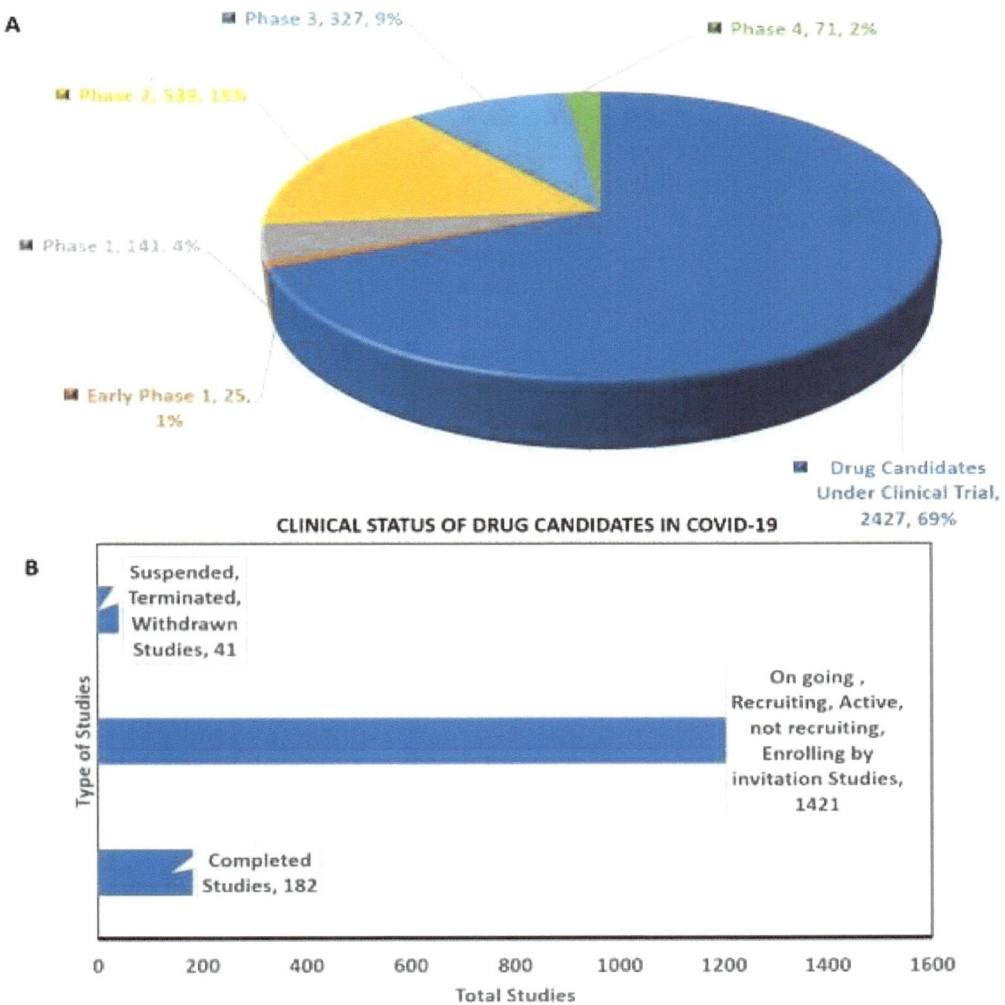

A

B

Fig. (7). (A) Pie-chart illustrates drug candidates in various stages of clinical trials for COVID-19 disease; **(B)** Bar graph represents drug candidates for COVID-19 signifying their clinical status.

Not only the small molecules but also vaccines or antibodies, natural products, and natural product derived chemicals have been actively tested for their potential in COVID-19 disease. The primary focus on the current scenario includes the use of these products/drugs to boost the immune system and provides preventative care in COVID-19 disease. Among various natural drug sources, ashwagandha has been found to boost immunity through modulation of host Th-1/Th-2. It may also be useful in inducing downregulation of TNFα, IL-1, IL-6, and other inflammatory mediators, which play a vital role in mediating cytokinin storm (Patwardhan *et al.*, 2020). Further, 17 organosulfur compounds from garlic have been reported to possess the inhibitory potential against host ACE2 protein and the main protease of SARS-CoV-2 (Thuy *et al.*, 2020). Other critical natural constituents like epicatechin gallate, quercetin, kaempferol, dimethoxy-curcumin, apigenin-7-glucoside, luteolin-7-glucoside, naringenin, catechin, allicin, oleuropein, curcumin, zingerone, and gingerol have been investigated as potent inhibitors of the Mpro, an essential protease possessing a role in SARS-CoV-2 translation (Khaerunnisa *et al.*, 2020). Additionally, Ayurveda Rasayana, such as *Asparagus racemosus* (Shatavari), *Phyllanthus emblica* (Amalaki), *Tinospora cordifolia* (Guduchi), *etc.* have immunomodulatory properties that may be beneficial against SARS-CoV-2 infection (Patwardhan *et al.*, 2020). Also, researchers and scientists involved in research on COVID-19 are exploring viral proteins to find some putative new leads or repurposed drugs through computer-aided drug design. Some of the important targets with their 3D structures are illustrated in Fig. (**8**). The thorough exploration of the active site of these proteins, including others involved in the SARS-CoV-2 life cycle, could be beneficial, leading to efficient drug design, and may speed up the quest to identify potent inhibitors shortly.

To summarize, SARS-CoV-2 was declared a pandemic by the WHO in 2020, leading to COVID-19 disease. Nevertheless, no drug or vaccine has been approved for the COVID-19 disease. Numerous clinical trials are undergoing in the quest to search for the best lead drug among the repurposed drugs. These drugs belong to diverse classes, which broadly include antiviral, anti-inflammatory, anticancer, antiparasitic, antiprotozoal, antifungal, antibacterial, RAAS-ACE-ARBs inhibitors, and natural products, along with other vital classes. These drugs importantly target the virus life cycle at different stages, and some are used as immunomodulators for developed cytokine storm with the progression of COVID-19 disease. As of now, most of the drugs in trials have exhibited good potential in a limited observational or non-randomized clinical study. The potential benefits are still awaited to come in the form of the first approved drug marking its presence for COVID-19 disease; the only remdesivir is gaining emergency authorization use to date. The authors believe that a multi-targeted approach to inhibit multiple targets involved in the virus life cycle using a combination of repurposed/new drugs explored through rational drug design would lead to significant results than monotherapy alone.

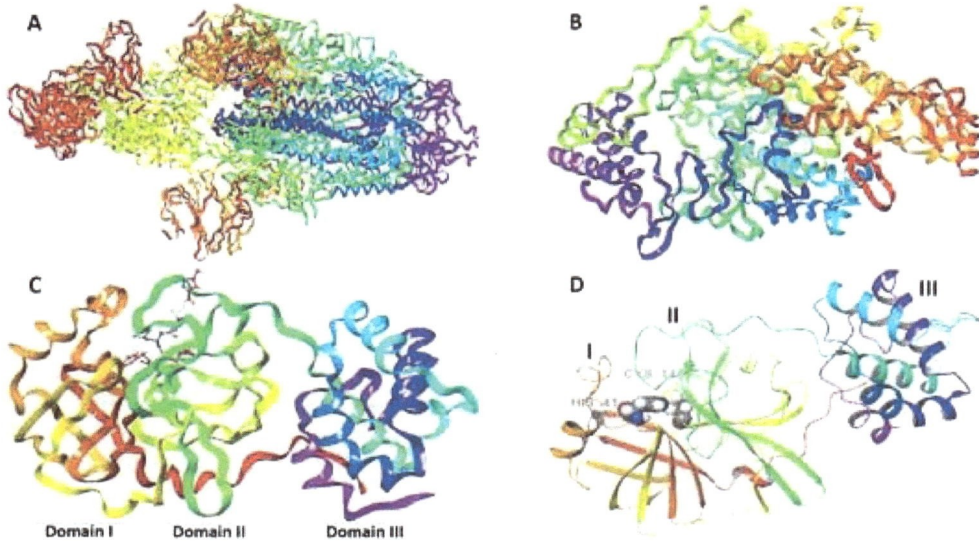

Fig. (8). Three-dimensional representation of SARS-CoV-2 molecular machines. **(A)** Ribbon diagram of the S protein (PDB ID: 6NB6). **(B)** Structural diagram of RdRp (Nsp12) (PDB ID: 6M71). **(C)** Illustration of 3Clpro in complex with its inhibitor N3 (PDB ID: 6LU7). **(D)** Three-dimensional structure of 3Cl pro showing amino acid residues CYS 145 and HIS 41 of the catalytic site and the domains I, II & III (PDB ID: 2BX4).

ABBREVIATIONS

ACE-RAAS –	Angiotension Converting Enzyme-Renin-angiotensin-aldosterone
ACE2-	Angiotensin-converting enzyme 2
CGRP –	Calcitonin gene-related peptide
COPD –	Chronic obstructive pulmonary disease
CPZ –	Chlorpromazine
HCQ –	Hydroxychloroquine
IL-6 –	Interleukin 6
iNO	inhalational Nitric oxide
MAPK-	Mitogen-activated protein kinase
JAK-STAT	Janus Kinase/Signal Transducer and Activator of Transcription
MERS-CoV –	The Middle East respiratory syndrome coronavirus
mTOR -	Mammalian target of rapamycin
NK-1 -	Neurokinin-1
NK-	Natural killer

PAH-	Pulmonary arterial hypertension
PDE-5-	Phosphodiesterase-5
RAAS-	Renin-angiotensin-aldosterone system
RBD-	Receptor-binding domain
RdRp -	RNA-dependent RNA polymerase
S1P -	Sphingosine 1-phosphate receptor
SARS-CoV-2-	Severe Acute Respiratory Syndrome Coronavirus 2
SGLT2 -	Sodium-glucose cotransporter-2
TNF-	Tumor necrosis factor

CONSENT FOR PUBLICATION

Not applicable.

CONFLICT OF INTEREST

The author declares no conflict of interest, financial or otherwise.

ACKNOWLEDGEMENTS

This work was supported by DST grant DST-SERB grant, New Delhi (EMR/2017/002702). MK thanks DST for providing JRF. SA thanks Bristol-Myer Squibb (grant no. 53803645), USA for providing the fellowship. Authors are also thankful to Honorable Vice-Chancellor, Central University of Punjab, Bathinda and Professor P. Ramarao, Dean Academic Affairs, Central University of Punjab, Bathinda for their relentless encouragement.

REFERENCES

Agostini, ML, Andres, EL, Sims, AC, Graham, RL, Sheahan, TP, Lu, X, Smith, EC, Case, JB, Feng, JY, Jordan, R, Ray, AS, Cihlar, T, Siegel, D, Mackman, RL, Clarke, MO, Baric, RS & Denison, MR (2018) Coronavirus susceptibility to the antiviral remdesivir (GS-5734) is mediated by the viral polymerase and the proofreading exoribonuclease. *MBio,* 9, e00221-18.
[http://dx.doi.org/10.1128/mBio.00221-18] [PMID: 29511076]

Akerström, S, Mousavi-Jazi, M, Klingström, J, Leijon, M, Lundkvist, A & Mirazimi, A (2005) Nitric oxide inhibits the replication cycle of severe acute respiratory syndrome coronavirus. *J Virol,* 79, 1966-9.
[http://dx.doi.org/10.1128/JVI.79.3.1966-1969.2005] [PMID: 15650225]

Alessandri, F, Pugliese, F & Ranieri, VM (2018) The role of rescue therapies in the treatment of severe ARDS. *Respir Care,* 63, 92-101.
[http://dx.doi.org/10.4187/respcare.05752] [PMID: 29066591]

Althouse, BM, Scarpino, SV, Meyers, LA, Ayers, JW, Bargsten, M, Baumbach, J, Brownstein, JS, Castro, L, Clapham, H, Cummings, DA, Del Valle, S, Eubank, S, Fairchild, G, Finelli, L, Generous, N, George, D, Harper, DR, Hébert-Dufresne, L, Johansson, MA, Konty, K, Lipsitch, M, Milinovich, G, Miller, JD, Nsoesie, EO, Olson, DR, Paul, M, Polgreen, PM, Priedhorsky, R, Read, JM, Rodríguez-Barraquer, I, Smith, DJ, Stefansen, C, Swerdlow, DL, Thompson, D, Vespignani, A & Wesolowski, A (2015) Enhancing disease

surveillance with novel data streams: challenges and opportunities. *EPJ Data Sci,* 4, 1-8.
[http://dx.doi.org/10.1140/epjds/s13688-015-0054-0] [PMID: 27990325]

Amici, C, Di Caro, A, Ciucci, A, Chiappa, L, Castilletti, C, Martella, V, Decaro, N, Buonavoglia, C, Capobianchi, MR & Santoro, MG (2006) Indomethacin has a potent antiviral activity against SARS coronavirus. *Antivir Ther,* 11, 1021-30.
[PMID: 17302372]

Arya, Rimanshee; Das, Amit; Prashar, Vishal; Kumar, Mukesh (2020) Potential inhibitors against papain-like protease of novel coronavirus (SARS-CoV-2) from FDA approved drugs. *ChemRxiv.*
[http://dx.doi.org/10.26434/chemrxiv.11860011.v2]

Aubé, J (2012) Drug repurposing and the medicinal chemist. *ACS Publications,* no. 3, 442-4.
[http://dx.doi.org/10.1021/ml300114c]

Baller, EB, Hogan, CS, Fusunyan, MA, Ivkovic, A, Luccarelli, JW, Madva, E, Nisavic, M, Praschan, N, Quijije, NV, Beach, SR & Smith, FA (2020) 'NeuroCOVID: Pharmacological recommendations for delirium associated with COVID-19'. *Psychosomatics,* 61, 585-96.
[http://dx.doi.org/10.1016/j.psym.2020.05.013] [PMID: 32828569]

Ben Salah, A, Ben Messaoud, N, Guedri, E, Zaatour, A, Ben Alaya, N, Bettaieb, J, Gharbi, A, Belhadj Hamida, N, Boukthir, A, Chlif, S, Abdelhamid, K, El Ahmadi, Z, Louzir, H, Mokni, M, Morizot, G, Buffet, P, Smith, PL, Kopydlowski, KM, Kreishman-Deitrick, M, Smith, KS, Nielsen, CJ, Ullman, DR, Norwood, JA, Thorne, GD, McCarthy, WF, Adams, RC, Rice, RM, Tang, D, Berman, J, Ransom, J, Magill, AJ & Grogl, M (2013) Topical paromomycin with or without gentamicin for cutaneous leishmaniasis. *N Engl J Med,* 368, 524-32.
[http://dx.doi.org/10.1056/NEJMoa1202657] [PMID: 23388004]

Bittmann, S, Luchter, E, Moschüring-Alieva, E, Villalon, G & Weissenstein, A C (2020) Camostat and The Role of Serine Protease Entry Inhibitor TMPRSS2. *J Regen Biol Med,* no. 2, 1-2.

Browning, DJ (2014) Pharmacology of chloroquine and hydroxychloroquine. *Hydroxychloroquine and Chloroquine Retinopathy.* Springer.
[http://dx.doi.org/10.1007/978-1-4939-0597-3]

Carr, AC & Maggini, S (2017) Vitamin C and immune function. *Nutrients,* 9, 1211.
[http://dx.doi.org/10.3390/nu9111211] [PMID: 29099763]

Chan, JF-W, Yao, Y, Yeung, M-L, Deng, W, Bao, L, Jia, L, Li, F, Xiao, C, Gao, H, Yu, P, Cai, JP, Chu, H, Zhou, J, Chen, H, Qin, C & Yuen, KY (2015) Treatment with lopinavir/ritonavir or interferon-β1b improves outcome of MERS-CoV infection in a nonhuman primate model of common marmoset. *J Infect Dis,* 212, 1904-13.
[http://dx.doi.org/10.1093/infdis/jiv392] [PMID: 26198719]

Chen, C, Huang, J, Cheng, Z, Wu, J, Chen, S, Zhang, Y, Chen, B, Lu, M, Luo, Y & Zhang, J (2020) Favipiravir *versus* arbidol for COVID-19: a randomized clinical trial. *MedRxiv.*
[http://dx.doi.org/10.1101/2020.03.17.20037432]

Chen, Z, Hu, J & Zhang, Z (2020) Efficacy of hydroxychloroquine in patients with COVID-19: results of a randomized clinical trial. *medRxiv,* 20040758.
[http://dx.doi.org/10, 22.20040758]

Chong, CR & Sullivan, DJ, Jr (2007) New uses for old drugs. *Nature,* 448, 645-6.
[http://dx.doi.org/10.1038/448645a] [PMID: 17687303]

Cupertino, MC, Resende, MB, Mayer, NA, Carvalho, LM & Siqueira-Batista, R (2020) Emerging and re-emerging human infectious diseases: A systematic review of the role of wild animals with a focus on public health impact. *Asian Pac J Trop Med,* 99.
[http://dx.doi.org/10.4103/1995-7645.277535]

Cure, E & Cumhur Cure, M (2020) Can dapagliflozin have a protective effect against COVID-19 infection? A hypothesis. *Diabetes Metab Syndr,* 14, 405-6.

[http://dx.doi.org/10.1016/j.dsx.2020.04.024] [PMID: 32335366]

D'Alessandro, S, Scaccabarozzi, D, Signorini, L, Perego, F, Ilboudo, DP, Ferrante, P & Delbue, S (2020) The Use of Antimalarial Drugs against Viral Infection. *Microorganisms*, 8, 85.
[http://dx.doi.org/10.3390/microorganisms8010085] [PMID: 31936284]

Devaux, CA, Rolain, J-M, Colson, P & Raoult, D (2020) New insights on the antiviral effects of chloroquine against coronavirus: what to expect for COVID-19? *Int J Antimicrob Agents*, 55, 105938.
[http://dx.doi.org/10.1016/j.ijantimicag.2020.105938] [PMID: 32171740]

Dong, L, Hu, S & Gao, J (2020) Discovering drugs to treat coronavirus disease 2019 (COVID-19). *Drug Discov Ther*, 14, 58-60.
[http://dx.doi.org/10.5582/ddt.2020.01012] [PMID: 32147628]

Dorlo, TP, Balasegaram, M, Beijnen, JH & de Vries, PJ (2012) Miltefosine: a review of its pharmacology and therapeutic efficacy in the treatment of leishmaniasis. *J Antimicrob Chemother*, 67, 2576-97.
[http://dx.doi.org/10.1093/jac/dks275] [PMID: 22833634]

Downes, SM, Leroy, BP, Sharma, SM, Sivaprasad, S & Dollfus, H (2020) *Hydroxychloroquine Hitting the Headlines-retinal Considerations*. Nature Publishing Group.
[http://dx.doi.org/10.1038/s41433-020-0934-9]

Ferner, RE & Aronson, JK (2020) *Chloroquine and Hydroxychloroquine in COVID-19*. British Medical Journal Publishing Group.

Food, U & Administration, D (2020) Fact sheet for health care providers: emergency use authorization (EUA) of hydroxychloroquine sulfate supplied from the strategic national stockpile for treatment of COVID-19 in certain hospitalized patients. https://www.fda.gov/media/136537/download

Forkuo, GS, Nieman, AN, Kodali, R, Zahn, NM, Li, G, Rashid Roni, MS, Stephen, MR, Harris, TW, Jahan, R, Guthrie, ML, Yu, OB, Fisher, JL, Yocum, GT, Emala, CW, Steeber, DA, Stafford, DC, Cook, JM & Arnold, LA (2018) A novel orally available asthma drug candidate that reduces smooth muscle constriction and inflammation by targeting GABAA receptors in the lung. *Mol Pharm*, 15, 1766-77.
[http://dx.doi.org/10.1021/acs.molpharmaceut.7b01013] [PMID: 29578347]

Fortis, S, Spieth, PM, Lu, W-Y, Parotto, M, Haitsma, JJ, Slutsky, AS, Zhong, N, Mazer, CD & Zhang, H (2012) Effects of anesthetic regimes on inflammatory responses in a rat model of acute lung injury. *Intensive Care Med*, 38, 1548-55.
[http://dx.doi.org/10.1007/s00134-012-2610-4] [PMID: 22711173]

Frei, B (1994) Reactive oxygen species and antioxidant vitamins: mechanisms of action. *Am J Med*, 97, 5S-13S.
[http://dx.doi.org/10.1016/0002-9343(94)90292-5] [PMID: 8085584]

Galiè, N, Ghofrani, HA, Torbicki, A, Barst, RJ, Rubin, LJ, Badesch, D, Fleming, T, Parpia, T, Burgess, G, Branzi, A, Grimminger, F, Kurzyna, M & Simonneau, G Sildenafil Use in Pulmonary Arterial Hypertension (SUPER) Study Group (2005) Sildenafil citrate therapy for pulmonary arterial hypertension. *N Engl J Med*, 353, 2148-57.
[http://dx.doi.org/10.1056/NEJMoa050010] [PMID: 16291984]

Gao, J, Tian, Z & Yang, X (2020) Breakthrough: chloroquine phosphate has shown apparent efficacy in treatment of COVID-19 associated pneumonia in clinical studies. *Biosci Trends*, 14, 72-3.
[http://dx.doi.org/10.5582/bst.2020.01047] [PMID: 32074550]

Ghasemiyeh, P & Mohammadi-Samani, S (2020) Iron chelating agents: promising supportive therapies in severe cases of COVID-19. *Trends Pharmaceut Sci*, no. 6, 65-6.

Gironell, A, Kulisevsky, J, Pascual-Sedano, B & Flamarich, D (2006) Effect of amantadine in essential tremor: a randomized, placebo-controlled trial. *Mov Disord*, 21, 441-5.
[http://dx.doi.org/10.1002/mds.20676] [PMID: 16229019]

Hieronymus, H, Lamb, J, Ross, KN, Peng, XP, Clement, C, Rodina, A, Nieto, M, Du, J, Stegmaier, K, Raj, SM, Maloney, KN, Clardy, J, Hahn, WC, Chiosis, G & Golub, TR (2006) Gene expression signature-based

chemical genomic prediction identifies a novel class of HSP90 pathway modulators. *Cancer Cell,* 10, 321-30.
[http://dx.doi.org/10.1016/j.ccr.2006.09.005] [PMID: 17010675]

Hoffmann, M, Kleine-Weber, H, Krüger, N, Mueller, MA, Drosten, C & Pöhlmann, S (2020) The novel coronavirus 2019 (2019-nCoV) uses the SARS-coronavirus receptor ACE2 and the cellular protease TMPRSS2 for entry into target cells. *bioRxiv.*
[http://dx.doi.org/10.1101/2020.01.31.929042]

Huang, C, Wang, Y, Li, X, Ren, L, Zhao, J, Hu, Y, Zhang, L, Fan, G, Xu, J, Gu, X, Cheng, Z, Yu, T, Xia, J, Wei, Y, Wu, W, Xie, X, Yin, W, Li, H, Liu, M, Xiao, Y, Gao, H, Guo, L, Xie, J, Wang, G, Jiang, R, Gao, Z, Jin, Q, Wang, J & Cao, B (2020) Clinical features of patients infected with 2019 novel coronavirus in Wuhan, China. *Lancet,* 395, 497-506.
[http://dx.doi.org/10.1016/S0140-6736(20)30183-5] [PMID: 31986264]

Huang, Z, Liu, Y, Qi, G, Brand, D & Zheng, SG (2018) Role of vitamin A in the immune system. *J Clin Med,* 7, 258.
[http://dx.doi.org/10.3390/jcm7090258] [PMID: 30200565]

Hurle, M, Yang, L, Xie, Q, Rajpal, DK, Sanseau, P & Agarwal, P (2013) Computational drug repositioning: from data to therapeutics. *Clin Pharmacol Ther,* 93, 335-41.
[http://dx.doi.org/10.1038/clpt.2013.1] [PMID: 23443757]

Imazio, M, Trinchero, R, Brucato, A, Rovere, ME, Gandino, A, Cemin, R, Ferrua, S, Maestroni, S, Zingarelli, E, Barosi, A, Simon, C, Sansone, F, Patrini, D, Vitali, E, Ferrazzi, P, Spodick, DH & Adler, Y COPPS Investigators (2010) COlchicine for the Prevention of the Post-pericardiotomy Syndrome (COPPS): a multicentre, randomized, double-blind, placebo-controlled trial. *Eur Heart J,* 31, 2749-54.
[http://dx.doi.org/10.1093/eurheartj/ehq319] [PMID: 20805112]

Jasenosky, L D, Cadena, C, Mire, C E, Borisevich, V, Haridas, V, Ranjbar, S, Nambu, A, Bavari, S, Soloveva, V & Sadukhan, S (2019) The FDA-approved oral drug nitazoxanide amplifies host antiviral responses and inhibits Ebola virus. *iScience,* no. 19, 1279-90.
[http://dx.doi.org/10.1016/j.isci.2019.07.003]

Jean, S-S & Hsueh, P-R (2020) Old and re-purposed drugs for the treatment of COVID-19. *Expert Rev Anti Infect Ther,* 18, 843-7.
[http://dx.doi.org/10.1080/14787210.2020.1771181] [PMID: 32419524]

Jeon, S, Ko, M, Lee, J, Choi, I, Byun, SY, Park, S, Shum, D & Kim, S (2020) Identification of antiviral drug candidates against SARS-CoV-2 from FDA-approved drugs. *Antimicrob Agents Chemother,* 64, e00819-20.
[http://dx.doi.org/10.1128/AAC.00819-20] [PMID: 32366720]

Khaerunnisa, S, Kurniawan, H, Awaluddin, R, Suhartati, S & Soetjipto, S (2020) Potential inhibitor of COVID-19 main protease (Mpro) from several medicinal plant compounds by molecular docking study. *Prepr,* 1-14.

Khalili, JS, Zhu, H, Mak, NSA, Yan, Y & Zhu, Y (2020) Novel coronavirus treatment with ribavirin: Groundwork for an evaluation concerning COVID-19. *J Med Virol,* 92, 740-6.
[http://dx.doi.org/10.1002/jmv.25798] [PMID: 32227493]

Khan, RJ, Jha, RK, Amera, GM, Jain, M, Singh, E, Pathak, A, Singh, RP, Muthukumaran, J & Singh, AK (2020) Targeting SARS-CoV-2: a systematic drug repurposing approach to identify promising inhibitors against 3C-like proteinase and 2'-O-ribose methyltransferase. *J Biomol Struct Dyn,* 1-14.
[http://dx.doi.org/10.1080/07391102.2020.1753577] [PMID: 32266873]

Khan, TA, Schnickel, G, Ross, D, Bastani, S, Laks, H, Esmailian, F, Marelli, D, Beygui, R, Shemin, R, Watson, L, Vartapetian, I & Ardehali, A (2009) A prospective, randomized, crossover pilot study of inhaled nitric oxide *versus* inhaled prostacyclin in heart transplant and lung transplant recipients. *J Thorac Cardiovasc Surg,* 138, 1417-24.
[http://dx.doi.org/10.1016/j.jtcvs.2009.04.063] [PMID: 19931670]

Kim, Y, Kim, H, Bae, S, Choi, J, Lim, SY, Lee, N, Kong, JM, Hwang, YI, Kang, JS & Lee, WJ (2013) Vitamin C is an essential factor on the anti-viral immune responses through the production of interferon-α/β

at the initial stage of influenza A virus (H3N2) infection. *Immune Netw,* 13, 70-4.
[http://dx.doi.org/10.4110/in.2013.13.2.70] [PMID: 23700397]

Kitchen, DB, Decornez, H, Furr, JR & Bajorath, J (2004) Docking and scoring in virtual screening for drug discovery: methods and applications. *Nat Rev Drug Discov,* 3, 935-49.
[http://dx.doi.org/10.1038/nrd1549] [PMID: 15520816]

Klein, R W, Van, C E, Wieten, L, Germeraad, W & Bos, G (2018) Influence of vitamin c on lymphocytes: An overview. *Antioxidants (Basel, Switzerland),* no. 7, 41.
[PMID: 32504543]

Lane, T (2020) Expression of concern: Hydroxychloroquine or chloroquine with or without a macrolide for treatment of COVID-19: a multinational registry analysis. *Lancet,* 395, e102.
[http://dx.doi.org/10.1016/S0140-6736(20)31290-3]

Lane, J C, Weaver, J, Kostka, K, Duarte-Salles, T, Abrahao, M T F, Alghoul, H, Alser, O, Alshammari, T M, Biedermann, P & Burn, E (2020) Safety of hydroxychloroquine, alone and in combination with azithromycin, in light of rapid wide-spread use for COVID-19: a multinational, network cohort and self-controlled case series study. *medRxiv.*
[http://dx.doi.org/10.1101/2020.04.08.20054551]

Li, G, He, X, Zhang, L, Ran, Q, Wang, J, Xiong, A, Wu, D, Chen, F, Sun, J & Chang, C (2020) Assessing ACE2 expression patterns in lung tissues in the pathogenesis of COVID-19. *J Autoimmun,* 112, 102463.
[http://dx.doi.org/10.1016/j.jaut.2020.102463] [PMID: 32303424]

Li, H, Zhou, Y, Zhang, M, Wang, H, Zhao, Q & Liu, J (2020) Updated approaches against SARS-CoV-2. *Antimicrob Agents Chemother,* 64, e00483-20. b
[http://dx.doi.org/10.1128/AAC.00483-20] [PMID: 32205349]

Liu, B, Li, M, Zhou, Z, Guan, X & Xiang, Y (2020) Can we use interleukin-6 (IL-6) blockade for coronavirus disease 2019 (COVID-19)-induced cytokine release syndrome (CRS)? *J Autoimmun,* 111, 102452.
[http://dx.doi.org/10.1016/j.jaut.2020.102452] [PMID: 32291137]

Liu, S, Zheng, Q & Wang, Z (2020) Potential covalent drugs targeting the main protease of the SARS-CoV-2 coronavirus. *Bioinformatics,* 36, 3295-8. b
[http://dx.doi.org/10.1093/bioinformatics/btaa224] [PMID: 32239142]

Journal of Young Pharmacists, D, Wadhwani, A & Krishnamurthy, P T (2019) Drug repurposing in antiviral research: a current scenario. *J Young Pharm,* no. 11, 117.
[http://dx.doi.org/10.5530/jyp.2019.11.26]

Mehra, MR, Desai, SS, Ruschitzka, F & Patel, AN (2020) Hydroxychloroquine or chloroquine with or without a macrolide for treatment of COVID-19: a multinational registry analysis. *Lancet.* S0140-6736, 31180-6.
[http://dx.doi.org/10.1016/S0140-6736(20)31180-6] [PMID: 32450107]

Mercorelli, B, Palù, G & Loregian, A (2018) Drug repurposing for viral infectious diseases: how far are we? *Trends Microbiol,* 26, 865-76.
[http://dx.doi.org/10.1016/j.tim.2018.04.004] [PMID: 29759926]

Mittal, A, Manjunath, K, Ranjan, RK, Kaushik, S, Kumar, S & Verma, V (2020) COVID-19 pandemic: Insights into structure, function, and hACE2 receptor recognition by SARS-CoV-2. *PLoS Pathog,* 16, e1008762.
[http://dx.doi.org/10.1371/journal.ppat.1008762] [PMID: 32822426]

Moffat, JG, Vincent, F, Lee, JA, Eder, J & Prunotto, M (2017) Opportunities and challenges in phenotypic drug discovery: an industry perspective. *Nat Rev Drug Discov,* 16, 531-43.
[http://dx.doi.org/10.1038/nrd.2017.111] [PMID: 28685762]

Martinez Molina, D, Jafari, R, Ignatushchenko, M, Seki, T, Larsson, EA, Dan, C, Sreekumar, L, Cao, Y & Nordlund, P (2013) Monitoring drug target engagement in cells and tissues using the cellular thermal shift assay. *Science,* 341, 84-7.

[http://dx.doi.org/10.1126/science.1233606] [PMID: 23828940]

Molina, JM, Delaugerre, C, Le Goff, J, Mela-Lima, B, Ponscarme, D, Goldwirt, L & de Castro, N (2020) No evidence of rapid antiviral clearance or clinical benefit with the combination of hydroxychloroquine and azithromycin in patients with severe COVID-19 infection. *Med Mal Infect,* 50, 384.
[http://dx.doi.org/10.1016/j.medmal.2020.03.006] [PMID: 32240719]

Mustafa, S, Balkhy, H & Gabere, MN (2018) Current treatment options and the role of peptides as potential therapeutic components for Middle East Respiratory Syndrome (MERS): A review. *J Infect Public Health,* 11, 9-17.
[http://dx.doi.org/10.1016/j.jiph.2017.08.009] [PMID: 28864360]

Nicastri, E, Petrosillo, N, Ascoli Bartoli, T, Lepore, L, Mondi, A, Palmieri, F, D'Offizi, G, Marchioni, L, Murachelli, S, Ippolito, G & Antinori, A (2020) 'National institute for the infectious diseases "L. Spallanzani", IRCCS. Recommendations for COVID-19 clinical management'. *Infect Dis Rep,* 12, 8543.
[http://dx.doi.org/10.4081/idr.2020.8543] [PMID: 32218915]

Gordon DE, Jang GM, Bouhaddou M, Xu J, Obernier K, White KM, O'Meara MJ, Rezelj VV, Guo JZ, Swaney DL, Tummino TA, Hüttenhain R, Kaake RM, Richards AL, Tutuncuoglu B, Foussard H, Batra J, Haas K, Modak M, Kim M, Haas P, Polacco BJ, Braberg H, Fabius JM, Eckhardt M, Soucheray M, Bennett MJ, Cakir M, McGregor MJ, Li Q, Meyer B, Roesch F, Vallet T, Mac Kain A, Miorin L, Moreno E, Naing ZZC, Zhou Y, Peng S, Shi Y, Zhang Z, Shen W, Kirby IT, Melnyk JE, Chorba JS, Lou K, Dai SA, Barrio-Hernandez I, Memon D, Hernandez-Armenta C, Lyu J, Mathy CJP, Perica T, Pilla KB, Ganesan SJ, Saltzberg DJ, Rakesh R, Liu X, Rosenthal SB, Calviello L, Venkataramanan S, Liboy-Lugo J, Lin Y, Huang XP, Liu Y, Wankowicz SA, Bohn M, Safari M, Ugur FS, Koh C, Savar NS, Tran QD, Shengjuler D, Fletcher SJ, O'Neal MC, Cai Y, Chang JCJ, Broadhurst DJ, Klippsten S, Sharp PP, Wenzell NA, Kuzuoglu-Ozturk D, Wang HY, Trenker R, Young JM, Cavero DA, Hiatt J, Roth TL, Rathore U, Subramanian A, Noack J, Hubert M, Stroud RM, Frankel AD, Rosenberg OS, Verba KA, Agard DA, Ott M, Emerman M, Jura N, von Zastrow M, Verdin E, Ashworth A, Schwartz O, d'Enfert C, Mukherjee S, Jacobson M, Malik HS, Fujimori DG, Ideker T, Craik CS, Floor SN, Fraser JS, Gross JD, Sali A, Roth BL, Ruggero D, Taunton J, Kortemme T, Beltrao P, Vignuzzi M, García-Sastre A, Shokat KM, Shoichet BK, Krogan NJ (2020) A SARS-CoV-2 protein interaction map reveals targets for drug repurposing. *Nature,* 583, 459-68.
[http://dx.doi.org/10.1101/2020.03.22.002386] [PMID: 32353859]

Olofsson, S, Kumlin, U, Dimock, K & Arnberg, N (2005) Avian influenza and sialic acid receptors: more than meets the eye? *Lancet Infect Dis,* 5, 184-8.
[http://dx.doi.org/10.1016/S1473-3099(05)70026-8] [PMID: 15766653]

Omrani, AS & Memish, ZA (2015) Therapeutic options for Middle East respiratory syndrome coronavirus (MERS-CoV) infection: how close are we? *Curr Treat Options Infect Dis,* 7, 202-16.
[http://dx.doi.org/10.1007/s40506-015-0048-2] [PMID: 32226324]

Orkin, C, Llibre, JM, Gallien, S, Antinori, A, Behrens, G & Carr, A (2018) Nucleoside reverse transcriptase inhibitor-reducing strategies in HIV treatment: assessing the evidence. *HIV Med,* 19, 18-32.
[http://dx.doi.org/10.1111/hiv.12534] [PMID: 28737291]

Patel, AB & Verma, A (2020) COVID-19 and angiotensin-converting enzyme inhibitors and angiotensin receptor blockers: what is the evidence? *JAMA,* 323, 1769-70.
[http://dx.doi.org/10.1001/jama.2020.4812] [PMID: 32208485]

Patwardhan, B, Chavan-Gautam, P, Gautam, M, Tillu, G, Chopra, A, Gairola, S & Jadhav, S (2020) Ayurveda rasayana in prophylaxis of COVID-19. *Curr Sci,* 1158-60.

Paumgartten, F. J. R., Delgado, I. F., Pitta, L. da R., & Oliveira, A. C. A. X. de. (2020). Drug repurposing clinical trials in the search for life-saving COVID-19 therapies; research targets and methodological and ethical issues. Health Surveillance under Debate: Society, Science & Technology (Vigilância Sanitária Em Debate: Sociedade, Ciência & Tecnología) – "Visa Em Debate", 8, 39-53.
[http://dx.doi.org/10.22239/2317-269x.01596]

Quintás-Cardama, A, Vaddi, K, Liu, P, Manshouri, T, Li, J, Scherle, PA, Caulder, E, Wen, X, Li, Y, Waeltz, P, Rupar, M, Burn, T, Lo, Y, Kelley, J, Covington, M, Shepard, S, Rodgers, JD, Haley, P, Kantarjian, H,

Fridman, JS & Verstovsek, S (2010) Preclinical characterization of the selective JAK1/2 inhibitor INCB018424: therapeutic implications for the treatment of myeloproliferative neoplasms. *Blood,* 115, 3109-17.
[http://dx.doi.org/10.1182/blood-2009-04-214957] [PMID: 20130243]

Rejdak, K & Grieb, P (2020) Adamantanes might be protective from COVID-19 in patients with neurological diseases: multiple sclerosis, parkinsonism and cognitive impairment. *Mult Scler Relat Disord,* 42, 102163.
[http://dx.doi.org/10.1016/j.msard.2020.102163] [PMID: 32388458]

Robertson, CE (2020) Could CGRP antagonists be helpful in the fight against COVID-19? *Headache,* 60, 1450-2.
[http://dx.doi.org/10.1111/head.13853] [PMID: 32386433]

Rogosnitzky, M, Berkowitz, E & Jadad, AR (2020) Delivering Benefits at Speed Through Real-World Repurposing of Off-Patent Drugs: The COVID-19 Pandemic as a Case in Point. *JMIR Public Health Surveill,* 6, e19199.
[http://dx.doi.org/10.2196/19199] [PMID: 32374264]

Rosen, DA, Seki, SM, Fernández-Castañeda, A, Beiter, RM, Eccles, JD, Woodfolk, JA & Gaultier, A (2019) Modulation of the sigma-1 receptor-IRE1 pathway is beneficial in preclinical models of inflammation and sepsis. *Sci Transl Med,* 11, eaau5266.
[http://dx.doi.org/10.1126/scitranslmed.aau5266] [PMID: 30728287]

Rossignol, J-F (2016) Nitazoxanide, a new drug candidate for the treatment of Middle East respiratory syndrome coronavirus. *J Infect Public Health,* 9, 227-30.
[http://dx.doi.org/10.1016/j.jiph.2016.04.001] [PMID: 27095301]

Sakuta, H, Inaba, K & Muramatsu, S (1995) Calcitonin gene-related peptide enhances cytokine-induced IL-6 production by fibroblasts. *Cell Immunol,* 165, 20-5.
[http://dx.doi.org/10.1006/cimm.1995.1182] [PMID: 7671321]

Sanders, JM, Monogue, ML, Jodlowski, TZ & Cutrell, JB (2020) Pharmacologic treatments for coronavirus disease 2019 (COVID-19): a review. *JAMA,* 323, 1824-36.
[http://dx.doi.org/10.1001/jama.2020.6019] [PMID: 32282022]

Sanseau, P, Agarwal, P, Barnes, MR, Pastinen, T, Richards, JB, Cardon, LR & Mooser, V (2012) Use of genome-wide association studies for drug repositioning. *Nat Biotechnol,* 30, 317-20.
[http://dx.doi.org/10.1038/nbt.2151] [PMID: 22491277]

Savarino, A, Di Trani, L, Donatelli, I, Cauda, R & Cassone, A (2006) New insights into the antiviral effects of chloroquine. *Lancet Infect Dis,* 6, 67-9.
[http://dx.doi.org/10.1016/S1473-3099(06)70361-9] [PMID: 16439323]

Scaglione, F, Donde, S, Hassan, TA & Jannini, EA (2017) Phosphodiesterase type 5 inhibitors for the treatment of erectile dysfunction: pharmacology and clinical impact of the sildenafil citrate orodispersible tablet formulation. *Clin Ther,* 39, 370-7.
[http://dx.doi.org/10.1016/j.clinthera.2017.01.001] [PMID: 28139291]

Shah, A (2020) Novel coronavirus-induced NLRP3 inflammasome activation: a potential drug target in the treatment of COVID-19. *Front Immunol,* 11, 1021.
[http://dx.doi.org/10.3389/fimmu.2020.01021] [PMID: 32574259]

Sharif-Yakan, A & Kanj, SS (2014) Emergence of MERS-CoV in the Middle East: origins, transmission, treatment, and perspectives. *PLoS Pathog,* 10, e1004457.
[http://dx.doi.org/10.1371/journal.ppat.1004457] [PMID: 25474536]

Shaughnessy, AF (2011) Old drugs, new tricks. *BMJ,* 342, d741.
[http://dx.doi.org/10.1136/bmj.d741] [PMID: 21307112]

Sinha, S, Cheng, K, Aldape, K, Schiff, E & Ruppin, E (2020) Systematic cell line-based identification of drugs modifying ACE2 expression. Preprints 22020030446.
[http://dx.doi.org/10.20944/preprints202003.0446.v1]

Smith, SB, Dampier, W, Tozeren, A, Brown, JR & Magid-Slav, M (2012) Identification of common biological pathways and drug targets across multiple respiratory viruses based on human host gene expression analysis. *PLoS One,* 7, e33174.
[http://dx.doi.org/10.1371/journal.pone.0033174] [PMID: 22432004]

Spinelli, FR, Conti, F & Gadina, M (2020) HiJAKing SARS-CoV-2? The potential role of JAK inhibitors in the management of COVID-19. *Sci Immunol,* 5, eabc5367.
[http://dx.doi.org/10.1126/sciimmunol.abc5367] [PMID: 32385052]

Stebbing, J, Phelan, A, Griffin, I, Tucker, C, Oechsle, O, Smith, D & Richardson, P (2020) COVID-19: combining antiviral and anti-inflammatory treatments. *Lancet Infect Dis,* 20, 400-2.
[http://dx.doi.org/10.1016/S1473-3099(20)30132-8] [PMID: 32113509]

Su, S, Wong, G, Shi, W, Liu, J, Lai, ACK, Zhou, J, Liu, W, Bi, Y & Gao, GF (2016) Epidemiology, genetic recombination, and pathogenesis of coronaviruses. *Trends Microbiol,* 24, 490-502.
[http://dx.doi.org/10.1016/j.tim.2016.03.003] [PMID: 27012512]

Takayama, K (2020) *In Vitro* and Animal Models for SARS-CoV-2 research. *Trends Pharmacol Sci,* 41, 513-7.
[http://dx.doi.org/10.1016/j.tips.2020.05.005] [PMID: 32553545]

Tan, KR, Magill, AJ, Parise, ME & Arguin, PM Centers for Disease Control and Prevention (2011) Doxycycline for malaria chemoprophylaxis and treatment: report from the CDC expert meeting on malaria chemoprophylaxis. *Am J Trop Med Hyg,* 84, 517-31.
[http://dx.doi.org/10.4269/ajtmh.2011.10-0285] [PMID: 21460003]

Thuy, BTP, My, TTA, Hai, NTT, Hieu, LT, Hoa, TT, Thi Phuong Loan, H, Triet, NT, Anh, TTV, Quy, PT, Tat, PV, Hue, NV, Quang, DT, Trung, NT, Tung, VT, Huynh, LK & Nhung, NTA (2020) Investigation into SARS-CoV-2 resistance of compounds in garlic essential oil. *ACS Omega,* 5, 8312-20.
[http://dx.doi.org/10.1021/acsomega.0c00772] [PMID: 32363255]

Totura, AL, Whitmore, A, Agnihothram, S, Schäfer, A, Katze, MG, Heise, MT & Baric, RS (2015) Toll-like receptor 3 signaling *via* TRIF contributes to a protective innate immune response to severe acute respiratory syndrome coronavirus infection. *MBio,* 6, e00638-15.
[http://dx.doi.org/10.1128/mBio.00638-15] [PMID: 26015500]

Touret, F, Gilles, M, Barral, K, Nougairède, A, van Helden, J, Decroly, E, de Lamballerie, X & Coutard, B (2020) In *vitro* screening of a FDA approved chemical library reveals potential inhibitors of SARS-CoV-2 replication. *Sci Rep,* 10, 13093.
[http://dx.doi.org/10.1038/s41598-020-70143-6] [PMID: 32753646]

Treon, SP, Castillo, JJ, Skarbnik, AP, Soumerai, JD, Ghobrial, IM, Guerrera, ML, Meid, K & Yang, G (2020) The BTK inhibitor ibrutinib may protect against pulmonary injury in COVID-19-infected patients. *Blood,* 135, 1912-5.
[http://dx.doi.org/10.1182/blood.2020006288] [PMID: 32302379]

Turgay, A (2005) Treatment of comorbidity in conduct disorder with attention-deficit hyperactivity disorder (ADHD). *Essent Psychopharmacol,* 6, 277-90.
[PMID: 16222912]

Vaduganathan, M, Vardeny, O, Michel, T, McMurray, JJV, Pfeffer, MA & Solomon, SD (2020) Renin–angiotensin–aldosterone system inhibitors in patients with COVID-19. *N Engl J Med,* 382, 1653-9.
[http://dx.doi.org/10.1056/NEJMsr2005760] [PMID: 32227760]

Velavan, TP & Meyer, CG (2020) The COVID-19 epidemic. *Trop Med Int Health,* 25, 278-80.
[http://dx.doi.org/10.1111/tmi.13383] [PMID: 32052514]

Veronese, N, Demurtas, J, Yang, L, Tonelli, R, Barbagallo, M, Lopalco, P, Lagolio, E, Celotto, S, Pizzol, D, Zou, L, Tully, MA, Ilie, PC, Trott, M, López-Sánchez, GF & Smith, L (2020) Use of corticosteroids in coronavirus disease 2019 pneumonia: A systematic review of the literature. *Front Med (Lausanne),* 7, 170.
[http://dx.doi.org/10.3389/fmed.2020.00170] [PMID: 32391369]

Vickers, NJ (2017) Animal Communication: When I'm Calling You, Will You Answer Too? *Curr Biol,* 27, R713-5.
[http://dx.doi.org/10.1016/j.cub.2017.05.064] [PMID: 28743020]

Virtanen, AT, Haikarainen, T, Raivola, J & Silvennoinen, O (2019) Selective JAKinibs: prospects in inflammatory and autoimmune diseases. *BioDrugs,* 33, 15-32.
[http://dx.doi.org/10.1007/s40259-019-00333-w] [PMID: 30701418]

Wang, C-H, Chung, F-T, Lin, S-M, Huang, S-Y, Chou, C-L, Lee, K-Y, Lin, T-Y & Kuo, H-P (2014) Adjuvant treatment with a mammalian target of rapamycin inhibitor, sirolimus, and steroids improves outcomes in patients with severe H1N1 pneumonia and acute respiratory failure. *Crit Care Med,* 42, 313-21.
[http://dx.doi.org/10.1097/CCM.0b013e3182a2727d] [PMID: 24105455]

Wang, M, Cao, R, Zhang, L, Yang, X, Liu, J, Xu, M, Shi, Z, Hu, Z, Zhong, W & Xiao, G (2020) Remdesivir and chloroquine effectively inhibit the recently emerged novel coronavirus (2019-nCoV) *in vitro. Cell Res* 269-71.
[http://dx.doi.org/10.1038/s41422-020-0282-0] [PMID: 32020029]

Wang, Y, Zhang, D, Du, G, Du, R, Zhao, J, Jin, Y, Fu, S, Gao, L, Cheng, Z, Lu, Q, Hu, Y, Luo, G, Wang, K, Lu, Y, Li, H, Wang, S, Ruan, S, Yang, C, Mei, C, Wang, Y, Ding, D, Wu, F, Tang, X, Ye, X, Ye, Y, Liu, B, Yang, J, Yin, W, Wang, A, Fan, G, Zhou, F, Liu, Z, Gu, X, Xu, J, Shang, L, Zhang, Y, Cao, L, Guo, T, Wan, Y, Qin, H, Jiang, Y, Jaki, T, Hayden, FG, Horby, PW, Cao, B & Wang, C (2020) Remdesivir in adults with severe COVID-19: a randomised, double-blind, placebo-controlled, multicentre trial. *Lancet,* 395, 1569-78. b
[http://dx.doi.org/10.1016/S0140-6736(20)31022-9] [PMID: 32423584]

Webb, DJ, Vachiery, JL, Hwang, LJ & Maurey, JO (2015) Sildenafil improves renal function in patients with pulmonary arterial hypertension. *Br J Clin Pharmacol,* 80, 235-41.
[http://dx.doi.org/10.1111/bcp.12616] [PMID: 25727860]

Westover, JB, Mathis, A, Taylor, R, Wandersee, L, Bailey, KW, Sefing, EJ, Hickerson, BT, Jung, K-H, Sheridan, WP & Gowen, BB (2018) Galidesivir limits Rift Valley fever virus infection and disease in Syrian golden hamsters. *Antiviral Res,* 156, 38-45.
[http://dx.doi.org/10.1016/j.antiviral.2018.05.013] [PMID: 29864447]

Wu, C, Chen, X, Cai, Y, Xia, J, Zhou, X, Xu, S, Huang, H, Zhang, L, Zhou, X, Du, C, Zhang, Y, Song, J, Wang, S, Chao, Y, Yang, Z, Xu, J, Zhou, X, Chen, D, Xiong, W, Xu, L, Zhou, F, Jiang, J, Bai, C, Zheng, J & Song, Y (2020) Risk factors associated with acute respiratory distress syndrome and death in patients with coronavirus disease 2019 pneumonia in Wuhan, China. *JAMA Intern Med,* 180, 934-43.
[http://dx.doi.org/10.1001/jamainternmed.2020.0994] [PMID: 32167524]

Yamaya, M, Shimotai, Y, Hatachi, Y, Lusamba Kalonji, N, Tando, Y, Kitajima, Y, Matsuo, K, Kubo, H, Nagatomi, R, Hongo, S, Homma, M & Nishimura, H (2015) The serine protease inhibitor camostat inhibits influenza virus replication and cytokine production in primary cultures of human tracheal epithelial cells. *Pulm Pharmacol Ther,* 33, 66-74.
[http://dx.doi.org/10.1016/j.pupt.2015.07.001] [PMID: 26166259]

Yang, N & Shen, H-M (2020) Targeting the endocytic pathway and autophagy process as a novel therapeutic strategy in COVID-19. *Int J Biol Sci,* 16, 1724-31.
[http://dx.doi.org/10.7150/ijbs.45498] [PMID: 32226290]

Yasuda, T, Yoshida, T, Goda, AE, Horinaka, M, Yano, K, Shiraishi, T, Wakada, M, Mizutani, Y, Miki, T & Sakai, T (2008) Anti-gout agent allopurinol exerts cytotoxicity to human hormone-refractory prostate cancer cells in combination with tumor necrosis factor-related apoptosis-inducing ligand. *Mol Cancer Res,* 6, 1852-60.
[http://dx.doi.org/10.1158/1541-7786.MCR-08-0012] [PMID: 19074830]

Ye, Y, Jia, X, Bajaj, M & Birnbaum, Y (2018) Dapagliflozin attenuates Na+/H+ exchanger-1 in cardiofibroblasts *via* AMPK activation. *Cardiovasc Drugs Ther,* 32, 553-8.
[http://dx.doi.org/10.1007/s10557-018-6837-3] [PMID: 30367338]

Yuan, X, Deng, Y, Guo, X, Shang, J, Zhu, D & Liu, H (2014) Atorvastatin attenuates myocardial remodeling

induced by chronic intermittent hypoxia in rats: partly involvement of TLR-4/MYD88 pathway. *Biochem Biophys Res Commun,* 446, 292-7.
[http://dx.doi.org/10.1016/j.bbrc.2014.02.091] [PMID: 24582748]

Yuen, HW & Becker, W (2020) https://www.ncbi.nlm.nih.gov/books/NBK459224/

Zhang C, Wu Z, Li JW, Zhao H, Wang GQ (2020a) Cytokine release syndrome in severe COVID-19: interleukin-6 receptor antagonist tocilizumab may be the key to reduce mortality. *Int J Antimicrob Agents*, 55, 105954.
[http://dx.doi.org/10.1016/j.ijantimicag.2020.105954]

Zhang, L, Sun, Y, Zeng, H-L, Peng, Y, Jiang, X, Shang, W-J, Wu, Y, Li, S, Zhang, Y-L & Yang, L (2020b) Calcium channel blocker amlodipine besylate is associated with reduced case fatality rate of COVID-19 patients with hypertension. *MedRxiv.*
[http://dx.doi.org/10.1101/2020.04.08.20047134]

Zheng, YY, Ma, YT, Zhang, JY & Xie, X (2020) COVID-19 and the cardiovascular system. *Nat Rev Cardiol,* 17, 259-60.
[http://dx.doi.org/10.1038/s41569-020-0360-5] [PMID: 32139904]

Zhong, J, Tang, J, Ye, C & Dong, L (2020) The immunology of COVID-19: is immune modulation an option for treatment? *Lancet Rheumatol,* no. 2, e428-36.

Zhou, D, Dai, S-M & Tong, Q (2020) COVID-19: a recommendation to examine the effect of hydroxychloroquine in preventing infection and progression. *J Antimicrob Chemother,* 75, 1667-70. a
[http://dx.doi.org/10.1093/jac/dkaa114] [PMID: 32196083]

Zhou, Y, Hou, Y, Shen, J, Huang, Y, Martin, W & Cheng, F (2020) Network-based drug repurposing for novel coronavirus 2019-nCoV/SARS-CoV-2. *Cell Discov,* 6, 14. b
[http://dx.doi.org/10.1038/s41421-020-0153-3] [PMID: 32194980]

Zhu, N, Zhang, D, Wang, W, Li, X, Yang, B, Song, J, Zhao, X, Huang, B, Shi, W, Lu, R, Niu, P, Zhan, F, Ma, X, Wang, D, Xu, W, Wu, G, Gao, GF & Tan, W China Novel Coronavirus Investigating and Research Team (2020) A novel coronavirus from patients with pneumonia in China, 2019. *N Engl J Med,* 382, 727-33.
[http://dx.doi.org/10.1056/NEJMoa2001017] [PMID: 31978945]

SUBJECT INDEX

www.ingramcontent.com/pod-product-compliance
Lightning Source LLC
Chambersburg PA
CBHW050839220326
41598CB00006B/401